Common
Musculoskeletal
Problems

Common Musculoskeletal Problems

Arun J. Mehta, MB, FRCPC

Associate Clinical Professor
Department of Medicine
University of California, Los Angeles,
    School of Medicine
Los Angeles, California
Physical Medicine and Rehabilitation Service
Veterans Affairs Medical Center
Sepulveda, California

HANLEY & BELFUS, INC./Philadelphia
MOSBY/St. Louis • Baltimore • Boston • Carlsbad • Chicago • London
Madrid • Naples • New York • Philadelphia • Sydney • Tokyo • Toronto

Publisher: HANLEY & BELFUS, INC.
               210 South 13th Street
               Philadelphia, PA 19107
               (215) 546-7293
               FAX (215) 790-9330

North American and Worldwide sales and distribution:

               MOSBY
               11830 Westline Industrial Drive
               St. Louis, MO 63146

In Canada: Times Mirror Professional Publishing, Ltd.
               130 Flaska Drive
               Markham, Ontario L6G 1B8
               Canada

Library of Congress Cataloging-in-Publication Data

Mehta, Arun J., 1935–
    Common musculoskeletal problems / Arun J. Mehta.
        p.   cm.
    Includes bibliographical references and index.
    ISBN 1-56053-173-8 (alk. paper)
    1. Musculoskeletal system—Diseases.   I. Title.
    [DNLM: 1. Musculoskeletal Diseases.   WE 140 M498c 1996]
    RC925.M44   1996
    616.7—dc20
    DNLM/DLC
    for Library of Congress   96-20354
                                                       CIP

COMMON MUSCULOSKELETAL PROBLEMS   ISBN 1-56053-173-8

Last digit is the print number: 9 8 7 6 5 4 3 2 1

Contents

Contributors

Andrew A. Fischer, M.D., Ph.D.
Associate Clinical Professor, Department of Rehabilitation Medicine, Mount Sinai School of Medicine, New York, New York; Chief, Physical Medicine and Rehabilitation Service, Veterans Affairs Medical Center, Bronx, New York

Steven M. Gnatz, M.D.
Associate Clinical Professor, Department of Physical Medicine and Rehabilitation, University of Missouri—Columbia; Rusk Rehabilitation Center, Columbia, Missouri

Stanley Marcus, M.D.
Clinical Professor, Department of Medicine, UCLA School of Medicine, Los Angeles, California

Arun Mehta, M.B., F.R.C.P.C.
Associate Clinical Professor, Department of Medicine, Division of Rehabilitation Medicine, UCLA School of Medicine, Los Angeles, California; Veterans Affairs Medical Center, Sepulveda, California

Trilok Monga, M.D., M.R.C.P.I., F.R.C.P.C.
Professor, Department of Physical Medicine and Rehabilitation, Baylor College of Medicine, Houston, Texas; Chief, Physical Medicine and Rehabilitation Service, Houston Veterans Affairs Medical Center, Houston, Texas

Aerie Rim, M.D.
Assistant Clinical Professor, Department of Physical Medicine and Rehabilitation, Mount Sinai School of Medicine, New York, New York; Bronx Veterans Affairs Hospital, Bronx, New York

Chadwick F. Smith, M.D.
Clinical Professor of Orthopaedic Surgery, University of Southern California School of Medicine, Los Angeles, California

Jay Subbarao, M.D., M.S.
Clinical Professor, Department of Physical Medicine and Rehabilitation, Loyola University of Chicago Stritch School of Medicine, Maywood, Illinois; Hines Comprehensive Rehabilitative Services, Hines Veterans Affairs Hospital, Hines, Illinois

Andrew Lun Wong, M.D., F.A.C.R.
Assistant Clinical Professor, Department of Rheumatology, UCLA School of Medicine, Los Angeles, California; Chief of Rheumatology, Olive View Medical Center, Sylmar, California

Preface

"The most valuable of all talents is that of never using two words when one will do."
Thomas Jefferson

Medical students have to cover a lot of ground during their studies, and musculoskeletal problems often do not get enough attention. Later, in practice, a physician's time and study can often be taken up by life-threatening conditions, and again non–life-threatening conditions are put on the back burner. However, musculoskeletal problems rank first among all disease groups in their effect on the quality of life as measured by the magnitude of the disability, handicap, and limitation of activity. Further, these problems represent 10–20% of all visits to a primary care physician and account for 20% of the days of all hospital stays. Yet there is not sufficient time to read very detailed descriptions of these disorders.

With these factors in mind we have written a book for physiatrists, family practitioners, general internists, orthopaedic surgeons, and medical students in a clear, concise format that is easy to read and review. Appropriate, simple line drawings, while not proportionally accurate, schematically illustrate and help explain the text. Each chapter includes a brief list of pertinent articles for further reading.

It is said that "What the mind does not know, the eyes do not see." At the beginning of each chapter a list of disorders (differential diagnosis) is presented so that the mind will know beforehand what the eyes and hands should be looking for.

Very few people read a medical book from cover to cover. Most of us read a chapter or less at a time and would like to see all the relevant material in one place. While writing a book for such use may lead to some repetition in different chapters, we have followed this approach since it is a practical and useful method of presenting the material.

I have been fortunate in having some very experienced clinicians contribute to this effort. I am very grateful to them all for sharing their knowledge and experience. It is my sincere hope that readers will find this book helpful in the diagnosis and management of common musculoskeletal problems. I will be obliged if anyone who has any suggestions for improvement will take the time to write to me.

Arun Mehta, M.B., F.R.C.P.C.
Associate Clinical Professor of Medicine
UCLA School of Medicine
PM & R Service (117)
Veterans Affairs Medical Center
16111 Plummer Street
Sepulveda, CA 91343

1

General Principles

Arun J. Mehta, M.B., F.R.C.P.C.

EPIDEMIOLOGY OF MUSCULOSKELETAL PROBLEMS

Patients present with musculoskleletal problems in many different types of medical practices. A reported 10–20% of the patients who visit a family practitioner have complaints related to the musculoskeletal system (Tables 1–1 and 1–2). Musculoskeletal problems account for 20% of the days of hospital stay. Among chronic conditions, two of the top three conditions in prevalence are arthritis and deformity/orthopedic impairment. Nearly one-third of all persons who are unable to perform a major activity of daily living relate this to some musculoskeletal impairment. These problems rank first among all disease groups in terms of their effect on the quality of life as measured by the magnitude of disability, handicap, and limitation of activities.

Even though musculoskeletal problems are very common, the cost of health care for these conditions is low as compared with the cost for others. They require less-expensive medical interventions. However, the economic effects due to lost function e.g., loss of work days—are enormous. The total economic impact of musculoskeletal conditions is estimated to be around 1% of the U.S. gross national product, or approximately $52 billion/year. They are one of the leading causes of time lost from work.

Despite this, time spent by a medical student in learning about these disorders is negligible. It is usually left to the discretion of the student to select an elective in orthopedics, rheumatology, or physical medicine and rehabilitation to learn about these very common disorders. The reason for this may be that the musculoskeletal diseases do not make the top 15 causes of death.

ANATOMY

The musculoskeletal system is made up of muscles, tendons, bones, cartilage, and ligaments. The joints are composed of bones, cartilage, and ligaments. All these structures are supplied by blood vessels and nerves, except for the articular cartilage, which has no blood vessels or nerves in it. The musculoskeletal system is derived from mesenchyme.

The bone, cartilage, ligaments, and tendons contain specialized cells that secrete an extracellular matrix. The cells of these tissues are separated by this matrix, and the unique

1

Table 1–1.   **Total Number of Physician Contacts per Year for Acute and Chronic Conditions**

Condition	No. in Thousands
Acute conditions	
Influenza	36,008
Common cold	32,157
Fractures/dislocations	24,453
Sprains/strains	24,184
Chronic conditions	
Hypertension	69,088
Deformity/orthopedic impairment	59,205
Arthritis	44,167

Data from Ries.[13]

property of each of these tissues depends on the property of the matrix. For example, bone is hard and supports all other soft tissues, whereas cartilage in the ear is flexible. The matrix is composed of amorphous ground substance and two types of fibers. The main constituent of the ground substance is proteoglycan. Physical properties of the ground substance vary. There are two types of fibers in the connective tissues — collagen and elastic. The collagen fibers contribute strength to the tissue but cannot be stretched (e.g., tendon), whereas elastic fibers, such as those in blood vessels, can be stretched and return to their original length.

Muscle

The ability of skeletal muscles to contract and change their length is utilized in performing various voluntary movements. All movements are controlled by the central nervous system via peripheral nerves. Each muscle is made up of individual contractile units called muscle fibers. The group of muscle fibers innervated by one anterior horn cell forms a **motor unit.** This is the smallest unit that can be controlled by volition.

Tendons and Ligaments

Tendons and ligaments have similar structure, consisting primarily of bundles of collagen fibers that are parallel to each other. Tendons transfer the contractile force from muscles to bone and generate or prevent movement. Ligaments attach bone to bone and prevent abnormal movements between two bones and are essential for stability of joints. Since both these structures are metabolically not very active, they have minimal blood supply. Injuries of ligaments and tendons heal with fibrous tissue and not by regeneration of the original tissue.

Table 1-2. **Principal Reasons for Visits to Ambulatory Care Physicians in 1985**

	No. in Thousands	% of all Visits
Pain in upper extremity	15,495	2.4%
Back pain	17,195	2.7%
Pain in lower extremity	22,332	3.5%
Arthropathies	16,239	2.5%
Sprains/strains	14,567	2.3%
All visits	636,386	100%

Data from Nelson and McLemore.[10]

Cartilage

Cartilage is found in immature bones, over joint surfaces, and in stuctures such as the nose, ear, and tracheal rings. The amorphous matrix of cartilage has small cavities which contain chondrocytes (cartilage cells). Under normal circumstances, these cells are not very active metabolically. The joint surface is covered by **articular cartilage,** which provides a very smooth lining for the bones to move on with least friction. The articular cartilage is an avascular structure and gets its nutrition from joint fluid by diffusion. Once damaged, it does not heal well.

Bone

The bone is a living tissue capable of changing its structure to meet the demands of function and capable of repairing itself after injury. The cells in bone are called osteocytes. **Osteoblasts** are specialized cells that form the osteoid matrix of bone. Later, hydroxyapatite crystals are deposited in this matrix. Resorption of bone is done by **osteoclasts.** Osteoblasts and osteoclasts are very active during the process of repair after fractures.

Joints

Joints are formed where two or more bones meet. The joints where bones move against each other have articular cartilage covering them. Fibrous capsule and ligaments prevent abnormal movements between the bones. Synovial membrane lines the inner side of the capsule and secretes synovial fluid. This fluid lubricates and nourishes the articular cartilage. These joints are called **synovial joints.** When movement is not an essential function of a joint, two bones may be held together by fibrous tissue or cartilage. These joints are called **fibrous** or **cartilaginous joints.**

EVALUATION

A systematic plan for evaluating patients is very important to ensure correct diagnosis and management. During evaluation, we should seek answers to the following questions:
1. Where is the pathology? (What anatomical structure is involved?)
2. What is the pathology?
3. What can I do to help this patient?
The process of evaluation starts from the time the patient walks into the office and then continues.

HISTORY

A detailed history plays the most valuable part in arriving at the diagnosis. The patient should be given full opportunity to narrate the history. Questions should be asked in simple language without medical jargon.
1. **Age** and **sex** are noted since some diseases are common in certain age groups, whereas the prevalence of some other diseases varies according to the sex.
2. **History of present illness. Chief complaint** is the main symptom for which the patient has gone to see the physician. How and when did it start (**onset**), and how long (**duration**) has it been present? Have the symptoms been present continuously or intermittently (**progression**)? Has the **severity** of symptoms varied over time? Details of each symptom (**other complaints**) are noted in **chronologic order.** Sometimes, it is necessary to mention negative findings, such as "there was no history of trauma." Informa-

tion about previous **investigations** or **treatments** carried out by another physician and the results of these attempts should also be requested. Which medications has the patient tried before? Were there any adverse reactions? Did he or she undergo any operations? Were any physical therapy modalities tried?

3. **Review of systems** is important for the diagnosis of systemic illness or associated medical problems. Some patients may present with more than one medical problem. A patient with inflammatory arthritis may also have diarrhea, dry mouth, or inflammation of eyes. This information helps not only in diagnosis but also in management.

4. **Past medical history** of illnesses, injuries, and operations may shed some light on the diagnosis and management of present problems. It is very important to find out if the patient is **allergic** to any medications.

5. **Personal history.** Smoking and alcohol abuse can give rise to many medical problems and affect the outcome in other unrelated illness. Information about occupation and avocational activites may suggest overuse injuries and help formulate management strategies.

6. **Family history** plays an important role in the diagnosis of hereditary and environmental illnesses.

7. **Functional ability** includes:
   a. **Activities of daily living** (ADL). ADLs concern difficulty with buttons, shoe laces, dressing, etc. How are these activities affected by the illness? Does the patient need any help with bathing or getting off a toilet seat? Some musculoskeletal conditions are progressive. Has there been any change over time? Does the patient live alone, or is there a family member who can help in any of the ADLs?
   b. **Vocational.** Can the patient do his or her job? Did he or she lose a job because of the medical problem?
   c. **Avocational** pursuits (recreational activities). Was the patient an avid skier or runner before the accident? How important is it for the patient to ski or run again?

8. **Psychosocial history** seeks to determine how the patient is coping with the effects of the illness. Is there any evidence of:
   a. Denial, anger, anxiety, or depression.
   b. Strained family relationships. Who is doing the chores that the patient used to do before the accident? Is there conflict with other family members because the patient is not able to drive?
   c. Is the patient experiencing any financial problems because of the illness?

Clinical Features

Some of the common symptoms of musculoskeletal problems are:

   Pain (the most common symptom of musculoskeletal problems—*see* Page 18)
   Swelling
   Deformity
   Neurologic symptoms (tingling, numbness, weakness.)

History and physical examination of these complaints are modified according to the list of differential diagnoses.

Physical Examination

1. **Preliminary.** Observe how the patient walks into the office, how he or she sits down, the facial expressions, etc. Does the patient fidget or sit quietly? If possible, watch how he or she undresses: how far and how easily does he or she bend down to untie shoe laces?

2. **Pulse** rate and **blood pressure** are noted.

3. **Regional**. The part of anatomy to be examined is exposed adequately. For examination of low back pain, the whole spine and both lower extremities should be available for inspection, palpation, and measurements. Sometimes, pain or other symptoms are referred to a distant part of the body, e.g., hip pain referred to the knee. Under these circumstances, findings on examination of the hip will be completely normal.
4. **Inspection.** The most important and often neglected part of the physical examination is observation of the affected area.
   a. **Skin.** Note color, scars, sinus, ulcer, etc.
   b. **Swelling.** Site, size, shape, and signs of inflammation.
   c. **Alignment.** Note the relation of the injured part with the rest of the body (e.g., relation of head and neck to the rest of the body). What is the relation between different subunits of the part under examination (e.g., relation between the elbow and arm to the forearm)? Posture and angular deformity are observed.
      i. **Varus**—Distal part of the extremity is more toward the midline than in the normal (Fig. 1–1).
      ii. **Valgus**—Distal limb is deformed away from the midline (Fig. 1–1).
   d. **Muscle atrophy** of muscles proximal to a swollen joint or supplied by an involved nerve.
5. **Palpation**
   a. **Temperature.** With the dorsal surface of the fingers, compare temperature of the involved part with the normal. This should be done before the part is handled for other tests.
   b. **Tenderness.** Are the superficial tissues tender, or are deep tissues involved? **Localized tenderness** is the most helpful sign in determining the anatomic structure involved. Exquisite tenderness is associated with infection.
   c. **Swelling.** Confirm the findings of inspection.
      Surface—smooth or knobby?
      Consistency—Soft, firm, or hard (bony)?
      Edge—Lipomas have a definite edge which slips under the finger.

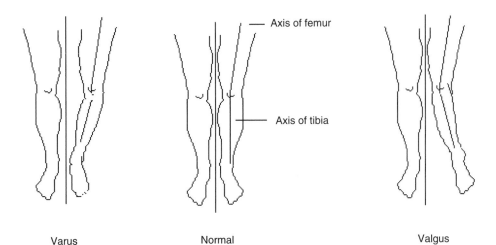

Varus   Normal   Valgus

Fig. 1–1 Varus and valgus deformity. In varus deformity, the distal part of the extremity is displaced toward the median plane, whereas in valgus deformity, the distal part moves away from the median plane.

Fluctuation—Fat (pseudofluctuation) or fluid?

Fixed or movable—Attached to skin or deeper structures?

Anatomic structure of origin—Does the swelling arise from skin, muscle, or bone?

Is it effusion in a joint?

Number—Is it a single swelling or multiple?

6. **Measurement**

   a. **Range of motion.** Is there any **pain** on movements? Palpate the joint for any **crepitation.** Joint movements are shown in Figure 1–2.

   i. **Active**—The patient performs ROM. Sometimes, the patient is asked to perform active movements **against resistance** offered by examiner's hand. This is done to elicit pain or measure muscle strength.

   ii. **Passive**—ROM is performed by the examiner. If the passive ROM is more than the active, then it is due either to weakness of the involved muscles, pain on movement, or injury to the muscles and tendons that carry out this movement.

   The ROM is measured in degrees of change in the angle from the neutral to the final position. **Fixed deformity** is measured by bringing the limb as close to the neutral as possible. For the knee joint, the leg is brought up to line up with the

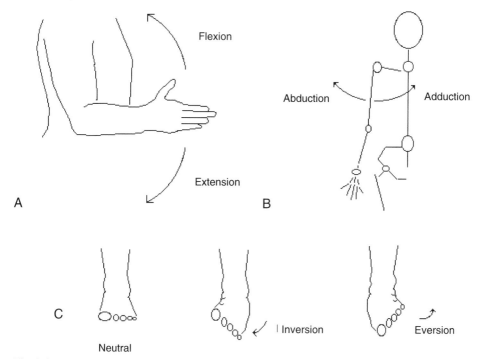

Fig. 1–2 Joint movements include flexion, extension, abduction, adduction, inversion and eversion. *A*, Flexion occurs when the distal part moves forward from the neutral position. The knee joint and spine are exceptions. For the knee joint, the leg moves backward during flexion; for the spine the proximal part (the head or trunk) moves forward. Extension occurs when the distal part moves backward. The knee and spine also are exceptions. *B*, Abduction occurs when the distal part moves away from the midline of the body or a predetermined axis (e.g., fingers and toes). Adduction is movement toward the midline of the body or a predetermined axis. *C*, Inversion and eversion are complex twisting or rotational movements of the foot. Inversion is movement toward the midline of the body, and eversion is movement away from the midline.

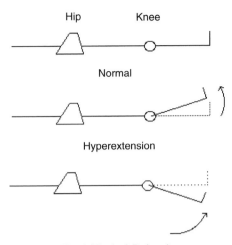

Fig. 1–3 Knee ROM. In a normal knee, the leg can be brought up to the same horizontal plane as the thigh (neutral position). If the leg can be extended beyond neutral, it is called hyperextension. When full extension is attempted but cannot be reached, the remaining angle is called fixed flexion deformity.

thigh. The angle between the neutral position and the closest possible position is the angle of fixed deformity (Fig. 1–3).

b. **Limb girth.** The diameter of the limb is measured at a definite distance from a bony point and compared with the opposite side. This is the best way to confirm atrophy of muscles.

7. **Special tests** are performed depending on the structure involved and differential diagnosis. Tests for ligamentous instability, McMurray's test, and others are included in this category.

a. **Neurologic examination** is necessary when a peripheral nerve or nerve root is affected or a central nervous system disease (CNS) is suspected.

i. **Sensation**—Touch, position, vibration, temperature, etc. are tested according to the symptoms and differential diagnosis.

ii. **Motor**—Muscle atrophy, tone, and strength are determined.

iii. **Reflexes**—Deep tendon reflexes and superficial reflexes such as plantar reflex help in localization of neurologic lesions.

b. **Gait** may be abnormal because of:

Pain

Joint stiffness

Muscle weakness

Neurologic disease

Leg-length discrepancy or deformity

The gait should be observed in all patients with lower extremity, back, and neurologic problems. Normal gait is smooth and symmetrical. The body's center of gravity, which is normally located just in front of the second sacral vertebra, moves up and down and from side to side about 2 inches. It is important to note any excessive or asymmetrical movement of any part of the body.

The gait cycle is described as starting from one heel touching the ground to the same heel striking the ground again (Fig. 1–4). At this point, one foot (**single stance phase**) or both feet (**double stance phase**) are in contact with the ground.

Stance phase

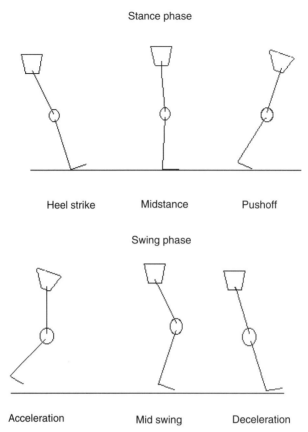

Heel strike   Midstance   Pushoff

Swing phase

Acceleration   Mid swing   Deceleration

Fig. 1–4   Normal gait cycle.

After the heel strike, the forefoot comes down smoothly. If there is weakness of the foot dorsiflexors, the forefoot comes down suddenly with a slap. Normally, the heel then rises off the ground, and the forefoot pushes downward and backward to propel the body forward. This movement requires strong gastrocnemius-soleus muscles. The foot is free to go forward until the next heel strike, which is called the **swing phase.** Does the patient spend equal time on both feet? If one side is painful, he or she will tend to cut short the weight-bearing time on that foot (**antalgic gait.**) Is the length of each step equal on both sides? Is he or she able to clear the ground well during the swing phase, or does the foot drag? Foot drop is usually due to previous stroke or peroneal nerve palsy. To avoid dragging the foot, the patient may have to lift the leg up high, as in **high steppage gait.** Observe each component of the body from foot and ankle to knees, hips, spine, shoulders, arms, and head, and see how each one of these parts moves in relation to the other. Does the patient walk with a lot of distance between the feet (**wide-based gait**)?

8. **Opposite side.** Always compare findings on the involved side to the similar structure on the opposite side. This is very useful if only one side is affected.
9. **Other Systems.** Examine the peripheral vasculature or abdomen as the circumstances demand. Is pain in the back secondary to systemic illness or abdominal malignancy?

Differential Diagnosis

The physician starts compiling a list of differential diagnoses while taking the history. Further questions are asked to rule out or confirm any of the differential diagnoses that are entertained. A similar process goes on during physical examination. It is important to think about the common problems first; then think about unusual manifestations of common problems; consider rare conditions last. Special tests in the physical examination are performed depending on the list of differential diagnoses.

INVESTIGATIONS

A list of differential diagnoses is compiled after the initial history and physical examination. This list should contain two types of problems:

1. The **most likely diagnoses** are on the top of the list—e.g., in a 60-year-old patient with knee pain for 6 months, degenerative arthritis should be the first consideration.
2. Diagnoses needing **immediate attention,** such as fracture or septic arthritis, are next on the list. Investigations are ordered immediately to rule out these conditions, as a delay in diagnosis will affect the outcome.

Tests are ordered according to the list of differential diagnoses. If after the first round of tests nothing turns up, then a list of more uncommon problems is made and tests are ordered to rule these out. The list of investigations should be as short as necessary to arrive at a diagnosis, prognosis, and prescription of appropriate treatment. However, in this day of legal and other threats, the list of investigations may become very long and expensive.

Two factors should be considered before ordering any test:

1. How **useful** will the test result be in the diagnosis and management of the patient. X-rays of the cervical spine in most of patients over age 60 will show changes of degenerative arthritis. Because these changes are so prevalent in this age group, cervical x-rays may not be very helpful in telling us whether the pain in the neck and shoulder is because of degenerative joint disease of the cervical spine or a trigger point. The x-ray finding may be a mere coincidence.

   An ideal test has a **sensitivity** of 100%, meaning the test will be positive in all patients with the disease (true-positive). The **specificity** of an ideal test will also be 100%, so that all those who do not have the disease will show a negative result (true-negative). However, there is no ideal test, and a certain percentage of results are always either false-positive or false-negative. If a very highly sensitive test is negative, it may help to rule out a disease. A very highly specific test when positive helps to confirm the disease.
2. The investigations should not be **harmful** to the patient. The patient should not be worse after a test than before. However, it is always difficult to predict outcome of any procedure in an individual patient.

Blood Tests

Complete blood count is useful in the diagnosis of anemia and infections.

Erythrocyte sedimentation rate (ESR) is a nonspecific test that, when abnormal, suggests diseases such as infection, inflammatory arthritis, or malignancy. The Westergren method is preferred. The normal range in males is 0–15 mm/hr, and for females, 0–20 mm/hr. It is higher in children and older individuals. It is useful in following the course of a disease and effectiveness of treatment in diseases such as giant cell arteritis.

Immunologic Tests

Rheumatoid factor (RF) is *not* diagnostic of rheumatoid arthritis. It is positive in 75–80% of rheumatoid arthritis patients and may be positive in other connective tissue diseases. RF is present in 15–50% of people over 60 years of age. A positive test should always be correlated with history and physical examination.

Antinuclear antibodies (ANA) are positive in most cases of systemic lupus erythematosus but may be positive in other connective tissue diseases and a small percentage of the normal elderly population. It is important to know the titer at which the test is considered positive.

Urine Tests

Urinalysis is done to check for proteinuria secondary to renal involvement or to follow a patient with nephropathy. A 24-hour excretion of uric acid helps in evaluating treatment of gout.

Diagnostic Imaging

Plain Radiographs

Plain x-rays are a very useful and commonly requested test. They are two-dimensional shadows and are usually done in two planes to get proper perspective of the structure being examined. **Anteroposterior** (AP) and **lateral** films are the standard views. Sometimes, **oblique** or special views are done for certain conditions. The intervertebral foramina in the cervical spine are visualized in oblique views only.

The density on a plain x-ray film depends on the atomic weight of the elements in the tissue and the thickness of the tissue. Since it is a negative image, the heavier (by atomic weight) and thicker tissues are seen as lighter, and lighter (by atomic weight) tissues are seen as darker on the film. From darkest to lightest on a plain film, it is gas > fat > muscle > cartilage > medullary cavity of a bone> bony cortex > metal (Fig. 1–5). These differences help to distinguish between different structures.

Plain x-rays are ordered almost routinely in the U.S. for anyone with musculoskeletal problems. It is important to know that degenerative changes in joints may be seen in an increasing percentage of people as they age. Just because some osteophytes are seen on x-rays of the cervical spine of a 60-year-old patient, it does not mean that the cause of pain is degenerative arthritis or the radicular pain is due to narrowing of the intervertebral foramen. Plain films are helpful in diagnosis and follow-up of bone and joint conditions.

1. **Indications.** X-rays should be ordered:
   a. After injury—When fracture or dislocation is suspected
   b. Osteomyelitis—Useful in diagnosis
   c. Malignancy—Useful in diagnosis
   d. Congenital abnormalities (e.g., spina bifida, clubfoot)—Provides information regarding bones and joints
   e. Inflammatory arthritis—Useful in diagnosis and to check progression
2. **Contraindications**
   a. Not useful in soft tissue problems, such as bursitis
   b. **Contraindicated in pregnancy**

Reading x-rays.

It is important to have a definite plan for observing x-rays. Always use a viewing box. If you are used to viewing the hand of a patient with his or her fingers pointing toward the

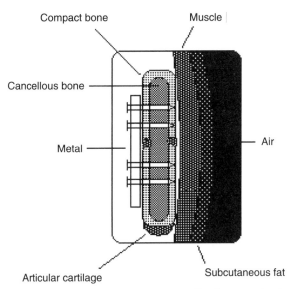

Compact bone   Muscle

Cancellous bone

Metal   Air

Articular cartilage   Subcutaneous fat

Fig. 1–5   X-ray density of different tissues. A plain x-ray film is a negative image of the x-ray's ability to travel through different tissues. Metallic implants stop most of the rays and are seen as the lightest, air is seen as the darkest shadow, and other tissues are seen as intermediate shades.

ceiling, then put the film on the viewing box in the same way. Try to visualize the anatomy of the structure you are studying. If you are writing a report, the part of the body being examined should be mentioned—e.g., "Plain x-ray of the right shoulder, AP and lateral views show . . . ."

Look at the film from a **distance** to get an idea of the whole picture. Observe the soft tisssues, general **density** of the bones, and **alignment** of bones and joints. Are the general **contour** and **proportions** of the bones normal?

Some structures are observed at a **closer** distance:

1. **Soft tissues.** Not enough attention is paid to soft tissues when viewing plain x-rays. **Swelling** of soft tissues is seen early in inflammatory arthritis. **Effusions** can also be seen on good plain film. **Calcification** may be seen in chronic rotator cuff problems as amorphous densities. Formation of organized bone in muscles is called myositis ossificans. **Gas** gangrene can be picked up as radiolucent areas in an extremity on plain x-ray.

2. **Joint. Soft tissue** surrounding the joint is observed first. The articular cartilage is less dense than bone, and this is seen as **joint space** on x-rays. In rheumatoid arthritis, there is uniform narrowing of this joint space, whereas in degenerative arthritis, the narrowing is irregular. Calcification of intra-articular cartilage (e.g., meniscus in the knee joint) is seen in chondrocalcinosis. **Bony surfaces** forming the joint are observed for any irregularities or erosions. **Osteophytes** are seen in degenerative arthritis near the margin of articular cartilage. The density of cortical and medullary bone near an inflamed joint is less (juxta-articular **osteoporosis**).

3. **Bone cortex.** Follow the margins of cortical bone, and look for any breaks, thickness, texture, erosions, new bone formation, or surface irregularities. The cortical bone is thin in **osteoporosis**. A break in the continuity of cortical bone is seen in **fractures. New bone** formation is seen in healing fractures, malignant tumors, and infections (osteomyelitis).

4. **Medullary cavity.** Is it larger than normal? Are cortical margins irregular? **Trabecular** pattern relates to muscle contraction and weight-bearing forces. Trabeculae are thinner or absent in osteoporosis and thicker in Paget's disease.

Computed Tomography (CT)

In CT, the x-ray images are manipulated by a computer to give more information about various anatomical structures. It involves exposing the patient to ionizing radiation. The CT scan can be done in a few seconds and is less distorted by movement than MRI. It also gives more details about the bone structure. For these reasons, it is more useful in acute trauma, especially of skull, spine, and pelvis. It is also useful in early cerebrovascular accidents to rule out hemorrhagic infarcts.

Magnetic Resonance Imaging (MRI)

The patient is placed in a strong magnetic field, and changes produced in this magnetic field create images of different tissues. The patient is not exposed to ionizing radiation. The images produced can be seen in different planes such as transverse, oblique, coronal, or sagittal to visualize anatomy and pathology. However, the patient must lie still within the magnet for a considerable time. New machines work faster, with less time required for imaging. Any implant with ferromagnetic material, such as a pacemaker, foreign body in the eye, or arterial clips, is a contraindication for this test.

MRI is more useful in delineating soft tissue pathology than CT. Tears of the cruciate ligaments and meniscus in the knee, protruded intervertebral discs, or rotator cuff tears in the shoulder are picked up much better by MRI than CT. The extent of tumor in the medullary cavity of the bone is determined better on MRI. However, distinguishing features of bony tumors is appreciated better on plain x-rays. Abnormalities of the CNS, such as cerebral infarcts, multiple sclerosis, tumors, and syringomyelia, can be diagnosed by MRI.

Electromyography and Nerve Conduction Studies

Electromyography and nerve conduction studies are useful in the diagnosis of a number of conditions (Table 1–3).

Electromyography (EMG) is done by inserting needle electrodes in various muscles. Normal muscle at rest shows no electrical activity; motor unit potentials are seen when a muscle contracts. Spontaneous electrical activity is seen in muscles whose nerve supply is

Table 1–3. Indications for Electromyography and Nerve Conduction Studies

Anatomical Site	Diagnosis
Anterior horn cell	Amyotrophic lateral sclerosis
Nerve root	Radiculopathy
Plexus	Brachial plexus injury
	Brachial plexitis
Peripheral nerve	Peripheral neuropathy
	Compression syndromes
	Nerve injuries
Myoneural junction	Myasthenia gravis
	Myasthenic syndrome
Muscle fiber	Muscular dystrophy
	Polymyositis
	Myopathy

damaged. These abnormal waveforms may be fibrillations, positive waves, or fasciculations. The diagnosis of nerve damage is arrived at by analyzing the type and distribution of spontaneous activity.

Nerve conduction studies (NCS) are carried out by stimulating peripheral nerves with electrical impulses, causing the muscle supplied by this nerve to contract. Electrodes placed over the muscle pick up the electrical changes and measure the time elapsed between stimulus and response. The time it takes for the impulse to travel along the nerve is determined, and hence, nerve conduction velocity is calculated. Sensory and motor nerves can be studied by this method. NCS is useful in peripheral neuropathy, compression neuropathy (e.g., carpal tunnel syndrome), and nerve injuries.

Aspiration of Joint Fluid (Arthrocentesis)

Normal joints contain very small quantities of fluid in the synovial cavity. This fluid is clear, yellow, and viscous. The joint space is a potential space that can accommodate a larger quantity of fluid under abnormal conditions. Fluid from a joint may be removed to determine the etiology of the joint effusion or as a treatment.

Indications for joint aspiration include:
1. **Diagnosis**
   a. **Infectious** or **inflammatory arthritis**—To confirm the diagnosis and identify the organisms and their antibiotic suceptibility.
   b. **Crystal-induced arthritis** (e.g., gout)—Diagnosed by observing urate crystals in the joint fluid
2. **Therapeutic** aspiration is done to remove the offending joint fluid and inject medications into the joint.
   a. Infection—Joint fluid is aspirated to remove harmful products that, if allowed to remain in the joint, may destroy the cartilage and ligaments.
   b. Trauma—Blood in the joint cavity (**hemarthrosis**) irritates the synovial lining and produces an inflammatory response. The degradation products of blood also damage the articular cartilage. After any injury, it is important to determine if the joint effusion is due to blood or excessive synovial fluid. Hemarthrosis suggests a fracture involving the articular surface, rupture of intra-articular ligament (e.g., cruciate liagament of the knee), or tear of the synovial membrane. It is also seen in bleeding disorders such as hemophilia.
   c. **Inflammatory arthritis**—Therapeutic substances like steroids are injected to control inflammation. Sometimes, fluid is removed so that large effusions do not lead to lax ligaments and deformity of joints.
   d. **Pain relief**—Acute distention of the joint by fluid is painful.

Contraindication. If there is infection near the site where the needle is to be inserted, then this infection may be carried into the joint. This complication should be avoided at all costs.

Technique

The technique of injection of an individual joint is described in that particular chapter. Thorough aseptic precautions are absolutely essential. The skin surrounding the site of injection is cleaned with iodine preparation and alcohol. Aspiration should be done in a clean environment with gloves and mask to prevent infection of the joint cavity.

Joint Fluid Examination

1. **White blood cell** (WBC) **count** is increased markedly in infections and to a lesser extent in inflammatory arthritis.

2. **Gram stain** is used to look for gram-positive or -negative organisms in suspected infections. If other organisms (e.g., tubercle bacilli or fungi) are suspected, then appropriate stains are used.
3. **Culture** and **antibiotic sensitivity** to antibiotics are important for treatment of joint infections.
4. **Crystals** of uric acid or calcium pyrophosphate, if seen on microscopy, are helpful in diagnosis and management.
5. **Rheumatoid factor** can also be tested in joint fluid.

Complications
1. **Septic arthritis** is the most dreaded complication. Pain, increased swelling, raised local and systemic temperature, and leukocytosis point to this diagnosis. If infection of a joint cavity is suspected, then joint fluid should be aspirated immediately; smear, culture, and sensitivity are done; and appropriate antibiotics started.
2. **Increased pain** is felt around the joint for a day or two after steroid injection. This usually subsides without treatment. The patient should be informed about this complication before the injection is given.
3. **Osteonecrosis** develops if too many steroid injections are given in the same joint. Any one joint should not be injected > 3 times in a year.

Biopsy
Biopsy is ordered for diagnosis of **tumors** of the bone or muscle or **deep-seated infection** of the bone. It is important to know the origin of the tumor and whether it is malignant or benign. A biopsy may be the only way to determine which organisms are causing the infection.

PRINCIPLES OF MANAGEMENT

All the efforts made in getting the history, examining the patient, and ordering investigations are ultimately to answer the question, "How can I help this patient?" Several factors should be kept in mind while coming up with a plan of treatment.
1. **Diagnosis.** The treatment is determined by the patient's medical problem.
   a. Does the condition need **immediate treatment?** If septic arthritis or fracture is the diagnosis, then the patient should be treated immediately to prevent damage to the joint or to control pain.
   b. Is there a **cure** for this condition? Is it possible to eliminate the pathology and restore complete function? The treatment for these conditions is usually definite, e.g., specific antibiotics for infection.
   c. Most musculoskeletal conditions do not fit in with either *a* or *b* above. The treatment plan for these conditions becomes more complicated. The exact etiology or pathology may not be known, nor can it be eradicated. Some physicians may give up when they see advanced degenerative changes on x-rays of the cervical spine. There is no real cure for this condition, and the osteophytes cannot be removed by surgery or the joints and discs cannot be replaced (yet) by artificial ones. Some patients, though, can benefit from other forms of treatment, including nonsteroidal anti-inflammatory drugs, (NSAIDs) local heat, and cervical traction.

2. **Prevention.** Some diseases can be prevented more easily than treated (e.g., poliomyelitis). If it cannot be prevented by a vaccine, then can its spread can be prevented (e.g., AIDS)? Can we do anything to stop its progress, or is it possible to prevent complications, such as deconditioning due to prolonged bedrest?
3. **Simple, innocuous measures first.** If plain acetaminophen can control the pain, narcotics should be avoided. If NSAIDs are effective, then it is better to avoid steroids. For most conditions, conservative therapy is preferable to surgery.

How to Plan a Treatment Program
1. **Problem List.** It is important to arrive at a diagnosis before planning a treatment program. For some musculoskeletal conditions, it is not enough to know the diagnosis, especially when the condition is not curable. After all the medical diagnoses are determined, a list of problems as perceived by the patient and the physician is made.

   For example, a patient with degenerative arthritis of the hip may have the problems identified in Table 1–4.

   It is important to make a list of all the problems (including small problems like putting on socks) and then fomulate a plan of treatment for each one. The greater the number of small problems one can solve, the more comfortable the patient will be. This type of approach requires evaluation and treatment by a multidisciplinary team. Depending upon the patient's needs and the available resources, the team may consist of a physician, physical therapist, occupational therapist, nurse, social worker, psychologist, and possibly others. Team meetings are held to discuss management and progress. After a reasonable time, a follow-up evaluation will help to determine if the treatments were effective.
2. **Goals.** For each problem, it is good to set a goal—what can be achieved by the proposed treatment?
3. **Plan.** The third step is to formulate a plan of action.

   Before starting any treatment, it is useful to ask several questions: What are the chances of the patient getting better without any treatment? Can we use a simple innocuous treatment? Is there any chance of the patient getting worse after potentially dangerous medication? Are complications of the treatment worse than the disease? What would we like to achieve with treatment?

Medications
Pain is the most common complaint, and medications for pain are prescribed most commonly. Drugs that are most effective and least toxic are given first preference. The inci-

Table 1-4. Planning a Treatment Program

Problem List	Plan
1. Pain on walking	Use cane in the opposite hand
2. Pain at night	NSAIDs
3. Difficulty tying shoelaces	Occupational therapy
4. Putting on socks	Occupational therapy
5. Getting into bathtub	Bench seat
6. Obesity	Diet to lose weight
7. Cannot walk long distance	Wheelchair
8. Job involves climbing ladders	Vocational counseling, desk job

dence of adverse reactions increases with dosage. Within reasonable limits, it is better to use the smallest dose that effectively controls the symptoms. However, for inflammatory arthritis, the patient may require a higher dose to control inflammation.

Ancillary Treatments

We often forget to use some of the simple measures.

Rest

Rest is required for healing of inflammation, infection, and trauma. It may be local or general. **Local** rest is provided by splints or cast and is prescribed for local injury or inflammation, e.g., deQuervain's disease. **General** rest for the whole body is necessary for acute flareups of rheumatoid arthritis or other systemic illnesses.

Physical and Occupational Therapy

The physical therapist (PT) provides local heat, cold, exercises, traction, ambulation training. The occupational therapist (OT) usually is involved with showing activities and exercises for the upper extremity, evaluating ADLs, and teaching patients how to be independent in ADLs. The OT also makes hand splints and suggests aids for independent living. It is important for the physician to know the academic background and training of PTs and OTs and to have good personal communication with them in order to obtain the best results for the patients. The therapist would like to know the medical diagnoses, any precautions to be aware of, and goals of treatment—i.e., what the physician would like to achieve.

Heat and Cold

Heat over the affected area helps to **relieve pain** for a short duration. It is often used before exercises in physical therapy to improve the patient's performance by reducing pain. It also helps reduce **muscle spasm.** Heat is **contraindicated** over skin with diminished sensation or with poor circulation because of fear of burns. Immediately after injury, heat may aggravate swelling and pain. In patients with bleeding tendency (e.g., hemophilia), heat is not indicated because of increased chances of bleeding into tissues.

There are mainly two types of heating modalities—superficial and deep. The **superficial** methods are electric heating pad, heat lamp, hydrocollator pack, or paraffin bath. The heating pad and lamp can be used at home for 20–30 minutes at a time, 3–4 times a day. It is important to instruct the patient in safe usage of these modalities. The paraffin bath is useful for subacute rheumatoid or degenerative arthritis of the hand. **Deep heat** is given by ultrasound or shortwave diathermy (SWD), usually by a physical therapist. SWD should *not* be used on a patient with a cardiac pacemaker or metallic implants.

Cold is used after acute trauma to a superficial musculoskeletal structure. It reduces posttraumatic pain, swelling, and muscle spasm. Some patients with acute exacerbation of inflammatory arthritis (e.g., gout), may prefer cold applications more than heat in relieving their pain. The cold packs are **contraindicated** in patients with poor circulation, Raynaud's phenomenon, or cryoglobulinemia.

Exercise

Exercise is a very important and commonly prescribed modality. It may be a preventive or therapeutic measure prescribed for achieving specific goals:

1. **Range of motion.** Exercises are used for maintaining or increasing ROM. All joints need to be moved through full ROM at least once a day to prevent contractures. Soft tissues, such as the joint capsule, ligaments, muscles, and tendons, are stretched by this type of exercises. Stretching exercises are also done as warmup before other vigorous exercises. Gentle, prolonged stretch is good for correcting contractures. These exercises may be passive, active-assisted, or active.
2. **Increase strength.** Muscles lose strength if they are not used, as seen in patients in casts or on prolonged bedrest. Many different types of exercises are used for strengthening, including isometric, isotonic with weights, isokinetic, and others. Isometric exercises are done by contracting the muscles but without moving any joint. The muscle length remains the same.
3. **Cardiovascular fitness.** During exercise, the increased heart rate is maintained for a certain length of time. This type of exercise increases endurance and has beneficial effects on heart and blood vessels.
4. **Improve coordination.** In some neurologic conditions, muscular coordination deteriorates.

   Types of exercises include:
1. **Passive.** The patient's body part is moved by the therapist. The patient does not actively contract any muscle. This type of exercise is done when the patient is unable to actively move the part.
2. **Active-assisted.** The work of moving the body part is done by both the therapist and patient.
3. **Active.** Exercises are performed by the patient.

   Exercise should be **stopped** or reduced if:
1. Pain is aggravated.
2. Swelling of a joint or extremity is increased.
3. New pain develops during exercise which lasts > 2 hours after exercise is discontinued.
4. Muscle spasm
5. Increased weakness, shortness of breath, or undue fatigue

Traction

Traction is used for reducing fractures and dislocations and also for treatment of painful neck and back problems. It may be given by manual method, fixed weight, or motorized traction unit. The motorized traction can be continuous or intermittent.

Hydrotherapy

1. **Whirlpool.** Mechanical agitation and medications in water help to clean ulcers. It is important to remember that the warmth of water and dependent position of the limb may aggravate edema. Warm whirlpools without any medications are used for relaxation.
2. **Hubbard tank.** This small tank of water, which is larger than a whirlpool but smaller than a swimming pool, allows a patient on a stretcher to be lowered into the tank. Patients with extensive burns or severe rheumatoid arthritis can be treated for ROM exercises and cleaning ulcers.
3. **Swimming pool.** Buoyancy of water reduces weight-bearing stress on joints such as the hip and knee. This form of therapy is very useful for various arthritides and after operations or fractures of the lower extremity. The hot and humid environment may put strain on the cardiovascular system, causing the patient to faint or go into congestive heart failure. It may also be dangerous for persons with a history of seizures.

Transcutaneous Electrical Nerve Stimulation (TENS)

TENS uses a small battery-operated unit to generate electrical impulses at variable frequency and intensity. The electrodes from this unit are placed on the skin over painful areas or trigger points. Stimulation of large-diameter sensory fibers inhibits pain sensation. TENS may be useful in relieving chronic pain syndromes such as back pain or acute postoperative or postherpetic pain. It should *not* be used in patients with cardiac pacemakers.

Splints and Braces

These external devices are prescribed to:
1. Support injured tissues, such as after partial rupture of ligaments
2. Prevent abnormal movements after complete rupture of ligaments
3. Assist weak muscle, as for a foot drop after a stroke. This helps to improve gait (improve function).
4. A lumbosacral corset or cervical collar may help to restrict movement of painful parts. This may be indicated after an acute episode or operation on the neck or back.
5. Relieve weight when full weight-bearing may damage a bone or joint

Activities of Daily Living

Most people who have no physical limitations do not realize the importance of being able to perform simple activities such as walking or picking up food from the plate and putting it into the mouth. The physical therapist usually teaches transfer training, gait training, and stair climbing. The occupational therapist teaches how to dress, bathe, and groom, as well as how to do simple activities in the kitchen.

Surgery

An operation to remove an offending structure, such as a protruded intervertebral disc, is always an option to be considered. However, surgery should be undertaken only when there are definite reasons and all other safer and equally effective options have been exhausted.

PAIN

Pain is a very complex, subjective sensation that is difficult to confirm or measure objectively. No tests can prove or disprove its presence.

A strong mechanical, thermal, or chemical stimulus may be felt as pain. The sensation of pain protects us from further tissue damage by telling us to withdraw from the painful stimulus or stop the activity that causes pain. Pain sensation can be modified by medications, acupuncture, surgery, or emotion. A football player may not feel the pain of a fracture while he is on the field. A detailed history of pain can give important information necessary for the diagnosis. Pain is one of the most common symptoms of musculoskeletal diseases. Long-standing pain may lead to depression.

Neuroanatomy

Any injury due to a strong mechanical, thermal, or chemical stimulus releases prostaglandins and leukotrienes (Fig. 1–6). These mediators activate free nerve endings called nociceptors. Two types of nerve fibers are involved in transmitting pain sensation to the spinal cord—the **A δ** small-diameter, myelinated fibers and **C** unmyelinated fibers. The A δ

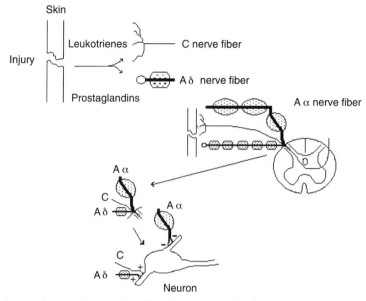

Fig. 1–6 Leukotrienes and prostaglandins released by injured tissues, generate impulses in un-myelinated C fibers and small-diameter A δ nerve fibers. Nerve impulses travel along these nerve fibers to the dorsal horn of the spinal cord. There, the nerve fibers form synapses with internuncial neurons. Further transmission of pain sensation can be inhibited by sensory input from large-diameter A α fibers.

fibers transmit nerve impulses faster than C fibers and convey sharp pricking type of pain sensation, whereas C fibers conduct long-lasting burning pain.

These fibers enter the spinal cord from the dorsal horn and form synapses with inter-nuncial neurons. The transmission of pain messages is inhibited at this level by sensations traveling along large-diameter A α fibers from the periphery. Descending fibers from the centers in brainstem and cortex are also capable of inhibiting pain sensation at this level. From the cells in the dorsal horn, the impulses travel along the spinothalamic and spin-oreticulothalamic tracts to the thalamus and from there to the cerebral cortex (Fig.1–7). The pain sensation is modified at both these levels. The sensory cortex posterior to the central gyrus in the parietal lobe is involved in pain sensation. The emotional aspect of pain is processed in the frontal lobe.

Pain sensation from superficial structures is very well localized by the nervous system. However, pain from deep structures is felt as a diffuse pain, and the patient is not able to localize the tissue of origin. The size of the area of this pain depends on the severity of pain. Sometimes, pain is felt in a part of the body away from its site of origin (**referred pain**). For example, pain due to the cholecystitis is referred to the right shoulder. The pain is re-ferred to the same segmental nerve distribution as the affected structure.[8] The diaphragm is supplied by cervical 3, 4, and 5 nerve roots, and the shoulder area is also innervated by the same cervical nerve root levels. The central nervous system is unable to localize the sen-sation exactly to upper quadrant of the abdomen, and the patient feels it in the shoulder.

Involvement of a nerve root, e.g., by a protruded intervertebral disc, gives rise to severe shooting pain along the course of that nerve. A **radiculopathy** may be confirmed by ab-

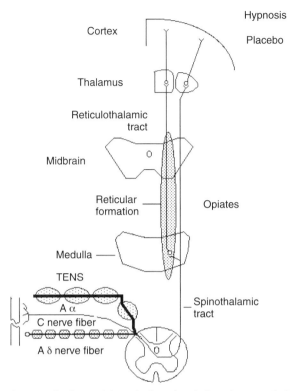

Fig. 1–7 From the posterior horn of the spinal cord, pain impulses travel along spinothalamic and reticulothalamic tracts to the thalamus and then to the cerebral cortex. Methods of inhibiting or moderating the painful stimulus are noted. TENS operates at the level of the synapses in the dorsal horn of the spinal column, where sensory impulses traveling on large-diameter A δ fibers block transmission from small-diameter A δ fibers. Opiates operate in the reticular formation. Hypnosis and placebo do not block pain transmission but modify their perception and the emotional response. Their site of action is the frontal cortex.

normal sensation (anesthesia or hyperesthesia), diminished muscle power, abnormal reflexes in the distribution of that nerve root, or electromyography.

History

1. **Onset.** Was the onset sudden or gradual? How did the pain start?
2. **Duration.** Date when the pain started.
3. **Precipitating causes.** Trauma, overuse, or other. Does the patient attribute the problem to any specific event?
4. **Site.** Location of the pain does not always coincide with the structure involved; e.g., pain around the knee joint may be referred from the hip joint. A **referred pain** is felt at a location away from the anatomical site of origin of the pain. Has the location of pain changed since its onset (**migration**)? This phenomenon may be seen in rheumatic fever.
5. **Character. Dull,** aching pain is usually from deeper structures. **Throbbing** pain is due

to an abscess. Severe **burning** may be due to nerve irritation. Has the character of the pain changed since its onset?

6. **Severity.** Depends on the pathology and the patient's threshold for pain. How does he or she react to pain ? Does the patient lie down, move around, or scream?

7. **Radiation.** When the pain starts in one place and radiates down or up to some other part of the body, it is described as radiation. Is it equally severe throughout its course? Does it radiate only at certain time or on certain movements? Radiation of pain is usually associated with involvement of a nerve root. For example, pain radiating down the thigh and leg along the sciatic nerve (**sciatica**) is thought to arise from involvement of one of the lumbosacral nerve roots forming the sciatic nerve.

8. **Aggravating factors.** Movements, position of the limb or body, coughing, or weather may affect the severity of pain. Did any previous treatment make the pain worse?

9. **Relieving factors.** Rest, local heat or cold, and body position may relieve the pain partially or completely.

10. **Course.** Has the pain been constant over a period of time, recurrent with exacerbations and remissions, or gradually progressive (getting worse)?

11. **Associated symptoms.** Right shoulder pain with fever and vomiting may be due to cholecystitis and not due to shoulder pathology.

Physical Examination

The physical examination depends on the region of the body involved. Regional examination is described at the beginning of chapters dealing with the individual part of anatomy involved.

1. **Inspection.** Does the skin over the painful area look normal? Is it red, or is there swelling in that region?

2. **Palpation.** Increased warmth and tenderness indicate **inflammation.** This is especially seen over a involved joint in inflammatory arthritis. Pain on light touch is seen in the acute stage of **reflex sympathetic dystrophy.**

3. **Range of motion.** All movements, active and passive, in all directions, are painful in septic or inflammatory arthritis. In degenerative arthritis, tendinitis, and bursitis, only certain movements are affected.

   a. **Active**—Movements are tested first without applying any resistance, and then they are performed against resistance. The patient is asked to carry out different movements. In subacromial bursitis, the patient may not be able to abduct his or her arm against resistance from neutral position but is able to abduct when no resistance is applied. Pain may be much worse when the muscle has to contract against resistance. There is no need to test passive ROM if a patient has full range of active movements without any pain.

   b. **Passive**—ROM tests are performed by the examiner. Movements are painful when the inflamed tissue is stretched. Passive ulnar deviation of the hand is painful in deQuervain's disease. All passive movements of the shoulder may be painful in adhesive capsulitis of the shoulder, but abduction and external rotation may be especially painful.

4. **Special Tests.** A **neurologic** examination is required to rule out nerve root involvement when a patient complains of radiating pain. Examination of the heart and an electrocardiogram may be necessary if myocardial infarction is suspected in a patient presenting with left shoulder pain.

Differential Diagnoses

Some anatomic structures or pathologic conditions give rise to characteristic pain, which may give a clue as to the structure involved.

1. **Abscess.** Severe, throbbing pain.
2. **Bone.** Sensory nerve endings are seen in the periosteum and around the blood vessels in the bone. Pain arising from diseases of the bone is described as deep and boring, and it is usually worse at night. It may be throbbing if it is due to infection such as osteomyelitis. Other common painful conditions are bone metastasis, osteoporosis, or Paget's disease. Pain due to fracture of a superficial bone is severe and well-localized. It is aggravated by movements and relieved, to some extent, by rest. Pain due to compression fracture of the lower thoracic or upper lumbar vertebrae (a deep structure) may be felt further down in the low back.
3. **Nerve.** Severe, burning pain and paresthesias radiating along the course of the nerve and in its distribution are felt in conditions affecting a peripheral nerve.
4. **Muscle ischemia.** Severe pain in a muscle may be due to ischemia or prolonged contraction (cramp). The pain of myocardial infarction or idiopathic muscle cramps are examples.
5. **Fibromyalgia.** Pain is felt at a distance from the trigger point and may mimic radicular pain by shooting down the extremity with paresthesias. Inflammatory conditions of muscles, such as polymyositis, give rise to localized muscle pain and tenderness.
6. **Degenerative arthritis.** There are no nerve fibers innervating the articular cartilage. Pain from superficial joints such as the knee is localized over the joint, but pain from the hip joint may be referred to the groin, thigh, or knee. It is worse during first 15–30 minutes after getting up in the morning, gets better after moving around, and then worsens again in the evening or after overuse.
7. **Inflammatory arthritis.** The pain is worse in the morning. The duration of morning stiffness and pain lasts much longer than the pain of degenerative arthritis and depends on the severity of disease.

Investigations

There is no specific test for pain. Thermography is believed by some to correlate with pain, but this is a controversial issue. Investigations for pain depend on the differential diagnosis.

Management

It is very important to remember that the complaint of pain is a symptom and not a diagnosis. Every effort should be made to arrive at a diagnosis. Treatment of pain depends on the diagnosis and whether the pain is acute or chronic. If the condition can be cured, then the management is for the specific pathology, e.g., an abscess needing drainage. Most of the common painful conditions of the musculoskeletal system, however, are not "curable." In that case, the following general guidelines should be followed. Reaction to pain is different at the extremes of age, i.e., in infants and children and in elderly patients.

Acute Pain

Medications for the treatment of acute pain are selected according to the diagnosis and severity of the pain. Drugs having the least chance of side effects and addiction are chosen—e.g., acetaminophen, aspirin, or an NSAID. Acetaminophen does not have any anti-inflammatory action, whereas aspirin and NSAIDs reduce the inflammatory response. For more severe pain, codeine may be considered, although side effects such as constipation and addiction should be kept in mind. Adequate control of pain during the acute stage is important so that the patient does not suffer too much and does not develop chronic pain syndrome. Musculoskeletal pain can also lead to muscle spasm, which in turn can give rise to more pain. This cycle of pain–muscle spasm–more pain should be broken by analgesics and muscle relaxants.

Simultaneous administration of two kinds of analgesics, such as aspirin and acetaminophen, can have an additive effect with better control of pain. During the acute stage, it is better to give analgesics at regular intervals around the clock than on an as-necessary basis (prn). The analgesic should be given before the pain becomes intolerable. Agents such as meperidine HCI (Demerol) are reserved for the immediate postoperative period and fractures. Methadone and hydromorphone HCI are also used for severe pain.

Acute Exacerbation of Chronic Pain

This pain is treated like an acute pain, with a work-up and follow-up for accurate diagnosis and appropriate treatment.

Chronic Pain

When pain has been present for a few months (usually $\geq$ 6 months), it is categorized as chronic. This group of patients has usually been to see many health professionals and received all sorts of treatments, including operations, NSAIDs, narcotics, physical therapy, and chiropractic treatments. They are in danger of developing depression and addiction to drugs and of losing their jobs and social status. On top of all these, their medical problem may not be curable.

The sensation of pain produces a different reaction from each individual patient. This subjective feeling of pain and the ability of each patient to tolerate it are different. In case of acute pain of short duration, analgesics help to relieve the pain. The patient gets a lot attention during the acute episode of pain and receives medications to control pain whenever he or she wants. This attention may be appropriate during that stage of illness, but if continued for a long time, it then reinforces drug-seeking and dependent behavior. After the acute stage, this behavior of the patient and the staff needs to change. The health professional should teach the patient about the disease and involve him or her in the treatment program. The patient takes responsibility for reducing the use of medications, and his or her level of activity is increased gradually.

Analgesics are not as effective in chronic pain as they are for acute pain. The patient may have been taking these drugs for a long time and may develop tolerance or addiction. These patients need a different approach. A multidisciplinary team evaluates the patient's medical condition and psychosocial effects. The treatment modalities may include local heat, exercises, transcutaneous electrical stimulation (TENS), hypnotherapy, relaxation techniques, acupuncture, biofeedback, behavior modification techniques, and others. These can be offered through a organized "pain clinic" setting.

INFLAMMATION AND REPAIR

Inflammation is the basic reaction of tissues to any injury. This response remains the same whether the trauma involves the bone or soft tissues. However, it differs in some of the details depending on the tissue involved. The common response is considered first, followed by how it differs in various musculoskeletal tissues. The purpose of the inflammatory response is to defend against further injury, remove debris, and repair the damaged tissue.

Etiology

A cell can be damaged by:
1. **Physical agents** such as trauma, excessive heat or cold, or ionizing radiation
2. **Chemical agents,** e.g., strong acids or alkali
3. **Biologic agents,** like bacteria, virus, or fungi
4. **Lack of oxygen** or other life-sustaining elements

Pathology

The inflammatory response attempts to reduce further injury, remove dead tissue, and repair the damaged tissue. It is initiated and maintained by **mediators** that are released from the damaged cells and from the blood. Histamine, prostaglandins, and lysosomal enzymes are liberated at the site of injury. They produce vasodilatation and increase vascular permeability. There is active migration of WBCs and exudation of fluid in the extravascular space. The clinical sign of redness is due to vasodilatation, local elevation of temperature is due to increased blood flow, and swelling is due to exudation of fluid in the extracellular space. Pain may be due to the mediators and/or swelling of the tissues. The inflammatory exudate is rich in protein and contains many polymorphonuclear leukocytes. Later, more mononuclear leukocytes (macrophages) are seen in the exudate. The macrophages engulf bacteria and dead cells and digest them. The enzymes in the exudate may destroy the normal cartilage of a joint. After the acute stage, the inflammatory process may lead to adhesions in a synovial joint or synovial sheath of a tendon and restrict motion.

   Repair is the last stage of the inflammatory reaction. New capillaries sprout from the edge of the necrotic area. Fibroblasts and new capillaries form granulation tissue. Collagen fibers are laid down to form scar tissue. Some tissues have great capacity for regeneration (e.g., bone), while others have very limited capability (e.g., muscle). After a fracture, the new bone resembles the original bone tissue, whereas damaged muscle fibers are replaced by fibrous tissue. Repair is delayed or deficient if there is infection or poor blood supply to the affected part or if the general condition of the patient is poor.

History

Pain is felt in the inflamed area and is due to chemical mediators of inflammation. The **swelling** and increased pressure on the nerve endings may also contribute. It is difficult to use the extremity because of pain (**loss of function**).

Physical Examination

1. **Inspection.** The inflamed region is **red** because of dilatation of blood vessels. The **swelling** is due to exudation of fluid in the extracellular tissue.
2. **Palpation.** Increased **warmth** is due to vasodilatation and increased blood flow through this area. The area is **tender** to touch and pressure.
3. **Range of motion.** All active and passive ROMs are restricted because of pain.

Management

Analgesics and **anti-inflammatory agents** help in relieving symptoms.

   Local **rest** to the affected part is provided by a splint or cast. Bedrest is prescribed when the inflammatory response is severe.

   Ice initially, followed by local **heat** later after the acute stage of the disease has subsided, is applied.

Bibliography

1. Anderson RE: Magnetic resonance imaging versus computed tomography—Which one? Postgrad Med 85(3):79–87, 1989.
2. Bassett LW, Gold RH: Magnetic resonance imaging of the musculoskeletal system. Clin Orthop 244(Jul): 17–28, 1989.
3. Cushmore FN, Kucharczyk W, Rodibaugh DL: MRI: When you can't afford not to. Patient Care Feb 28, 1989.
4. Doherty M, Hazelman BL, Hutton CW, et al: Rheumatology Examination and Injection Techniques. Philadelphia, W.B. Saunders, 1992.
5. Fields HL, Levine JD: Pain—Mechanisms and management. West J Med 141:347–357, 1984.
6. Health, United States, 1989. Washington, DC, National Center for Health Statistics, U.S. Department of Health and Human Services, 1990. [DHHS pub. 1 no. (PHS) 90–1232.]
7. Hoffman, MS: The World Almanac and Book of Facts. New York, World Almanac, 1991.
8. Kellgren JH: On distribution of pain arising from deep somatic structures with charts of segmental pain areas. Clin Sci 4:35–46, 1939.
9. Magid D: Computed tomographic imaging of the musculoskeletal system: Current status. Radiol Clin North Am 32(2):255–274, 1994.
10. Nelson C, McLemore T: The National Ambulatory Medical Care Survey: United States, 1975–1981 and 1985 Trends. Vital and Health Statistics series 13, no. 93. Washington, DC, National Center for Health Statistics, 1988. [DHHS publ. no. (PHS) 88–1754.]
11. Peterfy CG, Linares R, Steinbach LS: Recent advances in magnetic resonance imaging of the musculoskeletal system. Radiol Clin North Am 32(2):291–312, 1994.
12. Reuler JB, Girard DE, Nardone DA: The chronic pain syndrome: Misconceptions and management. Ann Intern Med 93:588–595, 1980.
13. Ries P: Physician Contacts by Sociodemographic and Health Characteristics, United States, 1982–1983. Vital and Health Statistics series 10, no. 161. Washington, DC, National Center for Health Statistics, 1987, [pp 14. DHHS publ. no. (PHS) 87–1589.]
14. Shmerling RH: Synovial fluid analysis. Rheum Dis Clin North Am 20(2):503–512, 1994.
15. Van de Streek PR, Carretta RF: Nuclear medicine approaches to musculoskeletal disease: Current status. Radiol Clin North Am 32(2):227–254, 1994.
16. Wernick R: Avoiding laboratory test misinterpretation in geriatric rheumatology. Geriatrics 44(2):61–77, 1989.

2

Pediatric Disorders

Chadwick F. Smith, M.D.

Musculoskeletal problems are very common in children and adolescents. Family physicians often see them before a specialist does. It is important for the primary care provider to recognize these conditions so that patients can be referred to a specialist at the appropriate time. Even among orthopedic surgeons, pediatric orthopedics is becoming a recognized subspeciality. Some pediatric problems are considered in other chapters:

4. Juvenile rheumatoid arthritis
5. Osteomyelitis
5. Infectious arthritis
12. Torticollis
13. Scoliosis (spina bifida)

18. Congenital dislocation of the hip
18. Slipped femoral epiphysis
18. Perthes' disease
20. Congenital clubfoot

General principles of history and physical examination mentioned in the first chapter are followed. It is important to know how the anatomy and pathology of the musculoskeletal system in infants, children, and adolescents differ from those in adults. Knowledge about the time of appearance of various epiphyses and their fusion with diaphyses is helpful in the diagnosis and treatment of injuries and other conditions.

Musculoskeletal trauma is fairly common in children. Bone and soft tissue injuries heal well and quickly and require little effort in rehabilitation. Some of the deformities due to malunion may correct on their own by the process of remodeling. On the other hand, injury to a growth plate may produce a deformity because of unequal growth. The possibility of child abuse should be kept in mind while examining a young patient with injuries. Abuse should be suspected if the parents are reluctant to talk about the injury or come up with conflicting stories. Recent and old bruises or burns on the same patient or fractures showing different stages of healing on x-rays also suggest child abuse.

GENU VARUM AND GENU VALGUM

Genu varum (bow legs) and **genu valgum** (knock knees) are the most common orthopedic complaints seen in children by primary care physicians. These deformities usually correct without treatment.

Anatomy

The long axis of the tibia is vertical, and the articular surfaces of its condyles are horizontal in the standing position. The femur forms an angle with the tibia which is $<180°$. This angle helps to accommodate the pelvis. Bow legs (genu varum) are normally present in infants and children up to age 3 years. This changes to knock knees (genu valgum) between ages 3 and 4 years. By the age of 5–7 years, the lower extremities become like those of the adult. Genu varum and valgum deformities of the growing years is called physiologic since most cases correct by themselves.

Etiology

The causes of **bilateral** genu varum and genu valgum deformities in children are:
1. Idiopathic
2. Rickets
3. Endocrine or other metabolic diseases

Unilateral genu varum is due to:
1. Injury to the epiphysis
2. Infection affecting the growth plate

Investigations

1. **Plain x-rays** of both lower extremities help to evaluate the degree of deformity and are useful in the diagnosis of conditions such as rickets.
2. **Calcium and phosphorus metabolism** is studied if any metabolic disease is suspected.

Genu Valgum

Knock knees is very common in children between the ages of 2–5 years. The deformity usually corrects itself by age 7, and no treatment is necessary.

Physical Examination and Investigations

1. **Special Tests.** The distance between the medial malleoli is measured while the child is standing and the knees are fully extended and touching each other. This is called the **intermalleolar distance.**
2. **Plain x-rays** of both lower extremities from hips to ankles are done with the child standing. The angle between the axis of the femur and that of the tibia is measured.

Management

A treatable condition such as rickets should be looked for and treated. Manipulative stretching, surgical epiphyseal stapling, closed osteoclasis, and open osteotomy have been tried in the past. In recent years, these conditions have been "left alone" to let nature take its course. In most cases, the mild to moderate degrees of valgus and varus resolve spontaneously. Mild bilateral deformity before the age of 6 years requires nothing more than regular followup to see if the deformity is increasing. Unilateral deformity and intermalleolar distance >10 cm in bilateral deformity should be investigated and may need surgical correction.

Genu Varum

Bow legs is very common in children younger than 3 years of age.

Physical Examination
Special Tests. The distance between knees is measured while the child is standing with his or her feet as close together as possible. If this distance is >5 cm, it is considered abnormal. The investigations and management are similar to those of genu valgum.

OSTEOGENESIS IMPERFECTA

Osteogenesis imperfecta, also known as **blue sclera, brittle bone disease,** or **osteitis fragilitans,** is the most common of the inherited diseases of connective tissue. It is characterized by multiple fractures in childhood and deformities as a result of malunion of fractures.

Etiology
Spontaneous mutations occur that affect the synthesis of type I collagen molecules, which results in formation of fragile bone. Transmission of osteogenesis imperfecta is usually autosomal dominant. The disease has many genetic and clinical variations. One of the more accepted classifications is listed in Table 2–1.

Pathology
The bones are shorter and thinner than normal. Since the shaft of the bone is thinner, the epiphysis looks bulbous. The periosteum is thick, and the cortex of the bone is thin. The transverse trabeculae are absent, and the vertical trabeculae are fewer in number and thinner. The medullary cavity is filled with fatty or fibrous tissue. The process of endochondral ossification in the epiphyseal plate stops at the stage of provisional calcification of cartilage. Further maturation is haphazard. The bones fracture easily, produce abundant callus, and heal easily.

History
The disease is usually fatal when it presents in the perinatal period. The later it presents in life, the better is the prognosis. Parents give a history of multiple fractures after minimal trauma. The child may not complain of pain.

Physical Examination
1. **Inspection. Deformities** result from malunion of fractures of the long bones. Spinal deformities such as scoliosis, kyphosis, or kyphoscoliosis are seen before the age of 8 years in more severe cases. The stature of the child may remain short because of these deformities. The sclera is translucent and appears **blue** instead of white in some patients. Deformity of the cornea (keratoconus) is seen occasionally.

Classification of Subtypes of Osteogenesis Imperfecta

Type I	Mild form of dominantly inherited disease, with fragile bones, blue sclera, and near-normal stature
Type II	Perinatal form; lethal; new mutation
Type III	Genetically heterogeneous with progressive deformities; severe spinal deformities
Type IV	Fragile bones, normal sclera, and short stature with mild to moderate deformities

2. **Palpation.** A callus may appear as a localized thickening of a long bone.
3. **Range of Motion.** There is excessive movement in joints because of laxity of ligaments. Contractures following a fracture may limit movements in some of the other joints.

Differential Diagnoses

Infants with the perinatal type (Type II) are stillborn or die in the perinatal period. The parents of a child presenting with multiple fractures may be suspected of child abuse. X-ray abnormalities of osteogenesis imperfecta may help distinguish between the two. Patients having the Type III variety with severe spinal deformities may survive only into their teens.

Investigations

Plain x-rays are helpful in diagnosis and management. The cortex of the long bones is thin. The bones are shorter and may show multiple deformities as a result of previous fractures. Abundant callus forms around the fractures. The vertical trabeculae are thin and less in number, and transverse trabeculae are absent.

Management

There is no specific systemic treatment for this condition. Genetic counseling may prevent some children being born with osteogenesis imperfecta. Orthopedic measures are required for treatment of fractures. Surgery is hampered by soft bone and bleeding tendency secondary to capillary abnormalities. Deformities of long bones are stabilized by intramedullary devices to maintain function. Progressive scoliosis is stabilized, even in a young child, by operative procedures.

MULTIPLE HEREDITARY EXOSTOSIS

Also known as **osteochondromatosis, metaphyseal aclasis,** or **diaphyseal aclasis,** multiple hereditary exostosis is characterized by bony outgrowths (**exostosis**) near the metaphyseal ends of long bones.

Etiology

Hereditary exostosis is an hereditary disorder transmitted as an autosomal dominant trait.

Pathology

The exostoses are seen most commonly around the knee (distal femur and proximal tibia and fibula), shoulder (proximal humerus), and wrist (distal radius and ulna). The epiphyses in these areas unite with the diaphyses late and are the growing ends of the bones. The exostoses are projections of bone from the shafts of the affected long bones (Fig. 2–1). The central part of the long bone is normal in shape and structure, but the metaphyseal end, between the exostosis and epiphysis, looks more rectangular with nearly parallel sides. It is larger in size with abnormal trabeculae. The exostosis may continue to grow as long as the affected bone is growing. Deformities of radius and tibia may occur because of unequal growth of the ulna and fibula.

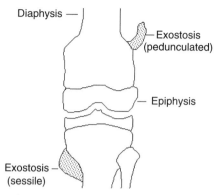

Fig. 2–1 An exostosis grows from the metaphyseal end of the diaphysis. Exostoses may be pedunculated or sessile. The metaphyseal end has nearly parallel sides.

History
The patient usually presents with a history of painless swelling around the knee, wrist, or shoulder. The swelling may be single or multiple. The patient may not have noticed some of the smaller swellings or minor deformities.

Physical Examination
1. **Inspection.** Some patients with multiple hereditary exostosis are shorter than normal. Only larger exostoses are visible as swellings. Abnormal curvature of the tibia or radius may be observed as a deformity.
2. **Palpation.** The exostoses are palpated as hard bony swellings fixed to the underlying bone and are nontender. The skin and other soft tissues are freely movable over the swelling.
3. **Range of motion** of the nearby joint is unaffected.

Investigations
Plain **x-rays** show the exostosis arising from the metaphyseal end of the diaphysis. Trabeculae and medullary cavity are covered by cortical bone. The bone between the exostosis and joint is more rectangular with an abnormal trabecular pattern.

Complications
The course is usually benign, but possible complications include:
1. Pressure on a nearby nerve, such as the common peroneal, may give rise to foot drop or pain.
2. Fracture of the exostosis presents with pain and tenderness.
3. A bursa may develop over the tip of the exostosis.
4. Malignant change into chondrosarcoma or osteogenic sarcoma is rare. It is suspected if there is pain and rapid growth of the tumor.

Management
Most patients do not require treatment. The exostosis is removed surgically if it presses on a nerve or interferes with movement of a joint. Malignant transformation is treated with appropriate measures.

ACHONDROPLASIA

In achondroplasia, also known as **chondrodystrophia fetalis,** the growth of long bones of the extremities is affected but not the trunk. The result is stunted growth with short limbs and normal trunk, i.e., an achondroplastic dwarf.

Etiology

It is an hereditary disorder transmitted in an autosomal dominant fashion. However, the vast majority (nearly 80%) of cases is due to new mutations.

Pathology

The long bones, especially the femur and humerus, are short and may be curved. The growth of the base of the skull is affected in the same way, and it remains smaller than normal. The vault of the skull develops normally, leading to depression at the base of the nose (saddlenose). Spinal deformities are common and spinal stenosis (narrow spinal canal) may cause neurologic problems in adult life. The process of proliferation and calcification of cartilage in the epiphyseal plate is abnormal, slowing the growth in length of long bones.

History

Parents may take the child to a doctor because of the short stature or deformities. Later in life, back pain or symptoms of spinal stenosis may be the presenting complaints.

Physical Examination

Inspection. The head looks large on a short person. The bridge of the nose is depressed. Both upper and lower limbs, especially the proximal parts, are short in comparison with the trunk. There is increased lordosis of the lumbar spine. Other spinal deformities, including scoliosis, kyphosis, and kyphoscoliosis, are often present.

Investigations

X-rays of the lumbar spine show that the distance between pedicles, especially in the 5th lumbar vertebra, is less than normal. The pedicles are short and thick. This reduces the space in the spinal canal considerably. The long bones are shorter in length and may be curved. They are not osteoporotic or abnormal in any other respect.

Course

Intelligence and other milestones are normal except for the height. Life expectancy is also normal.

Complications

Spinal stenosis. The anteroposterior diameter of the spinal canal is very small. Symptoms of spinal stenosis, such as low back pain, motor weakness in both lower extremities, and incontinence of bowel and bladder, appear relatively early in life, around 30–40 years. A prolapsed disk can cause sudden onset of neurologic deficit.

Management

Leg-lengthening procedures carry a very high morbidity and are performed only on a selected few patients with definite indications. Spinal stenosis and spinal deformities may require surgical correction.

Bibliography

1. Cohn DH, Byers PH: Osteogenesis imperfecta and other inherited disorders of structure and synthesis of type I collagen: Models for the analysis of mutations that result in inherited chondrodysplasias. Pathol Immunopathol Res 7:132–138, 1988.
2. Hanscom D, Bloom BA: The spine in osteogenesis imperfecta. Orthop Clin North Am 19:449–458, 1988.
3. Levine AM, Drennan JC. Physiological bowing and tibia vara. J Bone Joint Surg 64A:1158–1163, 1982.
4. Salenius P, Vankka E: The development of the tibiofemoral angle in children. J Bone Joint Surg 57A:259–261, 1975.
5. Scoles PV: Pediatric Orthopedics in Clinical Practice. Chicago, Year Book Medical Publishers, 1988.
6. Smith C: Current concepts review: Tibia vara, Blount's disease. J Bone Joint Surg 64A:630–632, 1982.
7. Vetter U, Maierhofer B, Miller M, et al: Osteogenesis imperfecta in childhood: Cardiac and renal mainifestations. Eur J Pediatr 149:184–187, 1989.
8. Vilarrubias JM, Ginebreda I, Jimeno E: Lengthening of the lower limbs and correction of lumbar hyperlordosis in achondroplasia. Clin Orthop 250:143–149, 1990.
9. Weiner DS: The natural history of "bow legs" and "knock knees" in childhood. Orthopedics 4:156–160, 1981.

3

Trauma

Arun J. Mehta, M.B., F.R.C.P.C.

Injuries to the musculoskeletal system are very common. It is important to know how to diagnose and treat simple injuries, which ones to refer to the specialist, how these injuries heal, and what complications may occur. Details of complicated and serious injuries are beyond the scope of this book.

Mechanisms of Injury
1. **Direct trauma.** The tissue damage occurs at the site of impact, e.g., where a car bumper hits the leg and results in fracture of the tibia.
2. **Indirect trauma.** Injury occurs away from the site of impact, e.g., when the clavicle is broken after a fall on a outstretched hand.

History
A detailed history of **how** the injury occurred is very important. It gives some idea about the structures that may be damaged. For example, the lateral ligament of the ankle is likely to be injured when the foot is inverted while walking. How much **force** was involved in the accident? If a large truck rams into a small car at high speed, the passengers in the small car are likely to suffer very severe injuries, whereas the truck driver walks away without a scratch. The **time** and other circumstances of the accident are also noted. Did the patient notice any **pain** or **swelling?** Was he or she able to walk or move the fingers? Loss of **function** of the affected part may be due to pain and swelling or to nerve, muscle, and tendon injury. It is very important to rule out nerve, muscle, or tendon injury before any treatment is started. Has the patient received any **treatments** for this injury?

Physical Examination
1. **Inspection.** The skin at the site of injury may have **abrasions, laceration,** or **discoloration.** The exact **location** and **size** of these abnormalities should be described. A laceration or breakdown in skin over a fracture site (especially of a subcutaneous bone) makes it an open (compound) fracture. The treatment of an open fracture is very different from that of a closed fracture. The injured extremity should always be compared with the opposite one to see if there is any **deformity.** If there is any angulation, rotation, or shortening; it should be described in detail.
2. **Palpation.** Localized **tenderness** is a very important sign for determining the anatomic structure involved. Tenderness is more diffuse when the trauma has affected a large area. Any **irregularity** of the surface of a subcutaneous bone (e.g., tibia) or tendon (e.g.,

Achilles tendon) is a very important clue to the diagnosis of injury (i.e., fracture of the tibia or rupture of Achilles tendon). Increased **warmth** suggests increased vascularity (e.g., inflammation or infection). The normal **consistency** of muscle is soft; it becomes firm when it is contracted. When there is bleeding or edema within the fascial compartment, muscle becomes very firm even without contraction. This sign, together with severe pain and neurovascular compromise, suggests **compartment syndrome.**

3. **Range of Motion.** ROM tests should be performed very slowly to cause the least amount of pain. There may be **abnormal movement** with crepitus at the fracture site. Since this is very painful, it should not be attempted deliberately. Abnormal movement without crepitus may be present when a ligament of a joint is torn.

   a. **Active**—If there is full range of active movements, passive ROM need not be tested. If there is pain or restriction of active movements, passive ROM should be tested. If a muscle or tendon is injured or inflamed, then active contraction, especially against resistance, is painful.

   b. **Passive**—Movements are painful if the joint being moved is inflamed or if the involved muscle, ligament, or tendon is stretched. If the biceps brachii muscle is injured, passive extension of the forearm is painful, but passive flexion is not.

4. **Special Tests.** Tests for involvement of nerves, ligaments, tendons, and muscles are described under various sections. These tests should be performed whenever indicated. If head trauma is suspected, a complete neurologic exam should be done. Injury to any viscera requires appropriate tests.

Investigations

1. **Plain x-rays** are the most often requested test to rule out fractures and dislocations.
2. **Stress x-rays** are useful when injury to ligaments of a joint is suspected. Abnormal movement of a joint under stress usually indicates rupture of a ligament.
3. **Bone scan** is sometimes ordered for stress fractures, which may not show up on plain x-rays. It is also indicated when infection or tumor of a bone is in the differential diagnosis.
4. **MRI** is useful in cases of ligament or tendon injuries, such as rotator cuff tears of the shoulder or cruciate ligaments of the knee.
5. **CT scan** is helpful when complex fractures or fractures of the spine are suspected.

Complications

A minor degree of **myositis ossificans** is a fairly common complication after injury to muscle near its origin. A hematoma forms near the bone which gets calcified and later ossified to form bone. If there is chronic irritation due to repeated trauma, then a sufficiently large part of the muscle is infiltrated with calcified tissue to restrict joint movements. This complication can be prevented by avoiding repeated trauma, forceful manipulation, and vigorous exercise in presence of pain. X-rays may be negative initially, but a fluffy calcification is seen near the bone which later becomes ossified. Early treatment consists of rest, local heat, and analgesics. Passive and forceful stretching should be avoided. Any surgical interference during the early phase is likely to aggravate the condition.

Management

Ancillary

1. A **cold pack** is applied to the injured part to reduce pain and swelling.
2. **Rest** and **protection** from further injury are provided to allow tissues to heal. Continu-

ous movement or use promotes inflammatory changes to become chronic. A plaster cast, elastic bandage, or bedrest is prescribed as necessary.
3. Local **heat** may be used after 48 hours to ease pain.
4. **Exercises** are prescribed for unaffected parts right from the beginning. These help maintain ROM and strength. Passive ROM exercises are started for the injured part and progressed through active-assisted, active, and exercise against resistance depending on the type of injury, treatment given (cast, operation, etc.), and the patient's response.
5. **Gait training** and **training in activities of daily living** (ADL) are provided by the physical and occupational therapists. Putting weight on the injured leg is an important decision in case of fractures and should be left to the orthopedic surgeon familiar with the case.

Surgery

Surgery may be necessary under the following conditions:
1. When a ligament or tendon is ruptured in an athlete
2. Compound fracture
3. Some fractures need open reduction and internal fixation to allow the patient to walk earlier (e.g., fractured neck of femur).

OVERUSE SYNDROMES

Sports-related injuries and **occupational overuse syndromes** are similar in some respects and are considered together in this section. Active participation in athletic activities has increased tremendously in last few decades, and this has resulted in a higher incidence of sports-related injuries. Society as a whole is also becoming more aware of musculoskeletal problems at the worksite. These injuries may be due to repetitive movements, poor posture, or unsafe working conditions. All of these have led to increased numbers of visits to physicians for musculoskeletal problems.

Etiology and Pathology

Injuries can be described as **macrotrauma** or **microtrauma.** When the individual suffers one incident of injury which results in, say, a fracture, then it is called a macrotrauma. On the other hand, if the individual performs the same task on multiple occasions, he or she may develop symptoms due to cumulative microtrauma sustained during each movement. An example is carpal tunnel syndrome in a typist due to tenosynovitis of the long flexors of the fingers or retrocalcaneal bursitis in a marathon runner.

Repeated small injuries or stress to any tissue leads to an **inflammatory reaction.** There is increased vascularity and outpouring of white blood cells from the capillaries. If trauma continues, new blood vessels are formed and fibrous tissue is laid down. Eventually, the tissue involved degenerates and breaks down, e.g., rupture of a tendon. A bone undergoing repeated stress may develop a stress fracture.

History

Pain is the most common symptom. Details about how it started, which activity brings on the pain or makes it worse, and where the pain is should be requested. Has there been any change at the worksite or in athletic activity? **Function** of the affected part is usually limited because of pain or restricted ROM. A tennis player may avoid backhand strokes because of tennis elbow.

Physical Examination

1. **Inspection.** Ideally, inspection should include the body part involved and also evaluation of the **working conditions** or actual **performance** of the sport in question. If the activity is running or walking, examination of **shoes** may give very important clues.
2. **Palpation. Localized tenderness** is a very helpful sign in pinpointing the anatomic structure affected. **Swelling** may be present in some conditions. Examination of the swelling should include location, size, surface, consistency, edges, tenderness, and tissue of origin.
3. **Range of motion.** Examination of ROM helps in diagnosis and management of the patient.
    a. **Active**—ROM, especially **against resistance,** is painful when the muscle or its tendon is affected. Active abduction of the arm against resistance is painful in supraspinatus tendinitis, whereas passive abduction may not be painful.
    b. Passive—**Stretching** of an inflamed structure is painful. For example, passive ulnar deviation of the wrist and thumb is painful in tenosynovitis of the long abductor and short extensor of the thumb (deQuervain's disease).
4. **Special tests** are carried out according to the structure involved.

Differential Diagnoses

Running or jogging
   Patellofemoral stress syndrome
   Shin splints
   Retrocalcaneal bursitis
   Achilles tendinitis
   Plantar fasciitis
   Pump bump
   Iliotibial tract friction syndrome
   Stress fracture of metatarsals, fibula, tibia, pubic ramus, or neck of femur
   Trochanteric bursitis
Tennis
   Tennis elbow
Golf
   Medial epicondylitis
Swimming
   Subacromial bursitis
   Bicipital tendinitis
Skiing
   Fracture of tibia and fibula
   Fracture thumb
Computer operator or typing
   Carpal tunnel syndrome
   Neck pain

Investigations

1. **Plain x-rays** are done for a suspected stress fracture. They may not show anything for a few weeks, and later there may be only a faint fracture line which can missed easily.

After some months, these fractures form a very thick callus and are sometimes diagnosed retrospectively.

2. **Bone scans** pick up stress fractures earlier than plain x-rays. There is increased uptake at the fracture site.

3. **Motion analysis** studies with video cameras, forceplates, and electromyography are sometimes employed to study sports-related injuries.

Management

Management of individual problems is considered in other chapters. It is important to avoid or completely stop the activity that aggravates pain and symptoms. NSAIDs and local heat help relieve pain. If these options fail, local injection of steroid is tried.

TENDONS

Tendons attach muscle to bone and move the bones and joints by muscle contraction. They can stabilize joints by simultaneous contraction of agonist and antagonist muscles. Injury to tendons is called a **strain.** The muscle, musculotendinous junction, tendon, or its attachment to the bone may be injured.

Anatomy

Tendons are made up of thick bundles of collagen fibers which are parallel to one another. They have very few elastic fibers in them and hence little elasticity. Because most of the fibers are parallel and few travel transversely, tendons do not hold sutures well and require a special technique of suturing. There are very few blood vessels and fibroblasts in this structure. Many tendons have a fibrous sheath; some have a synovial sheath with synovial fluid to facilitate movements. The patellar and Achilles tendons do not have a fibrous sheath, and they are the largest tendons in the body.

Etiology

A tendon may rupture because of:

1. **Trauma.** A sudden strong contraction of a muscle against tremendous resistance is a common cause of tendon rupture, especially in sports. The Achilles tendon may be damaged in a sprinter or jumper when the gastrocnemius-soleus muscles contract to propel the athlete.

2. **Inflammation.** In rheumatoid arthritis, rupture of the extensor digiti minimi tendon occurs because inflammation of the synovial sheath weakens the tendon.

3. **Degenerative.** If a tendon has to move against rough surface, it becomes frayed and eventually breaks. This may happen after a Colles' fracture and affects the long extensor of the thumb.

Pathology

Inflammatory response occurs at the site of injury, with new blood vessels invading from the surrounding connective tissue. If the tendon is covered by synovium where it is injured, the blood vessels grow from the synovial sheath. New collagen fibers are laid down by fibroblasts. The damage is repaired by scar tissue, which may anchor the tendon to the surrounding synovium. This may lead to **adhesions** and severely restrict movements of the tendon. The new collagen fibers can hold the ends of the tendon together by 7–10 days, and by the end of 3 weeks, the tensile strength is enough to overcome mild resistance. Later, the collagen fibers become longitudinally oriented. Scar tissue is not as strong as the original tendon, but the tendon heals with minimal scar if the ends are brought together by sutures. If the ends are not sutured, the two ends of the tendon retract and atrophy. Repair may become very difficult by a few weeks after the injury.

Classification

Tendon (and ligament) injuries are classified as:
1. **First degree** or *mild.* There is minor disruption of some of the fibers and some bleeding. The patient complains of some pain and limitation of movements. If pain is eliminated, the function of that muscle-tendon unit is not affected.
2. **Second degree** or **moderate.** The injury is between mild and severe.
3. **Third degree** or **severe.** There is complete tear of the tendon, and the muscle retracts. The muscle may be seen bunched up. When the long head of the biceps brachii muscle is torn at its origin from the glenoid, the muscle belly is seen in the lower arm.

History

The onset of a strain may be acute or chronic. In the **acute** variety, there is history of one episode of severe injury. In **chronic** cases, **pain** and **limitation of function** develop over a period of time during which the patient has been performing some repetitive movements. When a tendon ruptures, the patient may hear or feel a **snap** and develop sudden **pain** if the rupture is secondary to trauma. In degenerative and rheumatic conditions, the patient may have chronic, recurrent pain before the tendon ruptures, and the rupture itself may not cause more pain. The patient may notice that he or she is not able to extend the little finger or abduct the arm depending on the tendon involved.

Physical Examination

1. **Inspection.** There may be some swelling and discoloration of the skin after an acute strain. However, no abnormal signs may be present in chronic first and second degree strains. A **muscle bulge** may be seen after a complete tear, as in rupture of the long head of biceps.
2. **Palpation.** Localized tenderness helps identify the problem.
3. **Range of Motion**
   a. **Active**—Movement against resistance is painful in first and second degree strains (Fig. 3–1A) In the third degree or complete tear, a muscle-tendon unit is not able to initiate movement.
   b. **Passive**—Movement that stretches the injured tendon or muscle is painful. (Fig. 3–1B)
4. **Special tests** are performed according to the tendon or muscle involved.

Investigations

1. **Plain x-rays** are necessary after injury to rule out any fractures.
2. **MRI** can be useful in the diagnosis of complete or partial tears of tendons and ligaments. Rotator cuff tear may also be diagnosed by **arthrography** or **arthroscopy.**

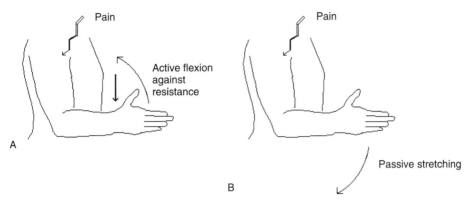

Fig. 3–1 *A,* Active flexion of the elbow against resistance requires contraction of the biceps muscle. This manuever is painful in bicipital tendinitis. *B,* Passive extension of the elbow stretches the biceps muscle and reproduces pain due to bicipital tendinitis.

Management

Management depends on the degree of injury. Most first and second degree tears can be treated conservatively. The initial treatment is with RICE (rest, ice pack, compression with elastic bandage and elevation). Gentle passive ROM exercises are started as soon as the patient can tolerate. Gradually increasing activity and exercises are allowed as pain and swelling subside. In the case of lower extremity injury, the patient is allowed to walk with gradually increasing weight-bearing with an appropriate walking aid. Surgical repair is indicated when the ruptured tendon affects the function, especially in a young athlete.

TENDINITIS

Inflammation of tendons or surrounding structures is a very common problem. It is called **tenosynovitis** if synovial sheath surrounding the tendon is inflamed. The inflammation of the surrounding structures of tendons without a sheath is called **peritendinitis** or **tendinitis.**

Etiology

The inflammation may be due to **overuse** or **degenerative** changes in the tendon. Inflammatory diseases such as rheumatoid arthritis or infection can also cause tenosynovitis.

History

The patient complains of **pain** on movements and is unable to perform certain functions because of pain. This may later lead to stiffness of the joint.

Physical Examination

Localized **tenderness** over the inflamed tendon helps localize the lesion. **Crepitus** may be palpated over a site of chronic tendinitis as the tendon slides over rough surfaces during movement. Pain can be elicited on active contraction of the muscle against resistance, e.g., pain on elbow flexion against resistance in bicipital tendinitis.

Differential Diagnosis
Acute or chronic infection should be ruled out.

Management
Treatment depends on the etiology. If tendinitis is caused by overactivity, the best treatment is to **stop or reduce the activity** that precipitated the problem. Rest and local ice help in relieving acutely inflamed and very painful tendinitis. Heat is used for chronic problems. If all these modalities fail, local **steroid injection** in the general area of the inflamed tendon should be considered.

LIGAMENTS

A ligament attaches two bones and prevents excessive or abnormal movements between them. Injury to a ligament is called a **sprain.** Tendons and ligaments have a similar structure, and and their injuries are classified in a very similar manner. The basic principles of treatment of injuries are also similar.

Anatomy
Ligaments, like tendons, are made up of thick bundles of collagen fibers which are parallel to one another, with very few elastic fibers. They provide resistance to stretching and pulling and thus prevent abnormal movement of the joints.

Etiology
The ligaments are usually injured while trying to prevent abnormal movement of a joint. The lateral ligament of the ankle joint is torn when the foot is twisted in inversion. A still stronger force would dislocate the joint.

Pathology
The inflammatory response and healing process are similar to those of a tendon. The ligaments of a small joint, e.g., finger, may heal within 3 weeks, whereas those of the hip joint may need 3 months. The scar tissue is not as strong as the original ligament, especially if there is a gap between the torn ends.

Classification
Ligament injuries are classified as:
1. **First degree** or **mild.** There is minor disruption of some fibers and some bleeding. The stability of the joint is maintained.
2. **Second degree** or **moderate.** The injury is between mild and severe.
3. **Third degree** or **severe.** There is a complete tear of the ligament. This type of injury may lead to instability of a joint.

BONE

Anatomy

Bone is a living tissue that is always undergoing changes. Like any other tissue, it has cells, which are called **osteocytes.** These cells are within small cavities or lacunae in the bone matrix. The bone matrix is secreted by osteocytes called **osteoblasts.** The matrix consists mainly (90%) of collagen fibers. Calcium salts (hydroxyapatite) are deposited in the matrix to give rigidity. The other type of cell found in bone is the **osteoclast,** which is involved in bone resorption. The process of bone formation and resorption goes on continuously. Under normal circumstances, there is good balance between these two activities, and the bone mass and structure is maintained. After fracture, there is increased bone formation, whereas there is increased bone resorption in senile osteoporosis.

All bones are covered on the outside by a vascular, fibrous membrane called the **periosteum.** The articular surface of the bone, however, is not covered by periosteum. Blood vessels enter the bone by passing through the periosteum. Under the periosteum is **compact bone,** which looks solid. However, under the microscope it is composed of units called the osteons or haversian systems. In the center of this unit is the haversian canal, which contains blood vessels. It is surrounded by concentric lamellae. The spongy or **cancellous** bone is within the shell of compact bone. It has larger cavities which contain blood vessels, blood-forming tissue, or fat. The trabeculae of spongy bone are laid down according to mechanical stress experienced by the bone. The proportion of compact bone and cancellous bone varies in different bones according to their function.

The part of the long bone that develops from a primary center of ossification is called **diaphysis.** This forms the shaft of the long bone. Secondary centers of ossification develop at the ends of the long bone. i.e, the **epiphysis.** A layer of cartilage cells separates the epiphysis from diaphysis during the period of growth. This is called the **epiphyseal plate,** or growth plate. The part of diaphysis near the epiphyseal plate is known as **metaphysis.** Bone increases in length as a result of activity in this region. It is very vascular during the period of growth and hence very susceptible to blood-borne infections (osteomyelitis).

Mechanisms of Injury

Normal bone is very strong and able to withstand considerable force before it breaks. The injury may be **direct,** e.g., a blow on the forearm, or it may be **indirect**, e.g., a fall on the outstretched hand causing fracture of the clavicle.

When the bone is abnormal, it can break during normal activities or after minimal injury. This is called **pathologic fracture. Metastasis** from lung, prostate, or breast cancer or infection of the bone (**osteomyelitis**) and osteitis deformans (Paget's disease) are common causes of pathologic fractures. Vertebral body, proximal femur, and proximal humerus are common sites for metastatic lesions. Fractures secondary to **osteoporosis** are very common and require relatively minor injury. **Stress** or fatigue fractures occur in normal bone subjected to repeated minor trauma. These fractures are commonly seen in metatarsal bones, fibula, or tibia. Long-distance walking or running are the usual causes.

If the fracture site communicates with the the atmosphere, then it is called an **open** fracture. This is a significant factor in treatment and prognosis for healing of the fracture, as chances of infection are much greater in this type of fracture. When there is no communication with the outside, it is called a **closed** (simple) fracture.

Pathology

A **hematoma** forms near the fracture site because of bleeding from torn blood vessels (Fig. 3–2). Soon after the injury, capillaries and osteogenic cells in the periosteum and endosteum start to proliferate. These cells gradually replace the hematoma, mature, and become osteoblasts. The intercellular matrix is laid down by osteoblasts. Later, calcium salts are deposited in this matrix. New trabeculae are formed. The new bone is called **callus** and replaces the hematoma. The callus is gradually replaced by mature bone. The callus near the outer surface of the bone is called external callus, whereas the callus near the medullary canal and cortex of the bone is called the internal callus (Fig. 3–2). The external callus may contain some cartilage. The cancellous bone is replaced by lamellar bone with near-normal bone structure.

When open reduction and internal fixation (ORIF) with a plate and screws is performed, little external callus is formed. If the plate and screws are removed too soon, the fracture can recur because of lack of protective callus. Fractures through the cancellous bone heal more readily than compact bone because of the abundant blood supply to the cancellous bone.

Union of fracture fragments is affected by the following conditions:

1. **Immobilization.** Movement at the fracture site promotes cartilage formation and nonunion. Sometimes a false joint (pseudarthrosis) forms. The fracture fragments should be fixed or immobilized until there is evidence of union.
2. Adequate **blood supply** is necessary for callus formation. Fractures of the neck of the femur and distal third of the tibia are good examples of a precarious blood supply affecting the outcome.
3. **Infection** in an open fracture may delay the union.
4. **Pathologic fracture** due to metastasis interferes with healing.
5. Bony union does not occur if there is muscle or other soft tissue interposed between fragments.

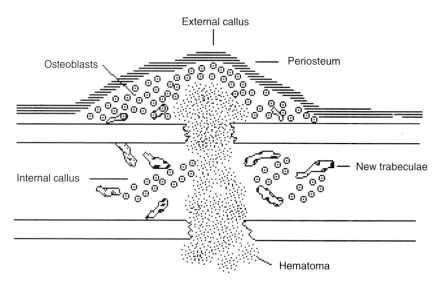

Fig. 3–2   Fracture healing.

History

There is usually a history of **injury,** a fall or forceful impact. A pathologic fracture can occur without any injury. **Pain** is very severe except in cases of stress fractures, when it may be present only on weight-bearing. The patient is not able to use the extremity immediately after the injury (**loss of function**). However, some patients are known to walk on an impacted fracture of the neck of the femur.

Physical Examination

1. **Inspection.** There may be **abrasions** at the site of injury. In the case of open fractures, a laceration or puncture wound is present. It may take few hours for **swelling** to appear and a day or two for the **bruise** to become visible. **Deformity** occurs in some of the fractures.
2. **Palpation.** Localized **tenderness** is present at the site of the fracture of subcutaneous bones.
3. **Range of motion.** All movements are painful and should be attempted slowly and carefully. **Crepitus** may be felt or heard, and there may be abnormal movement at the fracture site. It is not essential to do this test if there is extreme pain on any attempt to move the extremity.
4. **Special tests**
   a. **Circulation** beyond the fracture site should always be tested by palpating the pulse, checking the temperature of the skin, and checking capillary return. This should be done before any treatment, after reduction, and frequently after the cast has been applied.
   b. Sensation, muscle power, and reflexes are examined to see if there is any **nerve damage.** It is essential to rule out a spinal cord or cauda equina lesion in fractures of the spine.
   c. In case of multiple trauma, rib, or skull fractures, other **organ damage** should be ruled out. Rupture of the urinary bladder and urethra may occur with fractures of the pelvis.
   d. **Skin** at the fracture site is examined for any wounds that may be communicating with the fracture.

Investigations

X-rays are done whenever a fracture is suspected. At least two views at right angles to each other are taken (AP and lateral). Some fractures and dislocations may be missed if only one view is done. Films should include the proximal and distal joints of the involved bone. Other special views are ordered if necessary.

It is important to be familiar with the terms used by the radiologist and the orthopedic surgeon in describing fractures. The x-ray appearance of a fracture may be described in three different ways:

1. Appearance of the **fracture line** (Fig. 3–3)
   a. **Transverse** fracture through the shaft of a long bone may be stable.
   b. **Oblique or spiral** fractures are unstable, and reduction may be difficult to maintain in a cast.
   c. **Comminuted** fracture occurs when there are more than two fragments. These fractures are also unstable.
2. **Part of the bone** involved
   a. **Diaphyseal.** The shaft of the bone is fractured.
   b. **Metaphyseal.** Metaphyseal end of the diaphysis is involved.

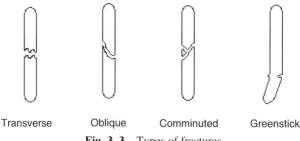

Transverse   Oblique   Comminuted   Greenstick

Fig. 3–3 Types of fractures.

   c. **Epiphyseal.** Occurs in children before the epiphysis is united with the diaphysis. This may interfere with growth of the bone.
   d. **Apophyseal.** The muscle attached to an apophysis tears off a piece of bone, e.g., avulsion of lesser trochanter by the psoas tendon. It is also called an **avulsion** fracture.
   e. **Intra-articular.** The fracture line extends into a joint. These fractures need accurate reduction and early mobilization of the joint. There is increased incidence of joint stiffness and degenerative arthritis of the joint.
3. **Deformity** as seen on x-rays
   a. **Undisplaced.** All bone fragments are in their normal position.
   b. **Angulation.** There is an abnormal angle between the axes of proximal and distal fragments. If the fracture heals with this angle, undue stress may be placed on joints with development of degenerative arthritis later.
   c. **Rotation.** The distal fragment is rotated in relation to the proximal fragment.
   d. **Lateral** displacement of fragments in the horizontal plane
   e. **Shortening.** When there is overriding of fragments, the extremity is shortened.
   f. **Compression.** Compression fracture occurs in the spine when a vertebral body loses some of its vertical height.
   g. **Greenstick.** Greenstick fracture is an incomplete fracture of a long bone in children. A part of the cortex is bent but not broken.
   h. **Fracture-dislocation.** A joint near the fracture site is dislocated. The treatment of this injury is complex, and outcome usually is not so good.
   i. **Impacted fracture.** The two fragments are pushed together. The patient may be able to walk on an impacted fracture of the neck of the femur for some time.

Course
Healing of a fracture may take anywhere from a few weeks to a few months. Some of the factors affecting the rate of bony union are:
1. **Age.** A fracture in an infant may heal in 4–6 weeks, but a similar fracture in an adolescent may take 6–10 weeks and in an adult, 12–20 weeks.
2. **Type of bone involved.** Fractures through cancellous bone, e.g., intertrochanteric fracture, heal well in about 3 months. Fracture of the neck of the femur near the head (subcapital) may take much longer.
3. **Type of fracture.** Impacted fractures heal well, whereas open fractures may take a long time to heal because of infection.
4. **Method of treatment.** Appropriate immobilization and accurate reduction of fracture fragments reduce the time it takes to heal.
5. **Other pathology.** Coexisting disease, such as severe osteoporosis or metastatic disease, also determine the rate of healing.

Complications

At the time of injury:

1. **Associated injury** to internal organs, blood vessels, nerves, and tendons should be ruled out.
2. **Shock** is common in multiple fractures, with excessive bleeding, and other traumas. A large amount of blood may be lost as internal hemorrhage in fractures of the pelvis or femur. It needs to be recognized and treated immediately.

Related to treatment:

1. A major nerve or blood vessel may be damaged at the time of manipulation or operation.
2. **Compartment syndrome** is due to increased pressure in a fascial compartment. It can happen after the injury or after application of a cast. The patient complains of severe pain in the extremity and numbness of all fingers or toes. If this pressure is not relieved, ischemic contracture of muscles may result.

Intermediate:

1. **Infection** may develop in the fracture site, especially in an open fracture.
2. **Fat embolism** is an uncommon but serious complication that occurs 2–4 days after the injury. There is sudden onset of respiratory and CNS symptoms, including breathlessness, confusion, or drowsiness.

Late complications:

1. **Joint stiffness** is common after prolonged immobilization or intra-articular fracture. Appropriate physical or occupational therapy can help to improve ROM.
2. **Malunion** occurs when bones unite in a deformed position with abnormal angulation or shortening. This places undue stress on joints, causing degenerative joint disease.
3. **Delayed union** occurs when healing takes longer than usual. Further immobilization may still bring about healing of the fracture.
4. **Nonunion** occurs when fibrous or cartilaginous tissue forms between the bone fragments and the ends of the bone become sclerotic. Bony union is not possible without surgical intervention.
5. **Avascular necrosis** is fairly common after fracture of the neck of femur and fracture of the scaphoid due to damage to blood vessels to one or both fragments.

Very late complications:

1. **Degenerative arthritis** is common after malunion and intra-articular fractures.

Management

Only broad principles of fracture management are mentioned here. Detailed descriptions are given in the textbooks cited in the bibliography.

The first aid management consists of maintaining an **open air way, stopping hemorrhage,** and temporarily immobilizing the fracture to prevent undue pain. The upper extremity can be bandaged to the chest and the lower extremity to the opposite lower extremity. The patient should then be transported to appropriate facility.

The diagnosis of fracture is confirmed by x-rays, and the type of fracture is determined. The deformity as seen on x-rays has a significant bearing on the treatment. The displacement of fragments and angulation with the normal position is noted as accurately as possible. If there is visceral injury or arterial bleeding, then these injuries are taken care of immediately. The treatment of open (compound) fractures is very different from that of closed variety. Thorough cleaning and debridement are done for an open fracture. The patient is given a tetanus shot and antibiotics. The fracture is then reduced and immobilized. A displaced closed fracture may need to be reduced and immobilized. An undisplaced fracture may only need to be immobilized.

The decision to **reduce a fracture** or not depends on several factors, including whether the deformity is acceptable, probable outcome of each treatment, and experience of the surgeon. A fracture can be reduced by manipulation, skeletal traction, or open reduction at operation. An internal fixation device is usually put in when open reduction is done (open reduction and internal fixation). Fractures require **immobilization** to reduce painful movement and prevent recurrence of deformity. It also helps in healing of the fracture. Immobilization can be achieved by plaster cast, traction, internal fixation, or external fixation device.

When a movable part, such as joint or tendon, is immobilized, adhesions form and stiffness develops. This is especially severe when there is bleeding inside the joint. The muscles that are unable to contract because of pain or are covered in a cast become atrophied and lose strength. Involvement by rehabilitation professionals is important to prevent and treat some of these complications. The number and type of professionals will depend on the complexity of problems. The patient may not be able to follow his or her vocational or avocational activities for a long time. Patients may become depressed because of financial and social problems that arise as a result of hospitalization and loss of job. The rehabilitation plan will depend on each patient's problem list.

STRESS FRACTURE

Stress fractures have been compared with "metal fatigue" seen in aircraft wings and other components which break down after repeated small stresses and movements. Each individual stress is not enough to break the bone, but the cumulative effect leads to a stress fracture. They are commonly seen in long-distance runners and occur in metatarsals, fibula, or tibia. The repeated stress of impact with the ground over time wears the bone out. They may also be seen in the pubic rami or femoral neck.

The initial **x-ray** may be negative, or the fine hair-line crack in the bone may be missed. Later x-rays show exuberant callus at the fracture site.

The activity that brought on the symptoms should be discontinued for 3–6 weeks, depending on the severity and persistence of pain. If the activity is resumed too soon, then symptoms may recur. Stress fracture of the neck of the femur may require the patient to stop weight-bearing on that extremity for fear of developing a displaced fracture. A displaced fracture of the neck of the femur may need open reduction and internal fixation.

JOINT DISLOCATION AND SUBLUXATION

Injury to a joint may result in effusion, hemarthrosis, rupture of ligaments, subluxation, dislocation, fracture-dislocation, or intra-articular fracture. Rupture of ligaments is considered in the chapter on tendons and ligaments. A swelling of a joint after any injury may be due to effusion in the joint or hemarthrosis (blood in the joint cavity).

Anatomy
A joint is maintained in its normal position by:
1. The shape of bones, e.g., hip joint with deep acetabulum surrounding the head of femur

2. Ligaments, as in knee or ankle joints
3. Muscles, e.g., deltoid and supraspinatus maintain the head of the humerus in contact with the glenoid despite gravity trying to pull it down. When these muscles are weak, as after a stroke, the shoulder tends to slide down and subluxate.

Etiology
Dislocation of joints can be classified according to the etiology:
1. **Congenital**—e.g., congenital dislocation of the hip. The patient is born with the defect or develops one soon after birth.
2. **Traumatic**—the most common variety
3. **Pathologic**—e.g., shoulder subluxation after a stroke

Classification
A joint is said to be **dislocated** when the articular surfaces are totally separated from each other. In **subluxation,** parts of the articular surfaces are still in contact with each other (Fig. 3–4).

History
In acute traumatic dislocation, the patient usually gives a history of severe **pain** immediately after an **injury.** He is not able to perform any **function** that involves the affected joint; e.g., a patient with a dislocated hip is unable to bear weight on the dislocated side and walk.

Physical Examination
1. **Inspection.** The **contour** around the joint is deformed. In dislocation of the shoulder, there is flattening of the normal rounded contour of the shoulder. A bruise may appear later.
2. **Palpation.** The injured area is very **tender** to touch. **Muscle spasm** is usually present. Bony landmarks are altered. In dislocation of the elbow, the relation between olecranon, medial, and lateral epicondyles is abnormal.
3. **Range of Motion.** Any attempt to move the joint is very painful, and movements are markedly **restricted**.
4. **Special tests.** Tests are performed to rule out neurovascular injuries.

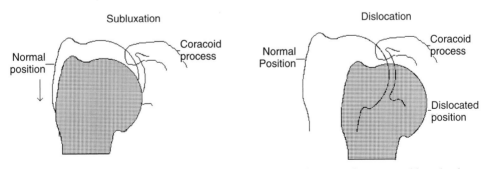

Fig. 3–4 In subluxation, parts of the articular surfaces of two bones are in contact with each other. There is no contact with articular surfaces in dislocation.

Differential Diagnoses

Fracture of nearby bones should be ruled out by x-rays. Presence of a fracture with dislocation requires special consideration in management because it makes the joint very unstable.

Investigations

X-rays in two planes (usually AP and lateral) are necessary. Dislocation of some joints, e.g., the shoulder, may be missed if only the AP view is done.

Complications

1. **Joint stiffness** occurs very frequently after a dislocation and requires rehabilitation therapy.
2. **Degenerative arthritis** may develop at an earlier age.
3. **Recurrent dislocation** or subluxation occurs when the ligaments or capsular attachment is torn, damaged, or too lax.
4. **Neurovascular injury.** The axillary nerve is commonly damaged in dislocations of the shoulder, and popliteal vessels can be injured in dislocation of the knee.

Management

These injuries should be treated as soon as possible because severe pain is experienced by the patient as long as the joint remains dislocated. If treatment is delayed it becomes increasingly difficult to reduce the joint because of soft tissue contractures. Most dislocations can be reduced by a **closed method**. Since this is very painful, some form of anesthesia is used. An **open reduction** may become necessary if:

1. Closed reduction fails
2. One of the ligaments is torn
3. Fracture-dislocation exists
4. Open (compound) dislocation exists (there is laceration of skin close to the dislocated joint).

The joint has to be immobilized until the soft tissues (capsule and ligaments) supporting the joint have healed. This may take 3 weeks for a finger joint to 3 months for the ankle. The period of immobilization should be as short as possible to prevent joint stiffness.

Ancillary treatment, including physical and occupational therapy, may be required to regain movements, strength, and function.

Bibliography

1. Adams JC: Outline of Fractures. Edinburgh, Churchill Livingstone, 1987.
2. Browner BD, Jupiter JB, Levine AM, Trafton PG, eds: Skeletal Trauma. Philadelphia, W.B. Saunders Co., 1992.
3. Buschbacher RM, Braddom R, eds: Sports Medicine and Rehabilitation: A Sports Specific Approach. Philadelphia, Hanley & Belfus, 1994.
4. Hoffman GS: Tendinitis and bursitis. Am Fam Physician 23:103, 1981.
5. Holder LE: Bone scintigraphy in skeletal trauma. Radiol Clin North Am 31:739–781, 1993.
6. Iverson LD, Clawson DK: Manual of Acute Orthopedic Therapeutics. Boston, Little, Brown and Co., 1987.
7. McRae R: Practical Fracture Treatment. Edinburgh, Churchill Livingstone, 1989.
8. Neviaser RJ: Tenosynovitis. Hand Clin 5:525–531, 1989.
9. Rockwood CA, Green DP, Bucholz RW, eds: Rockwood and Green's Fractures in Adults, 3rd ed. Philadelphia, J.B. Lippincott Co., 1991.
10. Smith NJ, Stanitski CL: Sports Medicine: A Practical Guide. Philadelphia, W.B. Saunders Co., 1987.
11. Sperryn PN: Sport and Medicine. London, Butterworths, 1985.
12. Walker LG, Meals RA: Tendinitis: A practical approach to diagnosis and management. J Musculoskel Med 6(5):24–54, 1989.

4

Inflammatory Arthritis

Arun J. Mehta, M.B., F.R.C.P.C., and Stanley Marcus, M.D.

RHEUMATOID ARTHRITIS

Rheumatoid arthritis is a chronic inflammatory disorder affecting the synovial joints. There are remissions and exacerbations of pain and swelling of joints and stiffness, especially in the mornings. Other manifestations of this disease which may be present include subcutaneous nodules, vasculitis, lymphadenopathy, and splenomegaly. The patient may develop deformities and difficulty in performing ADLs.

Epidemiology
Approximately 1% of the U.S. population suffers from rheumatoid arthritis, i.e., nearly 2.5 million people. The male to female ratio is 1:3, with maximum incidence occurring in **middle-aged females.**

Etiology
Some unknown factor or factors start the process of inflammation in the synovium of the joints. It is probably related to some bacterial or viral infection, though there is no definite evidence of this as yet. Genetic factors may make some individuals more susceptible to developing rheumatoid arthritis. Some environmental factors may modify the outcome or perpetuate the inflammatory reaction.

Pathology
The synovial membrane is the main target. There is an **acute inflammatory reaction** with vasodilatation, hyperemia, and exudation of fluid with cellular elements from the blood vessels. The exudate accumulates in the interstitial spaces of the synovial membrane and in the joint cavity. There are many polymorphonuclear leukocytes, lymphocytes, and plasma cells in the extravascular spaces of the synovial membrane and in synovial fluid. Focal necrosis of the synovial lining cells may be present. Chronic inflammation and effusion in the joint stretch ligaments and make them weak, predisposing the joint to develop **deformities.** Vasodilatation and hyperemia in the bone near the joint cause **juxta-articular osteoporosis.** The osteoporosis is aggravated by disuse and steroids.

    The normal inner lining of the synovial membrane is one to three cells thick. In chronic rheumatoid arthritis, the cells divide and become multiple layers thick. The **thickened synovial membrane** forms folds and villous projections. There are collections of mononuclear

51

cells in the loose connective tissue layer underneath the synovial lining. Lymphocytes and plasma cells collect around small blood vessels to form follicles. The superficial layer of the articular cartilage is destroyed by enzymes liberated from necrotic cells in the joint fluid and increased pressure in the joint due to effusion. On x-rays, this is seen as uniform narrowing of the joint space. The granulation tissue grows over the articular cartilage from the thickened synovial membrane (**pannus**). The articular cartilage under the pannus is eroded. When bone near a joint margin is eroded, it is called a marginal **erosion.**

Tendon sheaths are affected in a manner similar to the inflammatory process going on in the synovial membrane. There is hyperemia, exudation of fluid, and, later, thickening of the tendon sheath (**tenosynovitis**). The tendons may get displaced from their normal position and pull the bones and joints in an abnormal direction, causing **deformities.** Joint deformities commonly occur in metacarpophalangeal, metatarsophalangeal, interphalangeal, wrist, midfoot, and cervical joints. The inflammatory process may destroy the tendon, causing it to **rupture.** Tendon ruptures are seen over the dorsum of the hand, rotator cuff, or Achilles tendon. The synovial lining of bursae may get inflamed and develop **bursitis.** This is seen especially in olecranon, retrocalcaneal, and subacromial bursae.

The disease process can stop at any stage and become **quiescent.** The main goal of therapy of rheumatoid arthritis is to achieve this remission before there are any changes in the articular cartilage or erosions in the bone. Sometimes, remission occurs naturally, and sometimes, it may be brought about by the medications.

Inflammation of blood vessels (**vasculitis**) in various tissues is supposed to be the basis for formation of **rheumatoid nodules,** peripheral nerve involvement, and some skin changes. The rheumatoid nodule is formed by a necrotic center, surrounded by a second layer of elongated cells around its periphery, and a third, outermost layer of chronic inflammatory cells (lymphocytes and plasma cells). Vasculitis also gives rise to small, brown, splinter-shaped lesions in the nailfolds. This process may affect blood vessels in peripheral nerves such as the femoral or common peroneal (**mononeuritis multiplex**). The patient may present with weakness and atrophy of the quadriceps or foot drop due to weakness of the foot dorsiflexors.

Fibrosis is the end result of inflammation. The synovium of the joint capsule becomes fibrotic and limits movements of the joint. Fibrous tissue may form within the joint and between articular ends of the bones (**fibrous ankylosis**). Abnormal stress on the joint and damage to the articular cartilage leads to **degenerative arthritis** with subchondral sclerosis and osteophyte formation. The deformities seen in various joints are described in chapters on individual joints.

History

Onset of the disease is usually insidious. It can start at any age but usually occurs between the ages of 20 and 40 years. Females are affected more often than males (3:1 ratio). Most patients feel tired and lethargic and have aches and pains all over. This may progress to **painful swelling** of joints, usually of the hands, feet, wrists, elbows, shoulders, and knees (Fig. 4–1). In the hands, the metacarpophalangeal (MCP) and proximal interphalangeal (PIP) joints are commonly involved. The same joints on both sides are usually affected (**symmetrical** involvement).

Most patients experience **exacerbations** and **remissions** of symptoms and signs, with gradual deterioration over a period of months or years. The progression of the disease may stop at any time without any apparent reason. Initially, only a few joints are swollen and painful, but later, multiple joints are affected. The pain is aggravated by movements or weight-bearing.

About 20% of the patients may start with very aggressive disease—painful swelling of

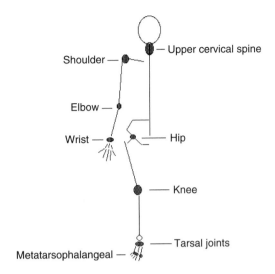

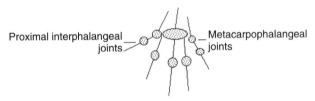

Fig. 4–1 Joints commonly involved in rheumatoid arthritis.

joints, severe morning stiffness, fever, and other signs. Some patients in this group may not have any remissions and deteriorate very rapidly. During exacerbations, the patient complains of feeling stiff all over after a period of inactivity, e.g., sleep. This **morning stiffness** usually lasts for > 1 hour. The severity of the disease can be judged by the number of hours the patient feels stiff in morning. During a very severe flareup, the patient may feel stiff throughout the entire day. Pain and stiffness interfere with activities like walking, writing, and others. During a remission, the patient has little or no pain in the joints, morning stiffness, fatigue, or malaise. There is no swelling or tenderness in the joints and no pain on movement of the joints. The ESR declines to within normal limits.

Physical Examination

1. **Inspection.** During acute exacerbation, the skin overlying the **swollen joints** may be slightly **red.** This erythema is noticeable over the superficial joints of the hands, feet, knees, ankles, and wrists. Later, **deformities** may be noticed (as discussed in chapters on individual joints). The **muscles** that act on the inflamed joints show **atrophy.** The skin may become very thin, shiny, and atrophic and may bruise very easily. This may be made worse by nonsteroidals or cortisone preparations given to reduce inflammation. The therapist who makes splints for these patients needs to take extra precautions to prevent skin breakdown.

Subcutaneous nodules are seen in about 25% of patients with rheumatoid arthritis. The most common site is over the subcutaneous border of the ulna near the elbow joint. Other sites are the occipital region and Achilles tendon. The nodules are believed to be due to pressure on the subcutaneous tissue over a bone. Presence of nodules is associated with severe disease, rapid progression, and positive rheumatoid factor. A nodule may decrease in size during remission and become painfully large during exacerbation. It may also ulcerate and take a long time to heal. Similar nodules are seen in rheumatic fever, sarcoidosis, and collagen diseases and are not diagnostic of rheumatoid arthritis.

2. **Palpation.** The skin over inflamed joints is **warm** and **tender.** An attempt should be made to distinguish between **swelling** due to fluid in the joint cavity and synovial thickening. In superficial joints such as the knee, the joint fluid can be displaced from one side to the other, which can be confirmed by aspiration of the joint. The joint fluid can spill over into nearby bursae that communicate with the joint cavity. If the synovium of the knee is thickened, the upper edge of it can be rolled against the femur. In some joints, both the fluid and thick synovium may contribute toward swelling.

3. **Range of motion.** All movements are painful during an exacerbation. When there is tenosynovitis, active movement against resistance or passive stretching of the involved tendon is painful.

4. **Special tests.**
   a. **Skin** is examined for rheumatoid **nodules.** These are usually seen over the subcutaneous border of the ulna near the elbow, in the occipital region, and over the sacrum. Nodules may increase in size and become tender during exacerbations and may become smaller during remissions.
   b. **Eye.** Dryness of the eyes and mouth due to reduced secretions from lacrimal and salivary glands is a complaint of some patients (**Sjögren's syndrome**). Corneal ulceration and inflammation of conjunctiva may result. Episcleritis is a benign condition that resolves on its own. There is pain and redness. Inflammation of sclera is more serious because it may lead to thinning and softening of the sclera.
   c. **Neurologic** exam may reveal common peroneal, radial, femoral, or other peripheral nerve involvement due to **mononeuritis multiplex.** The patient presents with a foot drop, wrist drop, or difficulty in getting off the toilet or chair. These complications may be an indication of vasculitis.
   d. **Felty's syndrome.** Some patients develop splenomegaly, enlarged lymph nodes, and pancytopenia (anemia, thrombocytopenia, and diminished neutrophil count). It is usually associated with fever, loss of appetite, and loss of weight.
   e. **Pulmonary.** Interstitial pulmonary fibrosis is seen in the majority of autopsy specimens.
   f. **Heart.** Occasionally, rheumatoid nodules develop in the myocardium or over heart valves. Acute or chronic pericarditis with adhesions in the pericardial cavity is also known to occur.

Differential Diagnoses

The diagnosis of rheumatoid arthritis is based mainly on the clinical picture since there are no diagnostic tests. It is difficult to be certain of the diagnosis in early stages of disease. The American Rheumatism Association recommends that at least 4 of the following 7 criteria be present for the diagnosis (the first 4 must be present for more than 6 weeks):

1. Morning stiffness in and around joints for more than an hour
2. At least three joints have soft tissue swelling or effusion at the same time
3. At least one joint area (MCP, PIP, or wrist) in hand

4. Symmetric involvement of joints on both sides of the body
5. Presence of subcutaneous nodules
6. Abnormal amounts of serum rheumatoid factor
7. Radiologic changes (erosions or juxtaarticular osteoporosis) in wrist and hand
   The following differential diagnoses should be ruled out:
1. **Degenerative joint disease** commonly affects distal interphalangeal joints (DIP), hips, and knees. Morning stiffness is usually < 0.5 hour. It is a chronic, slowly progressive disease. X-rays show irregular joint space narrowing with subchondral sclerosis and osteophyte formation.
2. **Infectious arthritis** involves signs of acute infection, such as increased temperature, red, painful swelling around the affected joint, and high leukocyte count with increased percentage of polymophonuclear cells. Gram stain and culture of the joint fluid are necessary to confirm the diagnosis.
3. **Crystal-induced arthritis.** Flareup of gout usually affects only one joint, commonly the metatarsophalangeal joint of the big toe. Joint fluid is examined for crystals.
4. **Spondyloarthropathies,** including ankylosing spondylitis or psoriatic arthritis, affect the sacroiliac joints and spine. The joint involvement is asymmetrical. In ankylosing spondylitis, proximal large joints such as the hips, shoulders, and knees are sometimes inflamed. In Psoriatic arthritis, the DIP and PIP joints of the hand and foot are affected. Plain x-rays of the sacroiliac joints, spine, hands, and feet are helpful. The rheumatoid factor test is negative in spondyloarthropathies.
6. **Systemic lupus erythematosus** may present with pain and joint swelling. Initial joint deformities are correctable. X-rays of joints show no erosions.

Investigations

1. **Hemoglobin** is slightly low, especially in chronic rheumatoid arthritis.
2. **ESR** is usually elevated and is a useful measure of disease activity.
3. **Rheumatoid factor** is an IgM immunoglobulin that can be detected by standard floculation tests in about 75–80% of patients with rheumatoid arthritis. This factor is present in about 1–5% of the normal population, but this percentage increases with age to about 10–15% in people over age 60 yrs. Rheumatoid nodules, severe disease, and systemic complications are usually associated with high titers of rheumatoid factor.
4. **X-rays.** During the early phases of disease, plain x-rays show **soft tissue swelling** around the inflamed joints because of effusion or edema. **Juxta-articular osteoporosis** is also seen. Later, there may be **uniform narrowing of the joint space** because of thinning of the articular cartilage (Fig. 4–2). In more severe cases, paraarticular erosions with destruction of contiguous bone may be seen. Comparison of yearly x-rays of selected joints is the best way to evaluate therapy.
5. **Synovial fluid** is yellowish in color. The **WBC** count is increased—2,000–100,000/mm.^{3} Higher counts may suggest infection in the joint; however, only the presence of **organisms** in the joint fluid confirms the diagnosis of infectious arthritis. If infection is suspected, fluid should be sent for culture and antibiotic sensitivity tests. The joint fluid examination also helps in diagnosis of crystal-induced arthritis, such as gout.

Course

The course of the disease in any patient is very variable and difficult to predict. Most patients have few mild exacerbations with prolonged remissions. A few have severe exacerbations and increasing residual signs of the disease and progressively deteriorating function.

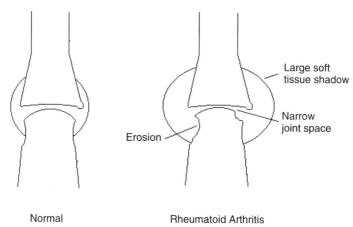

Normal   Rheumatoid Arthritis

Fig. 4–2   X-ray changes in rheumatoid arthritis.

A few patients have progressive disease without any remissions. These last two groups of patients are those seen as inpatients in hospitals and tertiary referral centers. The disease tends to be worse when it starts early in life and when rheumatoid factor test is positive.

Complications
Bones become **osteoporotic** because of inflammation, disuse, and use of steroids. This makes them vulnerable to fractures.

Management
Accurate diagnosis is very important but may be difficult in the early stages of disease. During a flareup, it is essential to rule out infection of the joint or crystal-induced arthritis since the treatment is so different.

Goals
1. Relief of pain
2. Control of inflammation
3. Prevent deformities
4. Maintain and/or improve function
   A patient who is aware of why he or she is following a particular therapy is more likely to cooperate and comply. This makes a **patient education** program a very important part of the management of this chronic, incurable condition. Mild cases can be managed with **NSAIDs** and local heat. Light exercises are prescribed to maintain ROM, and if these are tolerated, then exercises to strengthen muscles and increase endurance can be added. If one NSAID on its maximum recommended dose is not tolerated or does not control inflammation, then another NSAID of a different chemical group should be tried. Patients who continue to have trouble despite these simple measures may have to be referred to a specialist for disease-modifying drugs.
   There is a recent trend toward using multiple drugs of different classes—e.g., methotrex-

ate, sulfasalazine, hydroxychloroquine, and low-dose prednisone—at the same time. These patients need very close monitoring by a specialist.

Medications
1. **NSAIDs and nonacetylated salicylates.** Aspirin was the main nonsteroidal available for a long time, but now we have many NSAIDs of different chemical compositions that have superseded it. The pain and stiffness of rheumatoid arthritis are reduced in a few days by NSAIDs. However, joint swelling may take a few weeks to subside. Patients who develop an allergic reaction with one NSAID may show hypersensitivity to other NSAIDs. Prescribing two NSAIDs at the same time is not advisable because of increased risk of side effects. Elderly patients are especially susceptible because of borderline renal function, drug interactions with other medications, and greater chance of GI bleeding.
   Side effects of NSAIDs
   a. **GI upset,** bleeding, or aggravation of peptic ulcer symptoms are common complications of NSAIDs. All patients should be advised to take these pills after eating. Medications to neutralize or reduce secretion of acid and enzymes are added to reduce the chances of peptic ulcer.
   b. **Renal** adverse reaction may include interstitial nephritis with proteinuria and pyuria. Elderly patients and those with borderline renal function rarely present with renal shutdown.
   c. **Fluid retention** may precipitate congestive heart failure in some.
   d. Drug interactions with other medications may occur. The dose of **anticoagulants** and **antihypertensives** may have to be adjusted after starting on NSAID.
   e. Depression of liver function
   f. Confusion in some elderly patients
2. **Corticosteroids** have not been shown to definitely slow the progression of disease, and there is a definite risk of the patient becoming steroid-dependent. As time goes by, the patient may require higher doses and starts to develop complications of hypercortisolism. The main benefit of steroid preparations is in reducing the inflammatory reaction and temporary symptomatic relief. Before treatment is started with an oral corticosteroid or before injection of steroid preparation, infection in the joint or other systems should be ruled out. Steroids suppress the inflammatory reaction and may exacerbate and disseminate infection. A small dose of corticosteroid ($<$ 10 mg of prednisone for adult male and $<$ 7.5 mg for adult female) with a disease-modifying drug may be considered. Once a patient has been started on steroids, it is very difficult to discontinue them without a major flareup of disease.
   Local intra-articular injection of steroid preparation is given when there are one or two joints with persistent pain and swelling that have not responded to medications, rest, and physical therapy. The fluid from the joint is aspirated, infection is ruled out, and steroid injection given. The patient should be instructed to avoid overexerting the joint for a few days after the injection. The injection should not be repeated $>$ 3 times/year.
   Long-term use of corticosteroids ($>$ 10 mg prednisone/day) is indicated for **systemic involvement, vasculitis,** and other life-threatening complications. The disease-modifying drugs take up to 6 months to show any benefit. During this period, steroids may be used to control the disease for a few months. The steroids are gradually tapered off when other medications start acting.

3. **Disease-modifying drugs,** including antimalarials, gold, cytotoxic agents, and penicillamine, are used by specialists when other measures fail to stop the progression of disease, and there is early evidence of joint destruction (e.g., erosions, increasing functional disability, or systemic involvement). These medications may take from 4 weeks to 6 months to show any beneficial effect. They also have a greater potential for serious side effects.

   a. **Gold** has been shown to slow progression of disease in nearly 70% of patients. However, it has serious side effects such as skin rash, exfoliative dermatitis, membranous glomerulonephritis, nephrotic syndrome, thrombocytopenia, granulocytopenia, and aplastic anemia. It can be given as an injection once a week or orally. It may take up to 6 months to show benefit.

   b. **Antimalarials** such as hydroxychloroquine are considered relatively safe, working well with other medications, such as methotrexate and sulfasalazine. Minor side effects like skin rash and GI upset may occur. Rarely, some patients develop irreversible damage to the retina due to antimalarials. Patients should be checked by an ophthalmologist before starting the medication and then every 6 months thereafter.

   c. **Penicillamine** is not used very frequently because of significant side effects. Patients should be maintained on the smallest effective dose. Many patients complain of abnormal taste sensation. GI upset and skin rash are common side effects. Thrombocytopenia, leukopenia, and proteinuria may also occur.

   d. **Methotrexate** either alone or with sulfasalazine and/or hydroxychloroquine is an important agent in treating rheumatoid arthritis. They are useful in systemic involvement and vasculitis. Liver and kidney damage, bone marrow suppression, and increased risk of malignancy should be considered before starting these medications.

Ancillary

1. **Rest** is a very important aspect of care in rheumatoid arthritis, although it may not always be possible. **Bedrest** may be prescribed for severe flareup of multiple joints. If this is not possible at home, hospitalization may be necessary. Proper posture should be maintained during bedrest, with ROM exercises to prevent contractures. Fatigue and pain are used as indicators for determining the level of activity. Walking is curtailed to a minimum if there is inflammation of joints of the lower extremities and pain on weight-bearing. Local rest is provided by **splints** to immobilize joints. Activities are gradually increased as the patient improves. Later, periods of rest are prescribed between activities.

2. **Local heat,** in the form of paraffin baths for hands and hot packs for other joints or a warm shower, will help relieve pain for a short period of time and help the patient perform his or her exercises more easily.

3. **Exercises.** During an acute flareup, the therapist can perform **passive ROM** exercises to maintain ROM. The joints are likely to become stiff if this is not done. Later, as the patient improves, he or she is assisted in performing active ROM. **Isometric** exercises can be performed in a cast or splint to maintain or increase strength. Exercises against resistance are not advisable when the joint is inflamed and painful.

4. **Patient education** program is essential in getting the cooperation of the patient and family and in gaining their confidence. The patient should be taught about the disease, drugs and their side effects, the role of heat, exercises, splints, and assistive devices. The patient and spouse should be involved in counseling, including sex and general information about the disease. They are also shown a program of exercises and activities that the patient can and cannot do at home.

5. **Vocational rehabilitation** may be necessary if the patient is unable to carry on with a job and the employer is unable to make reasonable adjustments.

Surgical

1. **Synovectomy** is sometimes considered for chronic recurrent swelling of one or two joints that do not resolve with more conservative treatment. The synovial membrane regenerates in 2–3 years, and the inflammation usually recurs. This may give some time for the cytotoxic agents to take effect.
2. **Arthroplasty** to replace the joint surfaces is usually performed for the hip, knee, and small joints of the fingers if they are extensively damaged and painful.
3. **Tendon repair** or graft for tendon rupture

JUVENILE RHEUMATOID ARTHRITIS

Juvenile rheumatoid arthritis (JRA) is also known as **juvenile arthritis, chronic inflammatory arthritis of childhood,** and **juvenile chronic polyarthritis.** It is a chronic inflammatory arthritis starting during childhood and adolescence with different modes of presentation. This leads to difficulty in diagnosis. The spectrum of involvement may vary from only a few joints to multiple joints. There may be systemic involvement with fever, rash, lymphadenopathy, hepatomegaly, and splenomegaly.

Etiology

The exact etiology is not known. Streptococcal infection of the upper respiratory tract, genetic factors, and stress are suspected to play some role in the onset of JRA.

Pathology

Inflammation of joints, especially large joints, is the main feature of this disease. Unlike in rheumatoid arthritis, the affected joint is more likely to become ankylosed. JRA can also lead to premature closure of epiphysis. Stunted growth may result from administration of corticosteroids or early closure of the epiphysis. Other systems may be affected, giving rise to myocarditis, pericarditis, and pneumonitis. Hepatosplenomegaly and generalized lymphadenopathy are also found at times.

Clinical Features

The American Rheumatism Association divides this disease into three subtypes:

1. **Polyarticular.** There is chronic or recurrent episodes of inflammation in five or more joints with some systemic symptoms such as low-grade temperature and loss of appetite. This form is more common in girls. The onset may be insidious or sudden. The systemic symptoms are milder than in the systemic variety. Involvement of liver, spleen, and lymph nodes is not a major feature.
2. **Pauciarticular.** Four or fewer joints are inflamed. Knees and ankles in the lower extremity and wrists and elbows in the upper extremity are usually involved. This group of patients is particularly liable to develop iridocyclitis and cataracts. Since these eye complications may be completely asymptomatic, regular followup by an ophthalmologist is essential.

3. **Systemic.** The systemic symptoms and signs are more prominent than joint involvement. High fever, rash, and lymphadenopathy are common in this subtype. Liver and spleen may be enlarged, and there may be pleural and pericardial effusion. Inflammation of joints is transient, and a minor feature of the disease.

Management

Relief of symptoms and maintenance of function are the most important goals of treatment. The function of a joint can be maintained by preserving its ROM and muscle strength and by preventing deformities. Rehabilitation of these patients is a very important aspect of care. **NSAIDs** are commonly used to control inflammation. Corticosteroids are reserved for severe systemic involvement. An orthopedic surgeon may be consulted for correction of deformities.

SPONDYLOARTHROPATHIES

The diseases grouped under this heading include ankylosing spondylitis, psoriatic arthritis, Reiter's syndrome, and inflammatory bowel disease (which includes Crohn's disease and ulcerative colitis). They all test negative for rheumatoid factor but may include inflammatory arthritis as a component.

ANKYLOSING SPONDYLITIS

Also known as **rheumatoid spondylitis, Marie-Strümpell disease,** and **von Bechterew's disease,** ankylosing spondylitis is a fairly common inflammatory disease affecting the sacroiliac joints and spine. Peripheral joints such as the hips, shoulders, and knees may also be affected. Initial inflammation of structures around the joints is followed by ossification of ligaments and bony ankylosis of the involved joints. Ankylosing spondylitis is associated with histocompatibility antigen (HLA) B27.

Etiology

The exact etiology of the disease is unknown. It is possible that some environmental or infectious agent may make a genetically predisposed host susceptible to the disease. Ankylosing spondylitis is reported in about 0.1% of all whites. However, nearly 20% of individuals with HLA-B27 develop ankylosing spondylitis. HLA-B27 is present in 5–10% of whites, and 90–95% of persons with ankylosing spondylitis have this antigen. Prevalence of the disease varies among different races according to the incidence of HLA-B27 in that particular race.

Pathology

The **sacroiliac joints** are affected in almost all cases. Disease progresses later to involve the lumbar, thoracic, and cervical spine. The apophyseal, discovertebral, and costovertebral joints of the axial skeleton are involved in most patients. There is inflammation at the site of attachment of ligaments and joint capsules to the bone. The inflammatory changes in the synovium are very similar to those seen in rheumatoid arthritis, with infiltration by lymphocytes and plasma cells. The ligaments near the inflamed region ossify (which does not happen in rheumatoid arthritis). Ossification of the anterior longitudinal ligament gives rise to the appearance of "**bamboo spine**" on x-rays (Fig. 4–4). Bony ankylosis of sacroiliac and apophyseal joints occurs later. Peripheral joints, including the hip, shoulder, or knee, may be involved in one-third to one-half of cases. Other sites that may be affected are the eyes, aortic valve, and lungs.

History

Initial symptoms start between ages 15–35 years. The incidence of ankylosing spondylitis is the same in both sexes, but the disease is more severe in males than in females. Peripheral joints are affected more often in females, whereas the spine is more often involved in males. The onset of **pain** is insidious, usually in the sacroiliac region (in 75% of patients). Pain is more diffuse and may extend to the thoracic region and lower extremities. Pain radiating down a lower extremity (5–10% of all patients) may be mistaken for sciatica. Only a small percentage of patients complain of shoulder and hip pain during the initial stages. Nearly half of the patients have shoulder and hip involvement later. They complain of **morning stiffness,** which is relieved by heat and activity. It is aggravated by overactivity.

Constitutional symptoms include fatigue, weight loss, and low-grade fever and are present in some patients. Involvement of peripheral joints is more common in women, and this involvement may be mistaken as rheumatoid arthritis. Pain in the thoracic spine, radiating to the front of the chest, can mimic angina or pleurisy. It is aggravated by deep breathing. Pain in the heel is due to planter fasciitis. Acute and recurrent iritis may occur in 25% of cases. Pain shifts from the lumbar to the thoracic and cervical spine over a period of years. There may be exacerbations and remissions of pain and stiffness. The inflammatory process is self-limited, and symptoms subside on their own. Later, new symptoms develop secondary to complications of the disease.

Physical Examination

1. **Inspection.** In the early stages of the disease, the lumbar lordosis is lost and the lumbar spine becomes straight. Later, **kyphotic deformity** of the whole spine may occur. The extent of deformity can be measured by having the patient stand against the wall and measuring the distance of the occiput from the wall. If the knee or shoulder is involved, there may be **swelling** around these joints.
2. **Palpation.** There is **tenderness** over the sacroiliac and other inflamed joints. **Muscle spasm** may be palpable in the paraspinous muscles of the low back, thoracic, and cervical regions during exacerbation of the disease. An **effusion** may be palpable in a peripheral joint such as the knee or shoulder. Heterotopic ossification around a joint is more likely to occur after any operative procedure, e.g., arthroplasty of the hip, in ankylosing spondylitis.
3. **Range of motion.** ROM is limited during the initial stages because of pain or muscle spasm. Later, bony ankylosis prevents all movements. The lumbar spine is usually involved first. All movements—flexion, extension, lateral flexions and rotations—are markedly restricted in the affected area. Later, when the thoracic spine and costovertebral joints are involved, **chest expansion** is limited. **Flexion deformity** of the hip and knee may develop.

    Special tests are performed if other manifestations of ankylosing spondylitis are present:
    Plantar fasciitis
    Achilles tendinitis

Conjunctivitis, iritis, and uveitis (occurs in 1 out of 4 patients)
Costochondritis
Pulmonary fibrosis of the upper lobes (very late stages)
Aortic regurgitation (very late stages of disease)

Differential Diagnoses

Diagnosis of ankylosing spondylitis depends on the history, physical examination, and radiologic features. HLA-B27 is present in 90% of whites and 50% of blacks with ankylosing spondylitis. During the early stages, ankylosing spondylitis is difficult to diagnose because x-rays may be normal.

1. **Rheumatoid arthritis.** The clinical presentation in females may be similar to that of rheumatoid arthritis with inflammatory arthritis of the peripheral joints. Sacroiliitis and ossification of spinal ligaments on x-rays are present in ankylosing spondylitis and help distinguish these two conditions.
2. **Psoriatic arthritis.** Typical skin lesions of psoriasis are usually present, and x-rays of the hand may show changes of psoriatic arthritis.
3. **Reiter's disease.** Patients usually give a history of urethritis and skin lesions on the soles of the feet.
4. **Mechanical back pain** or **disc herniation.** Ankylosing spondylitis should be suspected in anyone presenting with low back pain in the late second or third decade of life. There may not be any x-ray changes in early ankylosing spondylitis.

    In **lumbar strain** or "mechanical back pain," there is:
    a. History of trauma or sudden onset of symptoms
    b. Pain that is aggravated by activity and relieved by rest
    c. No involvement of thoracic spine or chest wall
    d. No systemic symptoms like fatigue

    In **lumbosacral disc disease** with radiculopathy:
    a. In addition *a* to *d* above, there is radiating pain down one or both lower extremities.
    b. Neurologic signs of muscle weakness and abnormal reflexes
    c. Abnormal electromyogram

Investigations

1. **X-rays.** During early stages of the disease, the radiologic changes may be very subtle and can be easily missed. Initial changes are usually seen in the **sacroiliac joints.** The articular margins are fuzzy, and the joint space is irregular. There is **osteoporosis** of the surrounding bone. Later, *erosions* may develop along the articular margins. The disease process may involve only the sacroiliac joints and no other joints. Later, **bony ankylosis** may be seen with complete obliteration of joint space. When inflammatory arthritis occurs in other synovial joints, such as the hip, shoulder, or knee, there is uniform joint space narrowing with soft tissue swelling. **Lumbosacral** and **thoracolumbar spine** is involved early. Resorption of bone at the superior and inferior angles of the vertebral bodies leads to **squaring of the vertebral body** (Fig. 4–3). This is an early sign. Later, there is progressive ossification of outer fibers of the annulus fibrosus and anterior longitudinal ligament, giving rise to formation of bony bridges across the vertebrae and "**bamboo spine**" (Fig. 4–4).
2. **Blood tests**
    a. **Anemia** may be present in severe cases.
    b. **ESR** is raised.
    c. HLA-B27 test is supportive evidence in whites, but it is not necessary to perform this test in all patients.

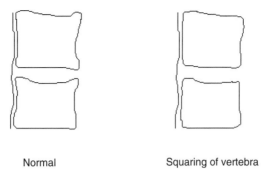

Normal   Squaring of vertebra

Fig. 4–3   Bone at the superior and inferior angles of the vertebral bodies is resorbed as a result of inflammation. This is seen on x-rays as squaring of the vertebrae.

3. **Pulmonary function tests** may show diminished vital capacity due to fusion of the thoracic spine and costovertebral joints.

Course
The disease usually starts in the sacroiliac region and in most cases remains confined to that region. After initial episodes of inflammation, the patient may not have any symptoms. An abnormal radiograph of the sacroiliac joints may be the only indication of the disease. In a smaller percentage of patients, it progressively involves the lumbar, thoracic, and cervical spine. There are **exacerbations** and **remissions** of the symptoms over a period of years. Finally, the spine fuses, and pain and inflammation subside. In others, the disease may progress without any exacerbations or remissions.

Complications
1. **Flexion deformity of the spine** can affect the whole spine. This is a preventable deformity, and every effort should be made to achieve a straight spine. Severe deformity makes ambulation difficult, and the patient may not be able to look straight ahead.
2. Flexion deformities of the hips and knees
3. **Fracture of the spine.** The spine becomes very rigid and fractures easily. Damage to the spinal cord may lead to paraplegia.
4. Limitation of chest expansion because of fusion of costovertebral joints and spine. The vital capacity is diminished. These changes and pulmonary fibrosis may lead to **respiratory difficulty.**
5. **Subluxation** of the atlantoaxial or other cervical joints may cause spinal cord compression.

Management
Goals of treatment are to:
1. Relieve pain
2. Prevent deformities
3. Maintain function
Control of pain is important for doing exercises to maintain ROM and prevent deformi-

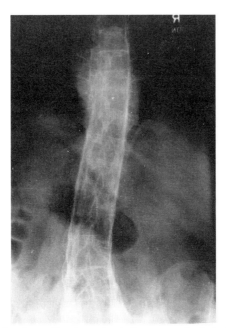

Fig. 4–4 Anteroposterior view of lumbar spine in late stage of ankylosing spondylitis shows ossification of anterior longitudinal ligament and margin of annulus fibrosus. It looks like the trunk of a bamboo treee and hence is called "bamboo spine."

ties and for maintaining function. This is achieved by medications and local heat. Patient education plays a very important part in managing this chronic disease, especially in preventing deformities and maintaining function.

Medications
1. **Indomethacin** is the drug of choice for many.
2. **Sulfasalazine** may now be the drug of choice, especially if peripheral joints are also involved.
3. **Phenylbutazone** is very effective, but chances of serious adverse reactions such as aplastic anemia are greater.
4. Other **NSAID**

Ancillary
1. Local **heat,** in the form of heating pad or warm shower, relieves the pain temporarily.
2. Sleeping on the back on a hard mattress without a pillow is recommended.
3. **Extension exercises** for the spine, similar to the cobra posture in yoga, helps in maintaining extension of the spine and preventing kyphosis. Swimming in a warm pool provides both heat and exercise.
4. **Proper posture** while sitting and at work
5. **Deep breathing exercises** to prevent rigid chest wall

6. Prevent flexion contractures of the hip by lying on the stomach and extending lower extremities

Surgical

1. Total replacement **arthroplasty** of the hip and, sometimes, of the knee is recommended if the articular cartilage is destroyed and the joint is very painful. Chances of heterotopic ossification are much greater after any operation in ankylosing spondylitis than in other conditions.
2. **Wedge osteotomy** of the spine may be necessary for very severe flexion deformities. Danger of paraplegia after this operation needs to be weighed before surgery.

Psoriatic Arthritis

Psoriasis is a common skin disease with erythematous scaling papules on the scalp and on arms and legs. About 5–10% of patients with psoriasis develop asymmetrical inflammatory arthritis involving the distal interphalangeal (DIP), proximal interphalangeal (PIP), and sacroiliac joints and the spine.

Etiology

Approximately 1–5% of the population has psoriasis, and of this, 5–10% develop arthritis. The exact etiology, however, is unknown. It is associated with HLA-B13, HLA-B17, and HLA–B39 histocompatibility antigens.

Pathology

Inflammation occurs in the synovial membrane of the joints. The inflammatory changes in the synovium are very similar to those seen in rheumatoid arthritis.

History

Skin lesions develop in the later part of the third or in the fourth decade. Arthritis develops a few months to a few years later. It affects both sexes equally. Unlike rheumatoid arthritis, there is **asymmetrical involvement** of joints, mainly **DIP** and **PIP** joints of the hands and feet. The patient complains of pain, limitation of movement, and diminished function in involved joints. Nearly half of the patients complain of back pain late in the course of the disease because of involvement of the spine and/or sacroiliitis. Systemic symptoms such as fatigue, fever, malaise, or generalized stiffness are not common. A few patients present with a clinical picture resembling rheumatoid arthritis, with symmetrical inflammatory arthritis and morning stiffness. There is a wide spectrum of symptoms and signs, ranging from very mild involvement of few joints to symmetrical arthritis of most of the joints and constitutional symptoms.

Physical Examination

1. **Inspection.** The **skin lesions** are maculopapular and vary in size. Sometimes, the skin lesions are not very obvious, and the examiner has to make special effort to look for them on the scalp or in the perianal region. The involved joint, usually a **DIP** or **PIP,** is swollen. Sometimes, the affected finger or toe may be diffusely swollen (**sausage finger**) because of DIP and PIP joint involvement and tenosynovitis of the flexor tendons. **Nails** show pitting, separation of nail from its bed (onycholysis), and subungual hyperkeratosis. Similar nail changes may also be seen in fungal infection, lichen planus, and other conditions. The psoriatic nail changes and DIP joint involvement usually occur in the same finger.
2. **Special tests.** Conjunctivitis, iritis, or episcleritis occurs in about a third of patients.

Differential Diagnoses

1. **Rheumatoid arthritis.** There is symmetrical involvement of metacarpophalangeal (MCP), metatarsophalangeal (MTP), and PIP joints. The test for rheumatoid factor is positive in 80% of the patients. The skin and nails are not affected.
2. **Gout.** There is a history of episodes of sudden onset of very painful swelling of joints. Blood uric acid levels are raised, and monosodium urate crystals are found in the joint fluid.
3. **Reiter's syndrome** is one of the seronegative spondyloarthropathies with large joint involvement. Usually the patient gives a history of urethritis and conjunctivitis.

Investigations

There are no diagnostic tests for this condition.

1. ESR is mildly elevated.
2. Joint fluid shows an increased number of polymorphonuclear cells, up to 12,000–15,000/mm^3.

X-rays of the hands and feet may show **soft tissue swelling** in early stages. Unlike rheumatoid arthritis, there is **no juxta-articular osteoporosis.** The tuft of terminal phalanx may be eroded. Maximum changes are seen in DIP joints. The joint space may be increased if there is destruction of subchondral bone. Narrowing of the joint space is seen if there is increased new bone formation. Marginal **erosions** extend to involve the central parts of the joint. This together with bony proliferation produce a picture described as **pencil-and-cup** (Fig. 4–5): bony erosions are seen at the posterosuperior aspect of the calcaneus and around the sacroiliac joint and ischial tuberosity. Large asymmetrical **bony spurs** are seen in the spine, especially in the thoracolumbar region. **Bony ankylosis** may be seen between interphalangeal joints and vertebrae.

Management

The treatment is symptomatic, and as with any chronic incurable condition, patient education plays an important role. NSAIDs help relieve some of the pain and reduce inflamma-

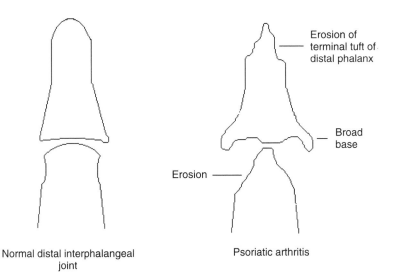

Normal distal interphalangeal joint

Psoriatic arthritis

Erosion of terminal tuft of distal phalanx

Broad base

Erosion

Fig. 4–5 X-ray changes of psoriatic arthritis seen in the distal interphalangeal joint.

tion. In a minority of patients, treatment of skin lesions may help the arthritis. Gold and antimalarials are useful but may aggravate the skin condition. Methotrexate may help the lesions and the joints but one must be vigilant for hepatic toxicity. The patient should receive instructions in ROM exercises and avoiding overuse. Local steroid injections are useful in the treatment of bursitis. Arthroplasty may be necessary for painful joints with destruction of articular cartilage.

Reiter's Syndrome
In Reiter's syndrome, a young adult develops inflammatory arthritis after an episode of urethritis, dysentery, or cervicitis.

Etiology
Sexual intercourse or dysentery usually precedes the inflammatory arthritis. GI infection may be due to *Salmonella, Shigella,* or *Yersinia.* Arthritis is supposed to be of a reactive nature. HLA-B27 is present in more than two-thirds of patients.

History
Recent studies suggest a male: female ratio of 5:1. Male patients present with burning **pain on micturition** and urethral discharge. Women may complain of symptoms suggestive of cystitis. Some patients may develop **conjunctivitis** or **circinate balanitis** (superficial ulceration on glans penis). Eye manifestations, including iritis, uveitis, and corneal ulceration, are seen in a small percentage of patients. **Keratoderma blennorrhagicum** consists of raised, papular or pustular lesions on the soles of the feet or, sometimes, palms of the hands. These start as vesicles and become firm and nodular. They may last for several weeks and then disappear. **Inflammatory arthritis** usually affects the knees and ankles. Sacroiliac joint involvement causes low back pain. Other peripheral joints of the hands and feet are sometimes inflamed. The joint involvement is **asymmetrical.** Systemic symptoms such as fever and weight loss are not common.

Physical Examination
1. **Inspection.** The inflamed joints are swollen. Eyes are examined for conjunctivitis, the soles of the feet and palms for keratoderma blennorrhagicum, and glans penis for balanitis circinatum.
2. **Palpation.** There may be tenderness at the site of insertion of the Achilles tendon and plantar fascia.
3. **Range of motion** of inflamed joints is limited.

Differential Diagnoses
Differential diagnosis is similar to that for psoriatic arthritis. **Gonococcal arthritis** should be ruled out by cultures because of urethritis associated with Reiter's syndrome.

Investigations
1. **Urine** may have polymorphonuclear leukocytes but is sterile on culture.
2. **ESR** is elevated.
3. **X-rays** of the sacroiliac joints may show **erosions** and **juxta-articular osteoporosis.** Later, there may be bony ankylosis. Fluffy new bone formation may be seen at the sites

of insertion of Achilles tendon and plantar fascia and over shafts of phalanges. The x-ray changes are asymmetrical. They may appear many years after the onset of symptoms.

4. **Joint fluid** may show 10,000–40,000 WBC/mm^3.
5. Evidence for chlamydial infection should be sought.

Management
Management is similar to that of psoriatic arthritis. Treatment of chlamydial infection may be beneficial.

Inflammatory Bowel Disease

Inflammatory bowel disease, including ulcerative colitis and Crohn's disease, are sometimes associated with inflammatory arthritis. It is not known whether some antigens affect both the gastrointestinal tract and joints or whether antigens produced in the bowel from infectious agents lead to arthritis. **Ulcerative colitis,** as its name implies, gives rise to ulcers in the colon. Patients present with diarrhea and blood in stools. There are exacerbations and remissions of the symptoms. In **Crohn's disease,** the terminal ileum and colon are involved. Inflammation affects all the layers of the intestinal wall, and patients complain of fever, abdominal pain, and diarrhea. Later, they may develop abscesses and fistulae.

About one in five patients with inflammatory bowel disease develop arthritis. The arthritis and bowel symptoms usually occur at the same time. There are exacerbations and remissions of joint symptoms, with migration of pain from one joint to another. The knee and ankle joints are usually affected. Nonspecific synovitis with joint effusion occurs. Inflammatory joint disease subsides with the bowel disease. The sacroiliac joints and spine are affected less often (in about 5%) than peripheral joints.

SYSTEMIC LUPUS ERYTHEMATOSUS

Systemic lupus erythematosus (SLE), also known as **lupus erythematosus,** is the most common connective tissue disease. Many organ systems are affected, and symptoms and signs can mimic any disease. This makes it very difficult to diagnose this disease, especially in its initial stages.

Etiology
Women are affected more often than men (10:1 ratio). SLE is more common among African-Americans than people of European descent. The onset of the disease is usually during the child-bearing years. Certain medications, such as procainamide, hydralazine, and isoniazid, are also believed to initiate SLE. These facts suggest that hormonal, environmental, and genetic factors may play some part in the etiology.

Pathology
There is increased production of antinuclear antibodies (ANA), especially anti-dsDNA (antidouble-stranded DNA). The antibodies and antigens form immune complexes, which are deposited in and around small blood vessels, glomeruli in the kidneys, and synovial membrane of joints. They initiate an inflammatory reaction and may lead to necrosis of

cells, including red blood cells and platelets. The number of organs affected and the severity with which each one is involved vary considerably. This produces a very variable clinical picture. Hematoxylin bodies stain blue on hematoxylin-eosin stain. These homogeneous, bluish masses are seen in most organs and are important in the diagnosis of SLE. Another characteristic is the **onion skin lesion** seen in the spleen, which consists of concentric layers of fibrous tissue around small arteries. Kidneys are involved in the vast majority of patients. In mild cases, there is thickening of mesangial matrix and proliferation of mesangial cells. The cells of the glomerular capillaries and Bowman's capsule also proliferate. Skin biopsy may show inflammation at the junction of dermis and epidermis with deposition of immunoglobin IgG.

Clinical Features

The disease may start with fever and malaise. Onset of the disease may be sudden and severe or gradual with episodes of exacerbations and remissions. Other symptoms and signs depend on the system involved. The extent and severity of involvement of different organs vary among different patients, giving rise to a very variable clinical picture. Prognosis is worse if the disease starts early in life and the course is more severe.

1. **Joints.** Pain and swelling of joints is very common. The joint involvement is symmetrical with morning stiffness. Rheumatoid arthritis should be considered as a differential diagnosis.
2. **Skin.** Edema of the skin and erythematous **rash** is seen during exacerbations and after exposure to the sun. The "butterfly" rash over the malar eminences (malar rash) is considered an important sign. Erythematous plaques with scales are seen on the scalp and face in discoid lupus. Atrophy of the skin and depigmentation occur in the central part. Superficial gangrene of the skin of fingertips and toes is seen as a result of vasculitis.
3. **Renal.** Proteinuria, hematuria, and casts are seen in a large proportion of patients with SLE. Renal insufficiency of varying grades occurs as disease progresses.
4. **Heart. Pericarditis** is seen in nearly 30% of patients. Arrhythmias and congestive heart failure can also occur.
5. **Lungs.** Shortness of breath may occur because of **pleural effusion,** interstitial lung disease, or myopathy of the diaphragm.
6. **Gastrointestinal. Oral ulcers** may occur during exacerbations.
7. **Central nervous system.** A wide spectrum of neuropsychiatric disorders is exhibited, ranging from mild depression and psychosis to seizures and stroke. Other presentations include transient ischemic attacks, migraine-like headaches, myelopathy, and peripheral neuropathy.

Complications

1. **Infections.** Patients treated with immunosuppressives and steroids are very vulnerable to infection. Pneumonia, septicemia, and renal failure are the usual terminal events.
2. **Avascular necrosis** of the head of the femur may occur in patients treated with high-dose steroids.

Management

Some of the medications used in the treatment have potentially dangerous side effects. It is important to balance the need for control of disease activity with the chance of developing a serious side effect to the medication. Patient education plays an important role in the management of SLE because of these factors. The patient should know about the disease and the medications used in its treatment. The patient and family should be able to recognize when to see a physician. Because infection is a very common and important complication, the patient needs to report fever, difficulty breathing, and other symptoms.

Medications

1. **NSAIDs** are prescribed to control arthralgia. The choice of NSAID depends on how effective it is in controlling an individual patient's symptoms, its cost, side effects, etc. Any NSAID that may affect renal function adversely should not be prescribed.
2. **Corticosteroids.** Topical steroids are used for skin rash. When minor symptoms are not controlled by NSAIDs, a low-dose corticosteroid preparation is given. It is advisable to give a single dose in the morning. As soon as symptoms are controlled, the dose is gradually reduced to a minimum. If the dose cannot be reduced below an acceptable level for long-term therapy (7 mg of prednisolone or equivalent), other agents such as immunosuppressives are added. Large-dose oral or intravenous corticosteroid bolus treatments are considered for major exacerbations involving the kidneys, vasculitis, or central nervous system. An intravenous bolus of 1 gm of methylprednisolone has the potential for very serious complications. High-dose oral prednisone treatments should not be continued for $>$ 6 weeks because of the risk of mortality from infection.
3. **Antimalarials** are especially effective against skin rash and arthritis.
4. **Immunosuppressives** are used when other drugs fail to control serious involvement of kidneys, CNS, or vasculitis.

POLYMYOSITIS–DERMATOMYOSITIS

Dermatomyositis and polymyositis are considered together because a large percentage of patients with polymyositis have the typical rash of dermatomyositis.

Etiology
Dermatomyositis and polymyositis are probably autoimmune diseases that are triggered by viral infection. Some medications, such as D-penicillamine, are also thought to trigger this disease. Polymyositis is more common in adults than dermatomyositis, whereas in children, dermatomyositis is more common.

Pathology
Lymphocytes and macrophages are seen surrounding the blood vessels and muscle fibers. The size of muscle fibers varies much more than in normal muscle. The nuclei of degenerated and necrotic muscle fibers move from the periphery to the center of muscle cells. Phagocytes remove necrotic muscle fibers, and atrophic fibers get replaced by fibrous tissue. There is some evidence of regeneration of muscle fibers. Polymyositis and dermatomyositis are associated with malignancy in about 15–20% of patients.

Clinical Features
1. **Muscles.** The onset is usually insidious, with weakness of proximal muscles, malaise, and loss of weight over a period of months. It may sometimes start suddenly with acute

symptoms and then may go on to remissions and exacerbations. The patient has difficulty getting up from a chair or toilet seat or going up and down stairs because of weakness of hip extensors. Involvement of shoulder girdle muscles makes it difficult to lift the arms above shoulder level. During acute exacerbations, the patient may have trouble lifting his or her head off the bed because of weakness of neck flexors. Weakness of muscles involved in chewing, swallowing, and respiration occasionally cause difficulty with these functions. Some patients complain of pain and tenderness over affected muscles.

2. **Skin.** Skin **rash** may precede muscle weakness by months or years. Erythematous, scaly plaques occur over the dorsum of proximal interphalangeal and metacarpophalangeal joints and exposed areas of the face and neck. There may be purple discoloration of the eyelid.

3. **Heart.** Congestive heart failure and arrhythmias are sometimes seen.

4. **Lungs.** Aspiration pneumonia and respiratory insufficiency may occur because of muscle weakness.

5. **Blood vessels. Vasculitis** (inflammation of blood vessel walls) can lead to intestinal perforation or Raynaud's phenomenon.

Differential Diagnoses

1. **Fibromyalgia.** The patient complains of aches and pains all over the body. There are tender points or trigger points in muscles. Muscle weakness is secondary to pain in the muscles. All laboratory tests, including ESR, muscle enzymes, and electromyogram (EMG) are negative.

2. **Polymyalgia rheumatica.** The patient complains of pain in muscles and fatigue. The ESR is markedly elevated but muscle enzymes are within normal limits.

3. **Myasthenia gravis.** The weakness is felt after activity or at the end of the day. Some patients complain of ptosis and difficulty in swallowing. The muscle enzymes are normal. Repetitive stimulation test and edrophonium test help in the diagnosis of myasthenia gravis.

Investigations

1. **ESR** is slightly elevated.

2. **Urine**—may show increased levels of myoglobin.

3. **Creatine kinase** (CK). The level of CK is a sensitive measure of muscle inflammation. It is useful in diagnosis of the disease and in following its course. Elevated levels of CK are not diagnostic of polymyositis and require corroboration by history, physical examination, EMG, and muscle biopsy. However, it is useful in determining whether the medications are effective or not and in diagnosis of a flareup.

4. **Electromyography** and **nerve conduction tests** (NCS). On EMG fibrillations and positive sharp waves are seen during exacerbations. The motor unit potentials are of small amplitude, short duration, and polyphasic in shape. EMG/NCS helps to rule out amyotrophic lateral sclerosis, peripheral neuropathy, myasthenia Gravis, and muscular dystrophy.

5. **Muscle biopsy** is helpful in determining the diagnosis and to rule out other conditions. The muscle selected for biopsy should not be completely atrophic or of normal strength. The fluorescent antinuclear antibody test is positive in about 80% of patients. Anti-Jo-1 autoantibody is very common.

6. **MRI** may help in demonstrating abnormality in muscles and in selection of muscle for biopsy.

Course
There are exacerbations and remissions. Women and African-Americans have a worse prognosis than males of European descent. Up to 80% of patients survive 7 years with proper management.

Management

Medications
1. **Prednisone.** The patient is started on prednisone, 1–2 mg/kg of body weight/day, until there is clinical improvement. The progress is judged by increase in muscle strength, improvement in symptoms, increasing ability to perform ADLs, and lowering of muscle enzyme levels. The prednisone dose is gradually reduced as tolerated by the patient.
2. **Cytotoxic agents.** Azathioprine or methotrexate is added to the therapeutic regimen if prednisone alone is unable to control the disease activity or its dose is more than acceptable levels for long-term maintenance.
3. Medications to prevent osteoporosis are prescribed when any patient is maintained on long-term corticosteroids.

Ancillary
Rehabilitation therapy. During acute exacerbation, the therapist performs passive ROM exercises to prevent contractures and stiffness of joints. Proper posture and rest are important during this stage. Later active exercises are added to gradually increase strength. It is important to avoid fatigue and excessive pain. The occupational therapist provides training in ADLs.

Bibliography
1. Bennett RM: Nonarticular rheumatism and spondyloarthropathies: Similarities and differences. Postgrad Med 187(3):97–99, 102–104, 1990.
2. Brick JE, DiBartolomeo AG: Rethinking the therapeutic pyramid for rheumatoid arthritis. Postgrad Med 91(2):75–91, 1992.
3. Bunch TW: When muscle weakness points to polymyositis. J Musculoskel Med 8(9):67–78, 1991.
4. Calabro JJ, Marchesano JM, Parrino GR: Juvenile rheumatoid arthritis: Long term management and prognosis. J Musculoskel Med 6(1):17–32, 1989.
5. Calin A: Management of ankylosing spondylitis. Bull Rheum Dis 31(6):35–38, 1981.
6. Cardenosa G: Ankylosing spondylitis. Am Fam Physician 42:147–150, 1990.
7. Dougados M: Diagnosis and monitoring of spondyloarthropathy. Compr Ther 16(4): 52–56, 1990.
8. Gladman DD: Psoriatic arthritis: Recent advances in pathogenesis and treatment. Rheum Dis Clin North Am 18:247–256, 1992.
9. Hay EM, Snaith ML: Systemic lupus erythematosus and lupus-like syndromes. BMJ 310:1257–1261, 1995.
10. McGuire JL, Ridgway WM: Aggresive drug therapy for rheumatoid arthritis. Hosp Pract 28(9):45–52, 1993.
11. Miller-Blair DJ, Robbins DL: Rheumatoid arthritis: New science, new treatment. Geriatrics 48(6):28–38, 1993.
12. Moll JM: Current thinking on spondyloarthritides. Compr Ther 14(1):60–63, 1988.
13. Porter DR, Sturrock RD: Medical management of rheumatoid arthritis. BMJ 307:425–428, 1993.
14. Ramanujam T, Schumacher HR: Ankylosing spondylitis: Early recognition and management. J Musculoskel Med 9(1): 75–92, 1992.
15. Reardon EV, Clough JD: Drug therapy in rheumatic diseases. Compr Ther 18(11):22–25, 1992.
16. Ries MD, Dennis DA, Clayton ML: Surgery in rheumatoid arthritis. J Musculoskel Med 9(10):29–46, 1992.
17. Tan EM, Cohen AS, Fries JF, et al: The 1982 revised criteria for the classification of systemic lupus erythematosus (SLE). Arthritis Rheum 25:1271-1277, 1982.
18. Targoff IN: Diagnosis and treatment of polymyositis and dermatomyositis. Compr Ther 16(4):16–24, 1990.
19. Wong AL, Weisbart RH: Rheumatoid arthritis: A review of current medical therapies. J Musculoskel Med 6(11):39–58, 1989.

5

Infections

Chadwick F. Smith, M.D.

OSTEOMYELITIS

Infection of bone by pyogenic organisms is called osteomyelitis. It may spread through the bone marrow and cortex or remain localized and become chronic. Chronic osteomyelitis is a fairly common disorder.

Anatomy
The metaphysis is the epiphyseal end of the diaphysis (Fig. 5–1). In children, osteomyelitis usually starts in the metaphysis because of the peculiarities of the blood vessels in this region. The nutrient artery divides into branches that travel to the metaphyseal end. There, they turn around, form a loop, and join the venous sinuses. The blood flow is slow, and hematogenous organisms have a chance to grow. The cartilaginous growth plate separates the metaphysis from epiphysis and keeps the infection on the metaphyseal side.

Etiology
Staphylococcus aureus is the most common infecting organism. However, *Haemophilus influenzae* and *Streptococcus* spp. may be found in children under 6 months of age. In most cases, the organisms are blood-borne. The bone may become infected from a wound or spread from adjacent structures, such as a joint or soft tissue abscess.

Pathology
Purulent exudate develops in the metaphysis and spreads into the medullary cavity or through the cortex to the underside of the periosteum (Fig. 5–2). It lifts up the periosteum and cuts off the blood supply to that part of the bone, which may cause a part of the bone to become necrotic. **Sequestrum** is a necrotic piece of bone that has separated from the living portion. The pus may become "walled off" by new bone formation, forming a chronic abscess (**Brodie's abscess**) inaccessible to antibiotics. If the metaphyseal end of the bone is within an articular capsule (as in hip, shoulder, and ankle), the pus may infect the joint (Fig. 5–3).

The usual sites for osteomyelitis in children are the proximal tibia, distal femur, and proximal femur. In adults, osteomyelitis starts in the epiphyseal region and spreads to in-

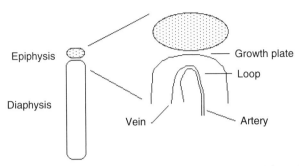

Fig. 5–1 Anatomy of the metaphysis. The epiphysis is separated from the diaphysis by a plate of cartilage (growth plate), which prevents the infection from spreading from the diaphysis to the epiphysis. The nutrient artery divides into branches that go toward the metaphysis, the epiphyseal end of the diaphysis. There, they form a loop and become a vein. The blood flow slows here, and blood-borne organisms get a chance to start a focus of infection.

fect the joint more often than in children. Osteomyelitis of the spine is associated with intravenous drug abuse. The tubercle bacillus also affects the spine. In adults, osteomyelitis may develop in an immunosuppressed host. An unusual predilection for *Salmonella* osteomyelitis is seen in patients with sickle cell anemia.

History
There may be little systemic reaction in infants and the very old. Children, on the other hand, may have a sudden onset of very high fever, chills, and toxic appearance (**explosive onset**). Adults may have a more gradual onset. Osteomyelitis is painful, and the child can not walk if any of the bones of the lower extremities are involved.

Physical Examination
1. **Inspection.** Swelling and discharging sinus are seen late in the course of disease.
2. **Palpation.** There is marked tenderness over the site of infection if the involved bone is superficial (e.g., proximal tibia or distal femur).
3. **Range of motion.** All movements of the adjacent joint are painful and limited.

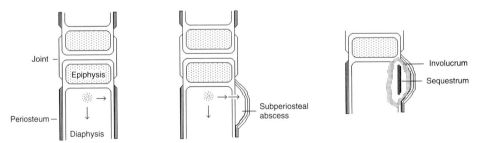

Fig. 5–2 Pathogenesis of bone infection. The infection may start in the metaphysis and spread to the subperiosteal region when the metaphysis is outside a joint capsule. There, it lifts up the periosteum and forms a subperiosteal abscess. Bone within an abscess cavity may become necrotic (sequestrum). It is denser than surrounding new bone, which is called involucrum.

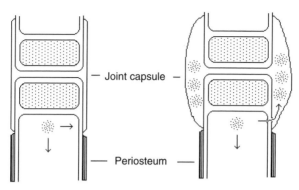

Fig. 5–3 When the metaphysis is within a joint capsule, the infection can spread to the joint cavity and lead to infectious arthritis.

Differential Diagnoses

1. **Infectious arthritis** and osteomyelitis are particularly difficult to differentiate in children. They both start near a major joint, such as the hip or knee, and have very similar systemic and local signs. There may be a sympathetic effusion in the joint secondary to osteomyelitis. In infectious arthritis, the swelling is limited to the joint, joint movements are markedly restricted, and there is muscle spasm.
2. A **fracture** is painful with swelling and loss of function. Plain x-rays usually help in distinguishing it from the infections.
3. A very malignant **tumor** may start with pain and swelling. X-rays show destruction of bone as in osteomyelitis. Ewing's tumor starts in the diaphysis and not the metaphysis and grows more slowly. Sometimes, a biopsy may be necessary.
4. In **rheumatic fever** there is a history of sore throat preceding involvement of multiple joints, and the onset is less acute.

Investigations

1. **X-rays** show **soft tissue swelling** within a few days. Bony changes may take 1–2 weeks. A radiolucent area without any definite margin appears. When the periosteum is lifted off the bone by underlying pus, it forms fluffy new bone (**involuerum**), which can be mistaken as a sarcoma. Later, a necrotic piece of bone (**sequestrum**) is seen as a separate, more dense area than the surrounding bone. A chronic abscess (Brodie's) within the bone has a sclerotic margin around a radiolucent area.
2. **Bone scan** shows increased uptake and may be useful in the early stages before x-ray changes.
3. **Blood.** ESR is increased, and there is marked leukocytosis. Blood cultures may be positive.
4. **Culture** and **sensitivity** testing of the isolated organisms is very important for selection of appropriate antibiotic treatment.

Complications

1. **Chronic discharging sinus** may result if the infection is not treated.
2. **Septicemia** and **death** can result in the very young and very old or in immunosuppressed patients.
3. The infection may spread to a nearby joint and cause **septic arthritis.**

Management

1. **Medications.** An appropriate antibiotic is the mainstay of treatment. The antibiotic is given intravenously for a few weeks and then continued orally.
2. **Ancillary.** The affected extremity is immobilized to reduce pain and prevent spread of infection.
3. **Surgical.** With the advent of antibiotics, incision and drainage is not absolutely essential. It is required if a joint is involved or there is fluctuant pus. Any necrotic pieces of bone are removed.

INFECTIOUS ARTHRITIS

Infection of joints occurs more often in infants and children than in adults. There is severe pain, local heat, redness, and swelling. It is often confused with noninfectious arthritis. Careful history, physical, and examination of joint fluid are necessary for accurate diagnosis. It is very important to arrive at a diagnosis as soon as possible and to start appropriate treatment; otherwise, the joint will be destroyed in a few days.

Etiology

The organisms reach the joint via:

1. The bloodstream (**hematogenous**). This is the most common method of development of septic arthritis. The organisms usually originate at some other site, such as pneumonia, decubitus ulcer, or abscess.
2. From a **wound** (puncture wound or laceration) over the joint. Sometimes, a puncture wound from a sliver of wood may not be obvious. Human bites over joints are particularly dangerous.
3. **Direct spread** from infection of a bone (osteomyelitis)

Common organisms that cause osteomyelitis in children include *Staphylococcus aureus, Haemophilus influenzae,* and *Streptococcus.* In sexually active adolescents and young adults, *Neisseria gonorrhoeae* is a common cause. In the elderly, postoperative infection after arthroplasty is becoming more common as the number of arthroplasties increases. Suppression of the immune system by steroids or cytotoxic agents makes the patient vulnerable to bone and joint infections. The hip and knee joints are the common joints that become infected.

Pathology

Often, one of the larger joints, such as the knee or hip, is affected. However, in the newly born and the very old, more than one joint can be involved. There is a violent **synovial reaction** with exudation of fluid and WBCs into the joint. Proteolytic enzymes from the breakdown of cells and increased pressure in the joint lead to **destruction of the articular cartilage.** Later, pus from the joint may discharge outside and form a sinus. The infection may resolve, and the newly formed fibrous tissue between the two bones (**fibrous ankylosis**) may severely restrict joint movements. If the infection is not controlled, toxemia and septicemia may cause death.

History

The child is brought in with a history of sudden onset of high **fever** and chills. Systemic symptoms may be minimal in infants and very elderly patients. If old enough, the child will complain of pain in the region of the joint. The patient avoids moving the affected extremity.

Physical Examination
1. **Inspection.** A **swelling** is seen around a superficial joint, such as the knee. The skin over it may be red.
2. **Palpation.** There is **warmth** and marked **tenderness** over the joint.
3. **Range of motion.** All active and passive movements are very painful and restricted.

Differential Diagnoses
1. **Fracture.** Intra-articular fracture can cause a very painful, warm, swelling of the joint. X-rays help to rule out a fracture.
2. Abscess or **cellulitis** of the skin overlying the joint is much more warm, edematous, and red. It is not restricted by the joint cavity and spreads beyond its limits.
3. **Osteomyelitis** can give rise to sympathetic effusion in a nearby joint. X-rays and bone scan may help in distinguishing it from septic arthritis. Joint fluid does not have a high WBC count or show organisms on Gram stain or culture.
4. Acute flare up of **rheumatoid arthritis** or **gout** may be difficult to distinguish from infectious arthritis. Finding monosodium urate crystals helps in diagnosis of gout. Sometimes, a joint in a patient with rheumatoid arthritis or gout may become infected. Demonstration of organisms in the joint fluid or on culture is necessary for diagnosis of infectious arthritis.

Investigations
1. **Blood.** There is a marked increase in **WBC** count with predominant polymorphonuclear cells. The **ESR** is also increased.
2. **X-rays** show **soft tissue swelling** in the early phase of the disease, which is due to effusion in the joint and edema of the surrounding structures. **Juxta-articular osteoporosis** develops as a result of increased vascularity. Narrowing of the joint space is seen when articular cartilage is destroyed. The treatment should be started before x-ray changes in bone are seen.
3. **Aspiration** of joint fluid is **the most important diagnostic test. Gram stain** and **culture** of the fluid helps in selecting appropriate antibiotics to control the infection. If gonococcal infection is suspected in a sexually active person, culture should be prepared at the bedside. Culture of specimens from the urethra, rectum, or pharynx is more likely to grow gonococci than those from joint fluid. Chronic, low-grade infections, such as tuberculosis or fungal infection, may require special culture methods, skin tests, or synovial biopsy. Uric acid and calcium pyrophosphate crystals should be looked for to rule out gout and pseudogout.

Course
Septic arthritis can destroy a joint within days. If the organisms are virulent and host immunity low, it can lead to **septicemia** and death. This may occur in the very old, the very young, or the immunosuppressed. In milder infections, pus may drain outside through a **sinus.** One of the sequelae is fibrosis in and around the joint, which restricts movement of the joint.

Complications

1. Damage to the growth plate can cause premature closure of the epiphysis with a short extremity or unequal growth and **deformity.**
2. Infection can spread to the bone (**osteomyelitis**).
3. Destruction of the articular cartilage may lead to early **degenerative arthritis.**
4. Fibrous or bony **ankylosis**

Prognosis for outcome depends on whether there was any delay in making the diagnosis. If the condition is diagnosed soon after onset and treated appropriately, then outcome is good. Infants and very old patients do not do so well. It takes longer to diagnose infection in a deep joint, and hence the prognosis is worse. Deep joints also are not as easily accessible for aspiration as superficial joints.

Management

All suspected cases of infection in a joint should be treated as an **emergency.** The joint fluid is **aspirated,** Gram stain performed, and the fluid sent for culture and sensitivity. Appropriate **intravenous antibiotics** are started and continued for 4–6 weeks. Intra-articular antibiotics are not usually recommended. The joint is immobilized. If fluid collects again in the joint, it is aspirated to reduce pressure in the joint and remove pus, breakdown products of bacteria, and WBCs. **Incision and drainage** is performed if the joint is deep (e.g., hip) or the pus becomes too thick and loculated to aspirate. If a joint gets infected after arthroplasty, the hardware needs to be removed. **Physical therapy** is required to regain ROM, strength, and function.

Bibliography

1. Cole WG: The management of chronic osteomyelitis. Clin Orthop 264:84–89, 1991.
2. Green NE: Early identification of gonococcal arthritis. J Musculoskel Med 8(3):83–86, 1991.
3. Fink CW, Nelson JD: Septic arthritis and osteomyelitis in children. Clin Rheum Dis 12:423–435, 1986.
4. Mikhail IS, Alarcon GS: Nongonococcal bacterial arthritis. Rheum Dis Clin North Am 19:363–377, 1993.
5. Scopelitis E, Martinez-Osuna P: Gonococcal arthritis. Rheum Dis Clin North Am 19:311–331, 1993.
6. O'Meara P, Bertal E: Septic arthritis: Process, etiology, treatment outcome. Orthopedics 11:623–628, 1988.

6

Metabolic Disorders

Andrew L. Wong, M.D., F.A.C.R., and
Arun J. Mehta, M.B., F.R.C.P.C.

GOUT

Monosodium urate crystals in synovial fluid cause an inflammatory reaction, and the patient presents with severe pain and swelling of one or more joints. There may be many such acute attacks over several years, after which the patient may end up in the chronic stage with multiple painful and persisteatly swollen joints. Gout is a clinical syndrome resulting from deposition of monosodium urate monohydrate or uric acid crystals in the joints and tissues.

Epidemiology

Gout has been called the "king of diseases" and the "disease of kings" because of its past association with rich diet. There is a direct correlation between the serum uric acid level and both the prevalence and incidence of gout. **Hyperuricemia** is defined as serum uric acid level > 7.0 mg/dl. About 10% of hyperuricemic men develop clinical gout. The incidence of gout increases with increasing levels of hyperuricemia. The prevalence of gout is high in the Maori of New Zealand, Polynesians, and Filipinos. It is also associated with obesity, hypertension, hypertriglyceridemia, and coronary artery atherosclerosis.

Etiology

Uric acid is the end product of purine metabolism. The enzyme uricase oxidizes uric acid (less soluble compound) to allantoin, which is more soluble. This enzyme is absent in humans. Uric acid, which is sparingly soluble, accumulates in the body fluids in humans, predisposing to uric acid crystal deposition disease (gout).

Uric acid level in blood may be high due to:

1. Excessive production of uric acid, due to defects in enzymes involved in purine metabolism or in myeloproliferative and lymphoproliferative diseases with increased turnover of nucleic acid.
2. Inability of kidneys to excrete enough uric acid in urine, which occurs in nearly 90% of patients with gout. Diuretics (e.g., thiazides and furosemide), low-dose aspirin, and alcohol affect renal tubular function and may precipitate an attack of gout. The serum uric acid level in women is lower because estrogens help in its excretion. It remains lower than in males until menopause.

Pathology

There is often long-standing hyperuricemia before clinical gout occurs. Monosodium urate crystals are deposited in the articular cartilage, epiphyseal bone, periarticular structures, and kidney. These deposits may produce local necrosis and a foreign-body giant cell reaction with proliferation of fibrous tissue. A gouty **tophus** consists of a core of urate crystals with a proteoglycan matrix, surrounded by mononuclear and giant cells and fibrous tissue.

The affected joints develop degeneration of articular cartilage, synovial proliferation, destruction of subchondral bone, and proliferation of marginal bone. Deposition of monosodium urate crystals in and around joints is believed to cause an acute inflammatory response. It is not clear how inflammation starts, because these crystals can be present even during a period of remission. In kidneys, it can sometimes cause gouty **nephropathy** or **uric acid stones.**

Collection of monosodium urate crystals in tissues is called **tophi.** Subcutaneous tophi may be seen over the subcutaneous extensor border of the ulna and the external ear. Tophi also may be found in the synovial membrane of joints and bursa, bone, and tendons.

Clinical Features

The **natural history** of gout generally passes through four stages:

1. **Asymptomatic hyperuricemia.** The serum uric acid level is elevated without any clinical manifestations. It occurs in 5–7% of Americans on at least one occasion during adulthood, but only one in five of these develop symptoms of gout. Asymptomatic hyperuricemia is treated by a low-protein diet, weight control, and avoidance of alcohol.

2. **Acute gouty arthritis** is the most frequent clinical manifestation of gout. It is predominantly a disease of the lower extremity, though any joint in the body can be affected. The **metatarsophalangeal (MTP) joint of the big toe** is the most frequently involved joint, seen in 60% of first attacks (**podagra**) and in 90% of patients at least once during the course of the disease. Other common sites are the ankle, knee, and tarsal joints. The wrist, fingers, and elbows may be involved years later in the course of disease.

   The first episode of acute gout typically begins abruptly in a single joint, often during the night, awakening the patient. The joint is swollen, red, warm to touch, and very tender. Fever, leukocytosis, and an elevated ESR may also be present. During the early course of the disease, acute attacks subside spontaneously in 2–10 days. After an acute attack, the patient may be completely well until the next episode, which may not occur for months or years. However, with time, attacks tend to occur more frequently, involve more joints, and last longer. Acute attacks may be triggered by trauma, surgery, infection, acute medical illness, alcohol, or dietary excess.

3. **Intercritical Gout.** The intervals between acute attacks are termed intercritical periods in gout. In most patients, a second attack occurs within 6 months to 2 years. In the beginning, the patient is usually asymptomatic during intercritical periods. Later in the course of disease, the patient may enter a phase of chronic polyarticular gout without painfree intercritical periods. A presumptive diagnosis of gout can be made during an asymptomatic intercritical period in about 70% of patients by demonstrating monosodium urate crystals in joint fluid from the knee and first MTP joint.

4. **Chronic tophaceous gout** is characterized by deposition of solid urate crystals (**tophi**) in articular and extra-articular tissues, leading to a destructive arthropathy. This occurs in fairly advanced stages of gout and is associated with earlier age of onset, frequent attacks, serum uric acid levels > 9 mg/dl, and a predilection for polyarticular and upper extremity involvement. With the advent of antihyperuricemic agents, the incidence of tophaceous gout has decreased considerably. The tophi occur most commonly in the he-

lix of the ear, olecranon and prepatellar bursa, ulnar aspect of the forearm, Achilles tendon, and hands and feet. The acute attacks become milder and may disappear altogether in the more advanced stage of disease.

Nearly one third of all patients with gout have hypertension and proteinuria, and renal failure accounts for up to 25% of deaths in patients with gout. There may be deposition of urate crystals in the papillae and pyramids of the kidneys. Uric acid stones can form in the urinary tract.

Differential Diagnoses
1. **Infectious arthritis,** especially gonococcal, should be ruled out by Gram stain and culture of joint fluid. Absence of organisms on Gram stain and culture and the presence of typical crystals are necessary criteria for definitive diagnosis of gout.
2. A patient with **fracture** will give a history of trauma, and plain x-rays will help confirm the break.
3. **Rheumatoid arthritis** may be suspected when multiple joints are involved as in the chronic stage of gout. Finding monosodium urate crystals in the joint fluid helps in distinguishing these two conditions. Rheumatoid factor is usually positive in rheumatoid arthritis.
4. **Pseudogout** has calcium pyrophosphate dihydrate crystals in joint fluid.

Investigations
1. **Joint fluid** aspiration and examination under the polarized light microscope shows needle-shaped, strongly negatively birefringent crystals of monosodium urate. They may be free-floating in the joint fluid or within WBCs. They may be seen even during a period of remission. These crystals also will be seen in the exudate from tophi. Demonstration of these crystals is essential for diagnosis.
2. **Serum uric acid** level may be elevated (> 7 mg/dl) or normal during an acute attack of gout. This test is not diagnostic, because it may be normal in patients with gout and can show abnormally high values in people who never had an attack of gout.
3. Increased **24-hour urinary excretion** of **uric acid** suggests increased production and greater risk of formation of uric acid stones.
4. **X-rays** show soft tissue swelling in early stages. Tophi may also be seen as soft tissue shadows. Joint space is maintained until the joint develops degenerative arthritis. Erosions near the joint (periarticular) with an overhanging edge of bone are seen later (Fig. 6–1). Unlike rheumatoid arthritis, the base of an erosion in gouty arthritis is sclerotic.

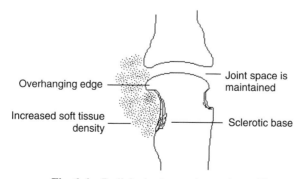

Overhanging edge

Increased soft tissue density

Joint space is maintained

Sclerotic base

Fig. 6–1 Radiologic changes in a patient with gout.

Course

Acute attacks occur with subsequent remission of symptoms which may last for months. Later, the periods of remission become shorter and the periods of pain and swelling last longer.

Management

Proper management can prevent or reduce the frequency of acute attacks of gout and deterioration of renal function. Acute gout is usually treated with **NSAIDs** like indomethacin or colchicine.

1. **NSAIDs** are very effective, and some specialists use them as the drug of first choice in acute attacks. Indomethacin is favored over others in treatment of gout.
2. **Oral colchicine** is given every hour until the patient develops symptoms of toxicity, such as abdominal cramps or diarrhea, or the symptoms of gout subside. The maximum dose allowed, as determined by body weight, should not be exceeded
3. **Corticosteroids** and **adrenocorticotrophic hormone** (ACTH) are also effective and may be used when NSAIDs and colchicine are contraindicated or ineffective. When used properly, corticosteroids and ACTH have minimal toxicity. Aspiration and intrarticular injection of corticosteroids in one of two affected large joints is a useful alternative after infection or septic arthritis has been excluded.
4. Long-term therapy with **uricosuric drugs** and **allopurinol** reduces the uric acid pool. This is given to patients with recurrent attacks of gout, visible tophi, or uric acid stones in the urinary tract. Probenecid increases the excretion of uric acid, whereas allopurinol reduces its production. Probenecid is preferred beause it has a lower incidence of severe drug reactions than allopurinol.
5. **Ancillary.** A weight-reducing diet low in purine content is sometimes recommended.

CALCIUM PYROPHOSPHATE DIHYDRATE CRYSTAL DEPOSITION DISEASE

This condition is also known as **pseudogout** and **chondrocalcinosis**. It is called pseudogout because patients may have attacks of acute inflammatory arthritis that mimics gout, but there are no urate crystals in the joint fluid. Because there is deposition of calcium crystals in the fibrocartilage and articular cartilage around various joints, this disease has earned the name chondrocalcinosis.

Etiology

The prevalence of calcium pyrophosphate dihydrate (CPPD) crystal deposition disease (CDD) increases with age. Up to 50–60% of people over age 80 may have asymptomatic CPPD-CDD. It may be associated with metabolic diseases such as hyperparathyroidism, hemochromatosis, and hypothyroidism.

History

CPPD-CDD is a disease of old age and affects both sexes equally. It may present in a variety of ways:

1. **Asymptomatic.** The patient may not have symptoms related to the joint but shows incidental findings of calcium deposition in cartilage on x-rays. This is very common.

2. **Pseudo-osteoarthritis.** Nearly half of all symptomatic patients present with symptoms similar to those of degenerative or osteoarthritis. They complain of pain on using the joint and mild swelling. However, unlike osteoarthritis, in CDD, wrist, metacarpophalangeal (MCP), elbow, and shoulder joints are also affected in addition to the knee and hip joints.
3. **Pseudogout.** About one-fourth of symptomatic patients will present with acute painful swelling in one or more joints, such as the knee. The pain may be as severe as in gout. The onset may be precipitated by a surgical procedure or injury to the joint.
4. **Pseudorheumatoid arthritis.** The patient presents with a symmetrical inflammatory arthritis involving multiple joints. The patient will often complain of morning stiffness and have an elevated ESR.

Differential Diagnoses
1. **Gout.** Joint fluid examination shows needle-shaped, strongly negatively **birefringent crystals** in WBCs or free-floating. Both conditions, gout and pseudogout, respond well to colchicine.
2. **Degenerative joint disease** does not affect the wrist, MCP, elbow, or shoulder joint. There are **no crystals** in the joint fluid.

Investigations
1. **X-rays.** Fibrocartilaginous structures, such as the meniscus of the knee, triangular cartilage of the wrist, and pubic symphysis, show fine punctate radiodensities. These cartilages may now become visible on x-rays. The articular cartilage of the hip and knee may be involved in a similar process. Degenerative changes are seen later in the joint. In the knee joint, the patellofemoral component shows more severe changes than the tibiofemoral condyles.
2. **Joint fluid** shows short and stubby rhomboid crystals in WBCs or free-floating. They are weakly positively **birefringent** under polarized light.

Management
Medications
1. NSAIDs are usually effective.
2. Aspiration of joint fluid and injection of corticosteroids should be tried if there is severe, acute inflammatory arthritis involving a large joint.
   Ancillary. Local heat and exercises to maintain ROM and strength may help relieve some symptoms.
   Surgical. Arthroplasty may be required for severe symptomatic degenerative arthritis.

OSTEOPOROSIS

Epidemiology
Osteoporosis is a disorder of too little bone of normal composition. It involves parallel reductions in protein bone matrix and mineral content and is defined as a bone mineral density or bone mineral content that is more than 2.5 standard deviations (SD) below the young adult mean (t score) value. It is the commonest metabolic problem affecting bone and af-

fects women six times more than men. Up to 20% of all women over 50 and up to 90% of all women over 85 years old will have osteoporosis. Osteoporosis results in considerable morbidity, mortality, and public health expenditures and accounts for up to 1.5 million fractures yearly in the United States, with almost half involving the vertebrae and one-fifth the hips. Hip fractures account for much of the increased morbidity and mortality. Osteoporosis is considered severe if it is accompanied by fracture.

Etiology

Osteoporosis is generally classified as primary or secondary. Primary osteoporosis is subdivided into involutional and idiopathic (<50 years old). There are two types of involutional osteoporosis: Type 1 (post-menopausal) affects people who are 50–70 and is characterized by a predominant loss in trabecular bone. Type 2 (senile) affects those older than 70 and is associated with a near equal loss in cortical and trabecular bone. Type 1 has a F:M ratio of 6:1 whereas type 2 has a near equal F:M ratio. Secondary osteoporosis can be due to non-estrogen-related endocrine causes, gastrointestinal causes such as malabsorption or chronic liver disease, medications such as corticosteroids, heparin, methotrexate, and thyroid, or chronic rheumatic conditions including rheumatoid arthritis and lupus. Second osteoporosis may account for up to 20% of cases of osteoporosis in women and 40% in men.

The following risk factors are implicated in the development of osteoporosis:

1. **Race.** Genetic factors are the most important determinants of peak bone mass. Caucasian people of northern European descent with blond hair and thin build and Asians with a small thin build are more likely to develop osteoporosis.
2. **Age.** Peak bone mass is reached at age 30–35 in females and then progressively declines about 1% per year. The peak occurs about 5 years later for males. In addition, women experience an accelerated phase of bone loss at menopause for 5–8 years.
3. **Menopause.** Lack of female hormones after menopause or a postsurgical early menopause after oophorectomy
4. **Lack of physical activity.** Due to an inactive lifestyle, paralysis, or immobilization.
5. **Slim body habitus.** Possibly due to decreased synthesis of estradiol in adipose tissue.
6. **Nutritional.** Inadequate intake of calcium as well as a high-protein, high-phosphate diet, smoking, alcohol abuse, and excessive caffeine intake may be contributory risk factors.
7. **Endocrine.** Ingestion of corticosteroids, Cushing's disease, hyperparathyroidism, hyperthyroidism, insulin dependent diabetes mellitus, and hypogonadism can cause generalized osteoporosis. Prolonged amenorrhea in young females is also an important, often overlooked risk factor for osteoporosis and may be secondary to anorexia nervosa or to excessive exercise, especially in female athletes.

Pathology

Bone is in a state of dynamic equilibrium, constantly being remodeled (resorption and formation). Bone remodeling is performed by osteoclasts and osteoblasts working together in a "coupled" fashion in remodeling units. In osteoporosis, there is an "uncoupling" phenomenon resulting in overall more bone resorption than formation. Bone biopsy reveals a decrease in bone mass with markedly reduced numbers and thickness of bony trabeculae. However, the ratio of bone matrix to mineral content is normal.

History

Patients with osteoporosis may present with:
1. **Back pain.** It may be diffuse pain in the thoracolumbar region, of gradual or sudden on-

set, due to a vertebral compression fracture.

2. **Fracture** of the wrist, distal end of the radius, hip, or neck of the femur after a fall. Patients with osteoporosis are prone to develop fractures even after minor trauma.

3. **No symptoms.** Osteopenia may be detected on routine radiographs where 25–50% of the bone mineral content may already be lost. Furthermore, up to one-half of vertebral fractures may be asymptomatic. Moreover, individuals with a positive family history or other risk factors for osteoporosis may request a bone densitometry measurement for screening purposes.

Physical Examination

1. **Inspection.** Examination of the spine may reveal kyphosis (increased forward curvature), abdominal protrusion, and loss of several inches of height in the patient. Other deformities also may be noted due to previous fractures.

2. **Palpation.** During acute episodes of back pain, paraspinous muscles may be firm and tender because of spasm. Local tenderness is usually present at the site of recent fractures.

3. **Range of motion.** All movements may be painful, especially after a recent fracture.

Differential Diagnoses

1. **Metastatic disease.** Serum calcium and alkaline phosphatase levels may be elevated. Identification of radiographic changes of primary or metastatic malignancy in affected bones or vertebrae is critical.

2. **Multiple myeloma.** Serum and urine immunoelectrophoretic patterns are abnormal. Radiographs may show multiple small (osteoblastic) radiolucent areas.

3. **Disorders** of adrenal, thyroid, and parathyroid glands should be excluded.

4. **Malabsorption syndromes** may result in secondary osteoporosis from nutritional causes, including deficiency of calcium.

5. **Osteomalacia.** Characterized by excessive unmineralized osteoid due to vitamin D-related abnormalities or deficiency, hypophosphatemia, or toxins.

6. **Other conditions,** including Paget's disease or genetic diseases such as osteogenesis imperfecta tarda

Investigations

Each patient's circumstances are considered, and necessary tests are performed for evaluation or treatment of osteoporosis or to exclude other causes of bone disease. People with an osteoporosis-related fracture should be investigated.

1. Serum levels, including calcium, phosphate, and alkaline phosphatase, and urinary levels, including hydroxyproline, are usually normal in typical involutional osteoporosis.

2. Radiographs of the spine and painful areas may be requested to exclude osteolytic or metastatic lesions. In osteoporosis, typically an increase in **kyphosis** in the thoracic region due to compression fractures resulting in diminution in the height and wedging of the anterior border of the vertebrae may be seen. The intervertebral discs in the lumbar region bulge out in the center and reduce the vertical height of the vertebrae, leading to **biconcave** (codfish) **vertebral bodies.** There is diffuse radiolucency with disappearance of trabeculae, especially of transverse trabeculae. The cortex of the bones may also become thin and indistinct.

3. Other tests are done to rule out hypercortisolism, hyperparathyroidism, hyperthyroidism, chronic renal or hepatic diseases, and chronic inflammatory arthritic diseases.

4. Serum and urine protein electrophoresis studies are ordered to rule out **multiple myeloma.**
5. Calcium intake/output studies may be helpful for optimizing calcium balance, such as the 24-hour urinary calcium excretion test where a low urinary level may suggest intestinal malabsorption while a high level may suggest hypercalciuria.
6. Bone-specific assays, vitamin D levels, and testosterone levels (in men) may be useful.
7. Measurement of bone density by single- or dual-beam photon absorptiometry (DPA), quantitated computed tomography (QCT), or dual energy x-ray absorptiometry (DEXA) may be beneficial for screening high-risk individuals and for monitoring of therapy. Bone density measurements are usually made of the lumbar spine or proximal femur.
8. An iliac crest bone biopsy may be considered in atypical or poorly responsive cases.

Complications

Fractures, including compression fractures of the spine, femoral neck fractures, and Colles' fractures, are common and may occur even after a minor fall or spontaneously in an osteoporotic individual. The incidence of these fractures seems to be increasing. Unfortunately, the morbidity and mortality associated with a hip fracture is high, frequently being a catastrophic event resulting in a 20% mortality within the first year, or often necessitating long-term nursing home care.

Management

Osteoporosis is preventable and treatments are available that are effective to decrease further fractures even in patients with severe osteoporosis. The goal in prevention is to increase peak bone mass and decrease the subsequent rate of bone loss. Adequate dietary calcium is important, especially during growth. Hormonal replacement therapy is probably the most effective preventative measure against osteoporosis. The goal of treatment in established or severe osteoporosis is pain control and decreasing the risk for further fractures. Pain relief is provided by analgesics and/or physical and local measures. Treatment of severe osteoporosis may include the following:

Medications

1. **Calcium.** Daily dose of 1,500 mg of elemental calcium supplements are recommended, especially for menopausal women whose dietary intake may be poor.
2. **Vitamin D,** 400–800 units/day, increases absorption of calcium.
3. **Thiazide** diuretics decreases urinary calcium excretion.
4. **Hormones.** Estrogen in females and testosterone in males with gonadal deficiency may be effective in decreasing the rate of bone loss and maintaining bone density.
5. **Anti-bone resorbers.** The bisphosphonates and calcitonins are potent inhibitors of bone resorption and may be an efficacious group of medications.
6. **Bone formers.** Low-dose fluoride and intermittent parathyroid hormone increases bone formation. Bone formers may be a group of medications with potential great promise.

Ancillary

1. **Diet.** Dairy products can be a good, nutritious source of calcium.
2. **Exercise.** Weight bearing or impact-loading and aerobic exercises, such as back extension exercises and jogging, can help to increase or maintain bone density.
3. **Sunlight.** Providing adequate sunlight for the elderly, especially during winter, may aid vitamin D synthesis.

4. **Avoid** smoking, alcohol, and high-protein, high-phosphate diets.
5. **Fall** prevention evaluation, including evaluating gait, balance, vision, arrthymias, hypotension, medications, and safety of the home environment.

Bibliography

1. Bonafede RP: Evaluating CPPD crystal deposition, an important disease of aging. Geriatrics 43(11):59–68, 1988.
2. Consensus Development Conference: Prophylaxis and treatment of osteoporosis. BMJ 295:914–915, 1987.
3. Consensus Development Conference on Osteoporosis. Am J Med 95(5A):1–75, 1993.
4. Doherty M, Dieppe P: Crystal deposition disease in the elderly. Clin Rheum Dis 12:97–116, 1986.
5. Einhorn TA: Evaluation and treatment methods in metabolic bone disease. Contemp Orthop 14(5):21–34, 1987.
6. Kaplan PS: Prevention and management of osteoporosis. Ciba Clin Symp 47:1, 1995.
7. Kanis JA: The diagnosis of osteoporosis. J Bone Miner Res 9:1132–1140, 1994.
8. Kelley WN: Gout and related disorders of purine metabolism. In Kelley WM, Harris ED, Ruddy S, Sledge CB (eds.): Textbook of Rheumatology, 3rd ed. Philadelphia, W.B. Saunders Co., 1989, pp 132–140.
9. Raiz LG: Local and systemic factors in the pathogenesis of osteoporosis. N Engl J Med 318:819–828, 1988.
10. Sinaki M: Osteoporosis. In DeLisa JA, Gans BM (Eds): Rehabilitation Medicine: Principles and Practice, 2nd ed. Philadelphia, J.B. Lippincott, 1993, pp 1018–1035.
11. Vawter RL, Antonelli MAS: Rational treatment of gout. Postgrad Med 91(2):115–127, 1992.
12. Williams RC Jr: Toe pain: Is it podagra or something else? J Musculoskel Med 8(12):31–42, 1991.

7

Neoplastic Diseases

Arun J. Mehta, M.B., F.R.C.P.C.

Tumors or neoplasms of the musculoskeletal system are not very common. Most tumors have a very gradual onset, and initial symptoms are vague. For these reasons, tumors may be missed until they are far advanced. It is important to keep this in mind for all patients with musculoskeletal complaints. When some aspects in the history and physical examination do not add up to a definite diagnosis, it is time to consider uncommon presentations of common diseases or an uncommon diagnosis such as tumor. Also, after treating a condition in which the outcome is not very satisfactory, it is time to revise the list of differential diagnoses.

Anatomy
Long bones grow in length by cellular proliferation at the **growth plate** (Fig. 7–1). This is a cartilaginous plate between the **diaphysis** and **epiphysis.** The diaphysis forms the shaft and epiphysis the articular end of the long bone. The part of the diaphysis close to the growth plate is called the **metaphysis.** This region is very well supplied by blood vessels, and many primary tumors of bone start here. It is also the area where osteomyelitis usually starts. After the bone growth stops, the growth plate (cartilage) disappears, and diaphysis and epiphysis become one continuous bone. The adult bone then has a diaphysis and articular end of the diaphysis.

Pathology
Most bone tumors are metastatic from a primary malignancy elsewhere. Common sites of primaries are the breast, prostate, lung, kidney, gastrointestinal tract, and thyroid. The primary tumor may remain occult, and metastatic disease may be the first indication of malignancy.

History
The patient may have trouble remembering the date or month when symptoms started, because these are usually very vague during the initial phases. It is more important to know the **rate of growth** than size of the tumor. Rapid increase in size of the tumor within a short period of time is suggestive of malignancy. **Pain** arising from bone is felt as deep boring pain and is poorly localized. It is worse at night when it is due to malignant tumors and osteoid osteoma. It may be throbbing when there is infection or if the tumor is very vascular. The pain of osteoid osteoma is well controlled by aspirin, whereas narcotics may be needed for pain due to malignant tumors. When the patient is not able to use his or her painful ex-

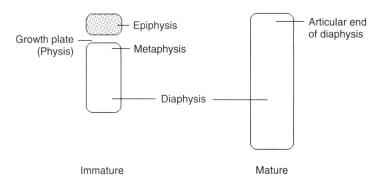

Fig. 7–1 In immature or growing bones, there is a cartilaginous plate, or *physis,* between the diaphysis and epiphysis. The diaphyseal end near the growth plate is called the metaphysis. In mature, adult bone, there is no growth plate or metaphysis.

tremity (**loss of function**), it should be considered a serious complaint and thoroughly investigated.

Swelling around the knee or other parts of any extremity may be noticed by the patient or parents. Sometimes, **minor injury** to the part draws attention of the individual and may convince the physician that trauma was the real cause of pain. This may delay the process of investigations and diagnosis. Minor injury can fracture a bone—**pathologic fracture**— which may bring the patient to the physician.

Because metastatic disease of the bone is more common than a primary tumor, it is very important to **review all systems** for any symptoms suggestive of primary malignancy. In the elderly male, nocturnal urinary frequency or dribbling may suggest prostatic enlargement. A long history of smoking, cough, and hemoptysis may be due to carcinoma of the lung. **Past history** of operation for cancer, chemotherapy, or radiation treatments can suggest recurrence of the tumor.

Physical Examination
1. **Inspection. Location** of the mass may give some indication of its structure of origin. The surface of the swelling should be observed—is it smooth or knobby? Visible **dilated veins** on the surface suggest a highly vascular tumor. **Erythema** is seen in infections and very malignant tumors.
2. **Palpation. Warmth** and **tenderness** are more marked in infections but may be present over a very vascular tumor. Abscess and cellulitis do not have a definite **border,** unlike a tumor. A benign tumor usually has a well-defined border (e.g., lipoma). A tumor with **soft consistency** and fluid inside its cavity is more likely to be benign, whereas a solid tumor with firm to hard consistency may be malignant. A tumor that is **adherent** to skin and/or deeper structures is also likely to be malignant.
3. **Range of motion.** Movements of a joint close to a tumor may be painful and restricted.
4. **Special tests. Neurovascular** exam of the distal part of the extremity helps in determining if these structures are damaged or compressed.

Clinical Features
The following factors should be considered in arriving at a diagnosis:
1. **Age.** Some tumors are more common during specific ages.

Osteosarcoma	10–25 yrs
Multiple exostosis	10–30 yrs
Giant cell tumor	20–40 yrs
Metastasis	>45 yrs
Multiple myeloma	>50 yrs

2. History of **pain at night** that keeps the patient awake should always be taken seriously.
3. **Pathologic fracture** is suggested by minor trauma that normally does not break any bones.
4. **Rate of growth** of the tumor
5. **Adherent** to deeper structures (bone and muscles)
6. Plain **x-rays.** The following findings suggest malignancy:
   a. Lack of definite **line of demarcation** between the tumor and normal bone
   b. Destruction of cortex and spread of tumor in surrounding **soft tissues**
   c. Periosteal **new bone formation** which is described as sunburst, hair-on-end, or onion-skin appearance.

Differential Diagnosis

1. **Infection.** An erythematous, warm, tender swelling without a definite border is suggestive of **cellulitis** or **osteomyelitis.** Acute infections come to medical attention after a very short course and are more likely to have high temperature, malaise, loss of appetite, and other systemic symptoms. It may take up to 2 weeks to see changes due to osteomyelitis on x-rays. Gallium scan may show an increased uptake in infections earlier than changes on plain x-rays.
2. **Fracture.** At times, history of injury may not be forthcoming. X-rays are useful in the diagnosis of most fractures, but they may be negative in the case of stress fractures. Technetium-99m bone scan is helpful in diagnosing stress fractures at that early stage, before they become obvious on plain x-rays.
3. **Myositis ossificans.** This occurs commonly around the elbow after an injury. The initial swelling may be due to hematoma. Later x-rays may show some calcification around the periphery of the soft tissue swelling.

Investigations

1. **ESR** and **WBC** count may be elevated in some malignancies.
2. **Alkaline phosphatase** is raised in metastatic carcinoma, osteogenic sarcoma, Paget's disease, and multiple myeloma.
3. **Serum electrophoresis** shows a typical pattern in multiple myeloma.
4. **Urine** exam shows Bence-Jones proteins in multiple myeloma.
5. **Plain X-ray** is the most useful test in diagnosis of bone tumors. The site of origin of the tumor in the vertical plane is described as epiphyseal, metaphyseal, or diaphyseal. Giant cell tumor and chondroblastoma arise from the epiphysis, whereas most other tumors arise from the metaphysis or diaphysis. The location of a tumor in a transverse plane is described as subperiosteal, intracortical, or intramedullary (Fig. 7–2). Determination of location helps in differential diagnosis of various bone tumors.
6. **Doppler studies** are done to see if the major blood vessels are involved in the tumor.
7. **Bone scan.** Increased uptake on bone scan indicates increased turnover—breakdown and repair—in the bone. There is increased uptake of technetium-99m in areas of increased vascularity due to neoplasm, infection, stress fractures, reflex sympathetic dystrophy, or inflammation. In case of tumors, it helps in determining local spread and in identifying bony metastasis all over the body. It is also useful during early stages when

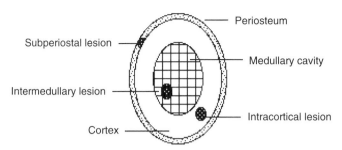

Fig. 7–2 Cross-section of a bone showing relationship of lesions with periosteum, cortex, and medullary cavity.

plain x-rays are negative in a patient with suspicious symptoms. Bone scan is not specific in identifying a tumor but is sensitive for abnormal circulatory changes. Multiple myeloma is an exception since there is no increased uptake in this condition.

8. **CT** is helpful in determining the spread of malignancy within the medullary cavity, destruction of cortex, and spread in soft tissues beyond the bone. Tumors of some bones, such as the spine, pelvis, and scapula, are difficult to assess on plain x-rays. CT of these sites gives more information about the extent of involvement of the bone and surrounding soft tissues.

9. **MRI** is very sensitive to changes in the marrow. Infiltration of bone marrow by metastasis, myeloma, leukemia, lymphoma, osteomyelitis, and avascular necrosis are seen well on MRI. MRI is better than CT in determining spread of tumor in the medullary cavity and in surrounding soft tissues. CT, on the other hand, is better in finding calcifications in the tumor. Neither MRI nor CT has any advantage over plain x-rays in evaluating benign tumors.

10. **Biopsy** is the definitive test to confirm the diagnosis, grade malignancy of the tumor, and formulate management.

BENIGN TUMORS OF BONE

Osteochondroma

Osteochondroma is the most common benign tumor of bone, comprising nearly half of all benign tumors of bone. They occur most commonly over the metaphyseal ends of the distal femur, proximal tibia, and proximal humerus. They occur between the ages of 10 and 35 years and continue to grow as long as the skeleton is growing. Osteochondromas may be a **single** tumor or **multiple.** The multiple form is hereditary (*see* Chapter 2).

Plain **x-rays** show a growth from the metaphyseal end of a bone, which may be pedunculated or sessile. Cortex of the bone is continuous over the cortex of the tumor, and its medullary cavity communicates with that of the bone. A cartilage cap, which is not visible on x-rays, covers the top of the tumor during the period of growth. The tumor is excised if there are complications, such as nerve palsy due to pressure of the tumor, pain, or fracture. Malignant change is not common in solitary osteochondroma but may occur in 10–15% of cases of multiple hereditary exostosis.

Benign Giant Cell Tumor

Benign giant cell tumor is also known as **osteoclastoma.** This slowly growing tumor starts in the epiphyseal region of long bones, particularly the distal end of the femur, proximal tibia, and distal radius. The tumor is vascular and locally invasive. It contains many large multinucleated cells—giant cells or osteoclasts. Other cells are smaller with one nucleus. These cells may show some characteristics of malignancy. The patient presents between the ages of 20–40 years with a painful swelling or pathologic fracture. He or she may have trouble moving the joint close to the tumor. Benign giant cell tumor is twice as common among females as males.

X-rays show a localized lytic lesion near the articular end of a long bone. There is a thin margin of cortical bone surrounding the tumor. X-rays do not show any new bone formation or sclerosis at the margins. Sometimes, the tumor breaks through the cortex and forms a soft tissue mass, or there may be a fracture through the tumor.

Treatment is by curettage, and the cavity is packed with cancellous bone graft. The recurrence rate for this tumor is very high. More radical treatment may be required if there is recurrence or infiltration of local soft tissues. Some surgeons advise more radical treatment from the very beginning.

MALIGNANT TUMORS

Malignant tumor of a bone may be a **primary tumor** arising from one of the various components of the bone or a malignant transformation in a benign condition (**secondary**). **Metastatic** tumors originate in some distant tissue and migrate to a bone. Malignancies also arise from blood-forming tissues in the bone. Some of the primary malignant tumors of the bone are osteosarcoma, chondrosarcoma, and Ewing's sarcoma. Multiple myeloma, leukemia, and Hodgkin's disease are examples of malignancies arising from the blood-forming tissues.

Osteosarcoma

Also known as **osteogenic sarcoma,** osteosarcoma is the most frequent variety of primary malignant tumor of the bone. Usually, it occurs between ages 10–25 years, with a peak incidence around 15–20 years. However, it is seen later in life as a complication of Paget's disease. As with most other bone tumors, the most frequent site is around the knee joint and proximal humerus. The tumor spreads in the medullary cavity and under the periosteum and grows into a fusiform mass. There are islands of cartilaginous and bony tissue within this mass as well as areas of hemorrhage and necrosis. As the periosteum gets lifted off the bone, it forms new bone at the margins of the tumor and also along the blood vessels that go from the periosteum to the cortex of bone.

Osteosarcoma is twice as common among males as females. The patient complains of vague **pain** in the region of the tumor. Sometimes, he may present with a **swelling** adherent to bone or a **pathologic fracture.** Unexplained pain in the metaphyseal region of long bone, difficulty walking, or a limp in an adolescent or young adult should suggest osteosarcoma. Fever and high WBC count may suggest infection and mislead the physician. Dilated veins on the surface of a swelling also suggest malignancy.

Plain **x-rays** show destruction of cortex and trabeculae. The periosteum, which is lifted up off the bone at the periphery of the tumor, forms new bone of triangular shape, described as **Codman's triangle.** The periosteum also forms streaks of new bone perpendicular to the shaft, giving a "sunray'" or "sunburst" appearance. At a later stage, the tumor breaks through the periosteum and invades the surrounding soft tissues. Some tumors form new bone and are seen as **sclerotic** lesions, whereas others are **osteolytic.** In the mixed type, both sclerotic and lytic areas are seen. **CT** helps in determining the extent of spread within the medullary cavity and surrounding soft tissues.

These tumors are treated by **surgical excision** and **radiation** therapy. They are very malignant, with fatal outcome in >80% of patients within 5 years.

Multiple Myeloma

Multiple myeloma presents after the age of 50 years. It is a malignant tumor of plasma cells and originates in the marrow of the skull, ribs, sternum, spine, and pelvis. **Deep-seated bone pain** which is aggravated by movements and weight-bearing is the usual complaint. Anemia and pathologic fracture are other presenting symptoms. Serum globulin is increased, and monoclonal IgG and IgA are seen on electrophoresis. Examination of urine shows Bence-Jones proteins.

Multiple well-circumscribed **osteolytic lesions** are seen in many bones on **x-rays.** These changes are observed all over flat bones such as the skull and pelvis and in medullary cavities of long bones. Unlike with metastatic lesions, the uptake of technetium-99m is not increased in these areas.

METASTATIC DISEASE OF BONE

Metastasis to bone probably occurs more often than to any other organ and is more common than any primary tumor of the bone. Common sites of primary malignant tumors that metastasize to bone are the breast, prostate, lung, kidney, intestines, and thyroid. The most common primaries in females are the breast and lung, and in males they are the prostate and lung. Usually, metastatic tumors spread from the primary site via the bloodstream. Common sites for bony metastasis are the thoracic and lumbar spine, proximal femur, pelvis, and proximal humerus. Primary tumors of the breast and lungs rarely metastasize to distal bones of the extremities.

Pathology

Nearly one-third of autopsies for malignant tumors show metastasis in bones. Most metastatic lesions are **osteolytic.** Sclerotic lesions are seen in metastases from the prostate and sometimes from the breast. They are irregular in shape and destroy the cortex.

History

The patient may complain of vague, deep-seated **pain** that is **worse at night.** Some patients may present with a **pathologic fracture. Hypercalcemia** due to multiple metastases causes nausea, vomiting, and loss of appetite. Other unusual presentations are peripheral neuropathy, corticocerebellar degeneration, herpes zoster, dermatomyositis, and recurrent thrombophlebitis.

Investigations
1. **Serum alkaline phosphatase** is elevated.
2. **Serum acid phosphatase** and **prostate specific enzyme** are elevated if carcinoma of prostate has spread beyond its capsule.
3. **Bone scan** shows metastatic lesion before it is seen on plain x-rays and is a very good screening test. It shows which bones are affected.

Management
The goals of treatment are to slow the process of further spread and treat symptoms to make the patient as comfortable as possible. **Pain** is the most common symptom. It is preferable to give adequate dosages of appropriate medications at regular intervals to control this pain rather than giving medications on an as-needed basis (prn). The fear of addiction and other side effects should not affect the selection of drugs. Sometimes, pain is due to hypercalcemia and is relieved by decreasing the blood calcium level.

For hormone-dependent carcinomas, hormonal therapy, oophorectomy, or orchiectomy are considered. Local radiation therapy, nerve blocks, or rhizotomy are other options.

Bibliography

1. Barbera C, Lewis MM: Office evaluation of bone tumors. Orthop Clin North Am 19:821–837, 1988.
2. Brown ML: Bone scintigraphy in benign and malignant tumors. Radiol Clin North Am 31:731–738, 1993.
3. Moser RP Jr (ed): Imaging of bone and soft tissue tumors. Radiol Clin North Am 31:237–447, 1993.
4. Weatherall PT: Benign and malignant masses: MR imaging differentiaton. MRI Clin North Am 3:669–694, 1995.

8

Degenerative Arthritis

Arun J. Mehta, M.B., F.R.C.P.C.

DEGENERATIVE JOINT DISEASE

Degenerative joint disease (DJD), also known as **osteoarthritis** and **osteoarthrosis,** is the most common disease of the joints. Patients complain of pain in the affected joints on weight-bearing or movements, morning stiffness lasting for <30 minutes, and difficulty in performing functions that involve the joint. It is a slowly progressive disease.

Etiology

DJD is present in almost everyone over age 65 years. These changes are seen on autopsy after age 20 years and on x-rays after age 40. The prevalence of the disease increases with age. It is more common in people of European and Japanese descent than in those of Chinese, African, or East Indian ancestry. The overall prevalence is equal in males and females. However, Heberden's nodes over the distal interphalangeal (DIP) joints are 10 times more common in females, and DJD of the hips is more common in males. This prevalence suggests a sex-linked genetic influence over these manifestations. DJD is more common in postmenopausal women because estrogens are believed to offer some protection. It is also more common among diabetics and patients with acromegaly, which suggests influence of other hormones. Genetic, hormonal, immunologic, mechanical, and biochemical factors probably play a part in the onset and progress of this disease.

DJD is usually classified in two types:

1. **Primary** or **idiopathic**—When no etiologic factor can be identified
2. **Secondary**—When disease develops as a result of another factor:
   a. Congenital or developmental **deformity,** such as congenital dislocation of the hip or slipped capital femoral epiphysis, places abnormal stress on the joints.
   b. **Injury** to the joint, e.g., Colles' fracture involving the articular surface of the radius or dislocation of the hip. Injury to ligaments (tear), subluxation, and abnormal mobility can also lead to DJD.
   c. **Inflammatory arthritis** leads to DJD in its late stages.
   d. **Infectious arthritis**
   e. **Sensory loss,** as in diabetic neuropathy, may lead to a neuropathic joint. The pathologic changes are like a markedly exaggerated form of DJD. Similar changes are seen in leprosy, syphilis, spinal cord injury, and syringomyelia.

Pathology

Primary or idiopathic DJD is considered to be a pathologic process and not part of normal aging. The articular cartilage normally has a very smooth surface, and when covered with joint fluid, it allows movements with very little friction. It consists of water (70%), collagen fibers, and proteoglycans. These proteoglycans form the matrix within which are cartilage cells called **chondrocytes.** Some fluid from the matrix is driven out into the joint cavity when pressure is applied to the cartilage, and it is reabsorbed when pressure is taken off. This is the mechanism by which cartilage gets its nourishment. The chondrocytes release enzymes as a result of some traumatic, inflammatory, biochemical, or immunologic event, which initiates some biochemical changes in proteoglycans and collagen fibers and leads to their breakdown during the early stages of DJD. The chondrocytes proliferate, and the water content of the matrix increases.

The articular cartilage loses its glistening white appearance and becomes yellow. **Fissures** develop in the superficial layers of the cartilage, and it becomes soft. Later, superficial layers of the cartilage are lost, and **erosions** appear on the surface. They gradually enlarge and deepen and destroy the whole thickness of cartilage up to subchondral bone. The subchondral bone thickens and is seen on x-rays as **subchondral sclerosis. Osteophytes** grow out from the margins of the joint. The synovial membrane thickens as a result of chronic inflammatory reaction, and a small effusion may form in the joint. The pain in DJD is probably due to inflammatory reaction of soft tissues since cartilage has no nerve endings, or it may be due to direct pressure on the subchondral bone without the protective covering of the articular cartilage.

History

Pain in the joint is the cardinal symptom and has a gradual onset. If it is from a superficial joint, such as the knee or fingers, it is well-localized. However, if it arises from a deep joint, such as the facet joints of the lumbar spine, then the patient feels it as a diffuse, poorly localized pain farther away from the affected site. Pain is aggravated by prolonged use and relieved by rest. Night pain is a sign of advanced disease.

The patient also usually complains of **joint stiffness** in the morning immediately after getting up from sleep, lasting for 10–15 minutes (<30 minutes). It is felt only in the affected joints and is not generalized as in rheumatoid arthritis. Injury or overuse may bring on an exacerbation of symptoms. Knee, hip, DIP, cervical and lumbar spine, and carpometacarpal joint of the thumb are commonly involved (Fig. 8–1) (*see also* individual chapters).

Primary generalized osteoarthritis affects the same joints but is a more severe form of arthritis with rapid progress. The x-ray changes are also more marked. A severe form of painful, inflammatory arthritis of the DIP joints is called **erosive osteoarthritis.** The joints are swollen and tender and later show flexion deformities. X-rays show erosions on both sides of the DIP joint.

Physical Examination

1. **Inspection.** There may be **swelling** around the joint because of effusion or soft tissue, cartilaginous, and bony swelling as is seen in Heberden's nodes. **Deformity** caused by DJD or that leading to DJD should be looked for. DJD of the medial compartment of the knee will show a varus deformity.
2. **Palpation.** Tenderness is seen over the joint line of a superficial joint such as the knee. Effusion in the joint is confirmed by special tests.

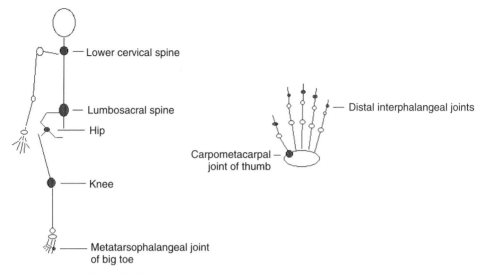

Fig. 8–1   Joints commonly involved in degenerative joint disease.

3. **Range of motion.** Limitation of the terminal few degrees of range is common. This may be due to soft tissue **contractures** or effusion. The patient complains of pain in the last few degrees of the range. **Crepitus** is palpable over the joint on movement. It can also be auscultated by a stethoscope.

Differential Diagnoses
1. **Rheumatoid arthritis** affects the metacarpophalangeal (MCP) joints and not the DIP joints. The distribution of joints affected is very different. There is usually a history of exacerbations and remissions of RA with morning stiffness lasting >1 hour. Involvement of joints is symmetrical and usually associated with systemic symptoms. The rheumatoid factor test is positive in 80% of patients. X-rays show juxta-articular osteoporosis, marginal erosions, and uniform narrowing of joint space. Examination of joint fluid shows greater numbers of WBCs.
2. **Crystal deposition disease.** Calcium pyrophosphate dihydrate or calcium hydroxyapatite crystal deposition diseases may mimic DJD. X-rays show calcification of the menisci of the knee or triangular cartilage of the wrist. Crystals are seen on examination of joint fluid.
3. **Psoriatic arthritis.** Patients have typical skin lesions, and x-ray changes are seen in sacroiliac, interphalangeal, metatarsophalangeal and MCP joints. The involvement is asymmetrical with joint space narrowing, erosions, osseous proliferation, and lack of osteoporosis.
4. **Reiter's syndrome.** Patients give a history of urethritis, conjunctivitis, and skin lesions over the soles of the feet.

Investigations
1. **Blood tests.** ESR, rheumatoid factor, and antinuclear antibody are all normal.
2. **X-rays.** Early symptoms of DJD and x-ray changes do not always correlate well.

Changes on x-rays are very common after age 55 years and do not necessarily suggest that pain is because of DJD. **Subchondral sclerosis** is seen early in the disease. Later, irregular **narrowing of the joint space** is observed. **Bone cysts** and **osteophytes** are seen near the joint margins (Fig. 8–2). Subluxation may occur later in the course of the disease.
3. **Bone scan** shows increased uptake because of inflammatory changes surrounding the joint.
4. **Synovial fluid analysis** shows a slight increase in the number of WBCs to 1,000/mm^3.

Course
The course is gradually progressive over years. Exacerbations may be due to injury or overuse.

Management
Prevention of DJD should be the aim in accurate reduction of intra-articular fractures and correction of deformities. Since there is no cure for the disease, treatment is directed toward symptoms. Ancillary and supportive treatment depends on joints affected and is covered in other chapters.
1. Medications.
   a. **NSAIDs** are very useful in controlling pain and inflammation. The dosage schedule of these drugs is not as high as in rheumatoid arthritis. If one NSAID is not effective within 2–4 weeks, another should be tried. This group of drugs may be combined with **acetaminophen** for better control of pain.
   b. **Intra-articular steroid** injection is given if one joint is painful and/or swollen despite NSAIDs. The injection should not be repeated >3 times in 1 year. After injection, the patient should protect that joint for a few days to avoid further damage.
2. Ancillary.
   a. **Rest** to the painful joint should be offered by cutting down the activities that require moving the affected joint. Use of a cane in the opposite hand takes a lot of weight off

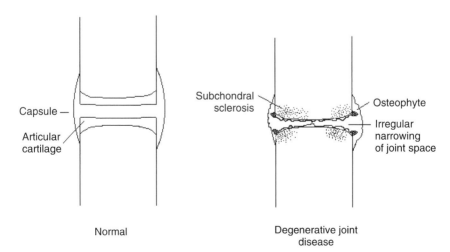

Fig. 8–2 Pathologic and x-ray changes seen in degenerative joint disease.

the hip joint while walking. Losing weight is also helpful for weight-bearing joints like the hip and knee.

b. Local **heat** helps relieve pain temporarily and allows the patient to perform exercises.

c. Stretching **exercises** help improve ROM. Isometric exercises are prescribed to maintain or increase strength. Exercises against resistance may aggravate the pain. Walking gradually increasing distance helps maintain function of the lower extremities.

d. For DJD of lower extremity joints, the physical therapist can instruct the patient in the proper use of a cane or crutches.

e. The occupational therapist can instruct the patient in energy-saving techniques, pacing activities, and equipment to improve function.

3. **Surgical** treatment is considered when conservative management fails to control pain, there is night pain, or the patient is experiencing severe limitation of function. **Osteotomy** or **arthrodesis** (fusion) of the joint are considered if the patient is young, and **arthroplasty** (replacement with artificial joint) if the patient is >60–65 years. Arthroscopic debridement and removal of loose bodies may be appropriate for milder cases.

Bibliography

1. Altaman RD: Osteoarthritis: Differentiation from rheumatoid arthritis, causes of pain, treatment. Postgrad Med 87(3):66–78, 1990.
2. Belhorn LR, Hess EV: Erosive osteoarthritis. Semin Arthritis Rheum 22:298–306, 1993.
3. Brandt KD: Should NSAIDs be used to treat osteoarthritis? Rheum Dis Clin North Am 19:29–44, 1993.
4. Schnitzer TJ: Osteoarthritis treatment update. Postgrad Med 93:89–95, 1993.

9

Geriatric Disorders

Trilok N. Monga, M.D.

MUSCULOSKELETAL DISEASES OF THE ELDERLY

Musculoskeletal diseases and injuries are very common in the elderly. About 50% of people over age 65 years have some form of musculoskeletal problem leading to limitation of ADLs.

The Aging Process

There is an increase in density and stability of collagen in all tissues except the skin, where collagen is decreased in the dermis. The elasticity of skin is decreased, and there is increased resistance to mobility. Aging also increases the time required for elastic recovery. The skin blisters easily, and loss of subcutaneous adipose tissue reduces its effectiveness as a thermal insulator. The water content of the elastic tissue decreases, and it undergoes fragmentation. Wound healing is prolonged and the chance of wound dehiscence is increased.

Muscle mass, strength, and endurance decrease with age, although this decline can be slowed by appropriate exercises. There is a decrease in the number and size of muscle fibers. The effective ROM (flexibility) is decreased because of reduction in length of muscle fibers and increase in the amount of connective tissue within muscles. Nutritional deficiency, reduced level of activity, and chronic diseases may all contribute toward a decline in muscle mass, strength, and endurance. Bone loss is a universal aspect of aging; however, its rate of loss varies among individuals. The rate of loss is higher in women and sedentary individuals. Decreased bone mass and altered mechanical properties of bone contribute to increased incidence of fractures.

Hyaline cartilage loses water as it ages, and its elasticity is reduced. The cartilage in weight-bearing areas becomes thin, which is reported on x-rays as narrowing of joint space. The intervertebral discs lose some height because of loss of water from the nucleus pulposus, resulting in reduced stature of the individual. An alteration in the relative proportions of the constituents of the musculoskeletal system can create problems for the elderly person who wishes to exercise and remain independent. Back and joint problems, sprains, tendon rupture, and fractures are due to changes in the properties of tissues involved. Other factors that may contribute are obesity, clumsiness, inadequate warm-up, a hard and uneven surface, and poorly fitting shoes.

Management

Most of these patients have multiple medical problems, such as coronary artery disease, diabetes, hypertension, and chronic obstructive pulmonary disease. The exercise prescription needs to be modified because of these problems. Other factors to be considered are deconditioning, poor flexibility, muscle weakness, and osteoporosis. **Exercise therapy** should start with stretching and ROM. Strengthening exercises should be paced with resting periods initially and gradually increased in duration and resistance. These patients become easily tired and cannot tolerate very long duration of exercises or activities. Even low-intensity, low-frequency, and short-duration exercises can benefit deconditioned and disabled persons.

Care should be taken in prescribing analgesics and anti-inflammatory medications. The incidence of gastrointestinal bleeding and other complications is higher in the elderly. Renal function also may be impaired, predisposing them to toxic drug levels in their blood.

Common Musculoskeletal Problems

Degenerative Joint Disease

Degenerative joint disease (DJD) is one of the most common diagnoses in the elderly (*see also* Chapter 8). Radiographic changes of degenerative arthritis are present in 85% of those between ages 75–79 years. However, the radiologic changes do not always correlate with clinical symptoms. The DJD may be primary (idiopathic) or secondary to trauma, metabolic disorders, or neuropathic disease. Degenerative conditions of individual joints are covered in the individual chapters on those joints.

Clinical Features. Symptoms are usually localized to the involved joints. The onset of disease is very gradual. Initially, pain occurs after excessive use of the extremity and is relieved by rest. Later, the patient may have pain at night. Lower cervical spine, lumbosacral spine, hip, knee, distal interphalangeal joints of the fingers, and the carpometacarpal joint of the thumb are commonly affected. In any individual patient, one or more joints may be involved. Degenerative arthritis of the knee and hip is a very common source of limitation of activities because of pain on walking. **Physical findings** include joint swelling, restricted ROM, crepitus, muscle wasting, and deformity. The patient has difficulty walking long distances, going up and down stairs, getting up from the toilet seat, and doing other activities.

Radiologic findings include irregular joint space narrowing, subchondral sclerosis, osteophyte and cyst formation, and subluxation. There are no characteristic abnormal findings on laboratory tests.

Management. Patient education plays a very important role in management. A physical therapist can show appropriate use of a cane, application of local heat, and ROM exercises. Pacing activities with rest periods and use of assistive devices can be taught by the occupational therapist. Weight loss helps relieve some pain in overweight patients. Prescription of **NSAIDs** requires special care because of a higher incidence of gastrointestinal bleeding and renal failure in the elderly. Intra-articular injection of **steroids** reduces pain and swelling of the knee or carpometacarpal joint of the thumb. Replacement arthroplasty of the hip and knee joints has become a fairly common procedure for patients who have exhausted all conservative measures and still have considerable limitation of function and pain at night.

Polymyalgia Rheumatica

The peak incidence of polymyalgia rheumatica occurs in 70- to 79-year-olds. It is almost unknown before age 50 years and is more common in females than males. The patient presents with a history of **sudden onset of pain** in the neck, back, and proximal parts of upper and lower extremities. This may be associated with morning stiffness. Some patients may have systemic complaints such as anorexia, weight loss, lassitude, and depression. Physical exam is usually negative. The ESR is elevated, often > 100 mm/hr. Other tests such as muscle enzymes, electromyography, and muscle biopsy are normal.

Response to **steroid** therapy is dramatic. If the patient does not respond favorably to steroids within 7–10 days, other diagnoses should be considered. An attempt should be made to prevent contractures and deconditioning by initiating appropriate ROM and strengthening exercises.

Giant Cell Arteritis
Giant cell arteritis is also known as temporal arteritis or cranial arteritis. It is sometimes associated with polymyalgia rheumatica and occurs in the same age group, i.e., > 50 years of age. It is a disease of medium to large-sized arteries. Patients may present with severe temporal headache, jaw claudication, transient diplopia, and acute unilateral blindness. Physical examination may reveal a swollen and tender temporal artery.

ESR is elevated, usually > 100 mm/hr, and is a good indicator of disease activity. Temporal artery biopsy reveals inflammatory changes with presence of macrophages, lymphocytes, and giant cells. The lumen of the artery is narrowed, and internal elastic lamina may be fragmented.

The patient is started on high-dose prednisone by mouth (40–60 mg/day). The dose is reduced as improvement in clinical signs and ESR occurs. Maintenance therapy with low-dose prednisone may be required for a very long time.

Lumbar Spinal Stenosis
The cross-sectional area of the lumbar spinal canal is reduced due to a variety of causes. The patient presents with a history of pain, numbness, or weakness in the buttocks or thighs. The symptoms are usually bilateral and brought on by walking or standing; they are relieved by flexion of the lumbosacral spine. The onset of disease is gradual with slow progression.

Physical examination may reproduce pain on extension of the spine. Absent or diminished ankle reflexes may be elicited immediately after the patient has walked a certain distance. CT scan or MRI is helpful in showing narrowing of the spinal canal. Electromyography may help to confirm the diagnosis.

NSAIDs and **physical therapy** are tried initially. Surgical decompression may be required for more severe cases.

Muscle Cramps
Idiopathic, involuntary, and painful muscle spasms in the legs are common in the elderly. Underlying neuropathy or metabolic disturbances should be excluded. The patient should be taught to stretch the involved muscle to relieve the spasm. Local heat may also help.

Shoulder Pain
Shoulder pain is very common in the elderly and is most likely due to underlying degenerative changes in the rotator cuff, bicipital tendinitis, or subacromial bursitis (*see* Chapter 15).

Pain in the shoulder region due to any cause may lead to adhesive capsulitis with marked restriction of joint movements. Elderly patients are especially susceptible to developing adhesive capsulitis. There is diffuse pain in the shoulder with restriction in ROM. Arthroscopic examination reveals loss of joint space.

It is very important to prevent adhesive capsulitis by keeping the period of immobilization of the shoulder joint to a minimum. Physical therapy modalities such as ultrasound and ROM exercises can usually help regain the movements. Judicious use of NSAIDs and intra-articular injection of steroids may relieve pain. Sometimes, manipulation under anesthesia is necessary to achieve functional ROM.

Foot Pain

Painful conditions of the foot are very common and make walking difficult. Proper footwear may prevent and relieve most of these problems. Usually, the shoes are too small for the forefoot. Broad shoes with an adequate toebox will benefit large numbers of patients. Plantar fasciitis with calcaneal spur, a common radiologic finding, is another common cause of pain in the foot.

Fractures

Fractures of the hip, spine, and wrist are becoming more common with the increasing number of elderly people. The primary involutional osteoporosis begins in middle age and becomes more common with advancing age (*see* also Chapter 6). These fractures are more common in postmenopausal osteoporotic women than in men. Hip fractures are associated with high morbidity and mortality. Most of these fractures occur as a result of a minor fall. It is important to eliminate causes of falls and thus prevent fractures in the elderly. Proper management of deteriorating vision and hearing and improving muscle strength and balance may reduce the incidence of falls.

The debate on how to prevent osteoporosis is ongoing. Loss of bone with advancing age is a universal phenomenon. However, it presents earlier in life in females than in males. There is a higher incidence of osteoporosis in sedentary people and also in extremities that are immobilized. Weight-bearing is probably the most important exogenous factor affecting bone development and in preventing osteoporosis. Prophylactic treatment with estrogens in women, adequate nutrition, and weight-bearing exercises are advocated for prevention of osteoporosis.

10

Miscellaneous Disorders

Arun J. Mehta, M.B., F.R.C.P.C., and Stanley Marcus, M.D.

FIBROMYALGIA

Fibromyalgia is also known as fibrositis, fibromyositis, nonarticular rheumatism, psychogenic rheumatism, myalgic spots, and myogelosis. It is a very common problem characterized by exacerbations and remissions of diffuse aching pain and tender points in affected muscles. The patient may also have generalized fatigue, morning stiffness, and sleep disorder. **Myofascial pain syndrome** is considered to be a different entity. Fewer tender points are restricted to one region of the body, and the syndrome may not be accompanied by fatigue, morning stiffness, and sleep disturbance.

Etiology
The exact etiology is unknown. Fibromyalgia may be associated with rheumatoid arthritis, degenerative joint disease, or thyroid disease.

Pathology
All symptoms and signs were previously thought to be due to localized inflammation in the muscle. However, there is no definite evidence of any pathology to support this hypothesis.

History
Fibromyalgia usually affects young females (F:M ratio of 4:1). The onset of disease is usually in the second or third decade. **Diffuse aching pain** in the muscles and/or joints is the common presenting symptom. The pain is not always well-localized and may be referred to a site away from the affected muscle. It is described as burning or stabbing in character. The neck, shoulder, low back, and hip are frequently affected. The patient also complains of generalized **fatigue** and **morning stiffness.** These symptoms are worse in cold and damp weather and also are aggravated by stress and overexertion. The patient feels better after local heat and aerobic exercises. Some patients wake up often during night and feel tired in the morning. Nearly one-third of the patients feel **depressed.** The patient may also complain of a feeling of swelling or numbness of an extremity, headache, or irritable bowel.

Physical Examination

1. **Inspection.** There are no visible abnormalities.
2. **Palpation.** There are definite, localized areas in muscles that are exquisitely tender to deep palpation (**tender points**). When the pain is referred to a distant area or radiates down one extremity, that tender point is called a **trigger point.** The trigger points are characteristically seen in **myofascial pain syndrome** rather than in fibromyalgia. Common sites of tender points are shown in Fig. 10–1. There should be 11 tender points out of a total number of 18 for diagnosis of fibromyalgia (according to the American College of Rheumatology). A "knot" or band of tight muscle may be palpable. A muscle twitch (contraction) can be observed at times when the tight band is snapped briskly (**twitch response** or jump sign).
3. **Range of motion.** There is no restriction of movements, even though the patient feels stiff.

Differential Diagnoses

Connective tissue diseases such as rheumatoid arthritis can be ruled out by absence of joint swelling, negative blood tests, and negative x-rays. In **myofascial pain syndrome,** the tender points are more localized, and there are no constitutional symptoms.

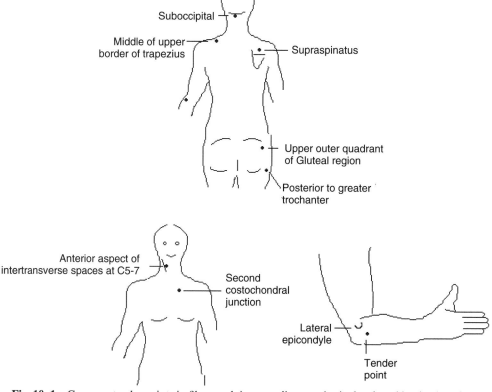

Fig. 10–1 Common tender points in fibromyalgia, according to criteria developed by the American College of Rheumatology, 1990.

Investigations

All blood tests and x-rays are normal in fibromyalgia. Routine blood tests, including complete blood count and Westergren ESR, should be ordered. Thyroid hormone levels (especially thyroid-stimulating hormone) are checked to rule out hypothyroidism. If signs and symptoms suggest degenerative joint disease or rheumatoid arthritis, appropriate x-rays and blood tests are ordered. It is important to keep in mind that tender points may coexist with these diseases.

Course

The course is marked by **exacerbations** and **remissions,** and almost 85% of patients continue to have symptoms for years.

Management

Most patients are worried and anxious, and some may be **depressed.** For many years, they may have been going from physician to physician or other health professionals without relief. Telling them that fibromyalgia is not a life-threatening illness and that it will not cripple them helps a lot. They should be started on a regular program of stretching and aerobic **exercises.** An **NSAID** is usually prescribed by most practioners, even though studies have shown that NSAIDs are not effective in most cases. **Amitriptyline** or cyclobenzaprine at bedtime help improve the sleep pattern and relieve symptoms. A low dose (10–25 mg) of amitriptyline is effective in most patients, although up to 300 mg/day may be required in a depressed patient. It may take up to 2 months to notice any improvement. Injection of **local anesthetic** or long-acting steroid preparation in trigger points is also an option. Relaxation therapy, stress management, and changing lifestyle should be considered if symptoms persist.

COMPARTMENT SYNDROMES

Compartment syndromes comprise a group of conditions in which circulation to the muscles and nerves confined within an osseofibrous compartment is compromised. The severity of symptoms varies from pain after strenuous physical activity to contractures and nerve palsies (e.g., **Volkmann's ischemic contracture**). When large volume of muscle tissue is damaged, as in **crush syndrome**, shock and renal failure can be important features of the clinical picture. These conditions are also described by the compartment involved (e.g., **anterior tibial syndrome**).

Anatomy

The deep fascia covering muscles of the leg and forearm do not have much elastic tissue. The fascia together with the bones form osseofibrous compartments that contain muscles, nerves, and blood vessels. Any sudden increase in volume within the compartment leads to increased pressure because of the unyielding nature of the deep fascia. The anterior compartment in the forearm and four compartments in the leg are the common sites of **neurovascular compression syndromes.** The symptoms and signs vary according to the contents of the compartment involved.

Etiology

An abnormal increase in intracompartmental pressure is the main cause. Normal pressure in the forearm or leg compartment is 0–4 mm Hg. As this pressure increases, it occludes venous return. This, in turn, encourages exudation of fluid from the capillaries, increases volume within the tight compartment, and leads to further increase in pressure. Ultimately, impaired arteriolar circulation results in ischemia of muscles and nerves.

Some of the causes of compartment syndrome are:

1. **Unaccustomed physical activity** leads to swelling of the muscles. It can happen to untrained athletes or to soldiers during basic training.
2. **Trauma** causing fractures and bleeding inside the compartment is another factor. A tight, unyielding bandage or cast can contribute toward increasing the pressure. Fractures of the tibia and forearm bones are common precursors of compartment syndromes.
3. In **crush injury,** an extremity or a large mass of muscles is compressed for a prolonged period of time, and the blood circulation to the muscles and nerves is impaired. When the external pressure is relieved, there is exudation of fluid within the compartment, and pressure within the compartment rises. This injury can happen to a drug addict or alcoholic who has been lying on his or her arm on a hard floor for a prolonged time or to someone trapped in a collapsed building.

Pathology

Prolonged ischemia of muscles and nerves leads to **necrosis.** The amount of time these cells can survive without oxygen depends on the amount and duration of pressure exerted on them. Nerve and muscle cells are more sensitive to ischemia than fibrous tissue. The necrotic muscle is gradually replaced by fibrous tissue. **Contractures** develop over a period of weeks. Nerve damage, paralysis of muscles, and shortening of fibrous tissue and ligaments of joints result in **deformities.**

History

There is usually a history of a precipitating event, such as unaccustomed activity or trauma to the forearm or leg. The patient complains of severe, continuous, diffuse pain in the affected area. There may also be tingling and numbness of fingers or toes.

Physical Examination

1. **Inspection.** The capillary circulation in the skin of fingers and toes is maintained until very late stage. The skin may be discolored. If the extremity is not in a cast, the **swelling** of the forearm or leg is usually visible.
2. **Palpation.** There is marked **tenderness** over the affected compartment, and it feels very **tense.** Increased pressure in the compartment may obliterate blood flow in the arterioles to the muscles and nerves but not in the main arteries of the limb. Presence of palpable **peripheral pulse** does not exclude compartment syndrome and may be misleading.
3. **Range of motion**
   a. **Active**—All active movements are painful and avoided by the patient.
   b. **Passive—Passive stretching of affected muscles is very painful** and is the most important sign indicating impaired circulation to the muscles.

4. **Special tests.** Diminished **sensation** over tips of fingers or toes or in the distribution of involved nerves should be sought.

Clinical Varieties

1. **Volkmann's ischemic contracture.** The anterior compartment of the forearm is involved (Fig. 10–2). Contractures of the flexor group of forearm muscles and ulnar and median nerve palsies develop if it is not detected and treated in time.
2. **Anterior tibial compartment syndrome of the leg.** This condition is also known as anterior tibial syndrome and traumatic necrosis of pretibial muscles (Fig. 10–3A). Some clinicians also include this as one of the causes of **shin splints.** Excessive physical activity is the usual precipitating cause. Other causes include fracture of the tibia, contusion of the leg, crush syndrome in drug addicts, or postoperative complication after vascular reconstruction of the femoral artery. Pain of varying severity is felt over the anterior aspect of the leg. The anterior muscle compartment feels tense and is tender. Skin over it is pink and warm. The patient is unable to actively dorsiflex the foot and complains of severe pain on passive plantar flexion.
3. **Deep posterior compartment of the leg.** This compartment contains posterior tibial muscle and vessels, flexor digitorum longus, and flexor hallucis longus muscles (Fig. 10–3B). Fracture of the tibia is the usual precipitating cause. The flexors of the toes are weak, and passive extension of toes aggravates the pain. Sensation may be impaired over the tips of toes and sole of the foot.
4. **Peroneal compartment syndrome.** This condition usually occurs after unaccustomed physical activity. Pain is felt over the lateral aspect of the leg and is aggravated by passive inversion of the foot. The patient may have diminished sensation over the lateral aspect of leg and foot (Fig. 10–3C).

Investigations

1. Measurement of **intracompartmental pressure** is a useful test. Normal pressure is 0–4 mm Hg. **Fasciotomy** is indicated if the pressure goes above 30 mm Hg.

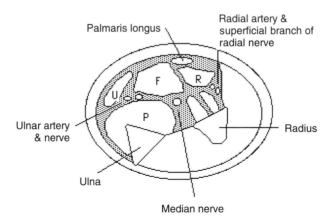

Fig. 10–2 Fibro-osseous compartment of the forearm. (U = flexor carpi ulnaris; F = flexor digitorum superficialis; P = flexor digitorum profundus; R = flexor carpi radialis.)

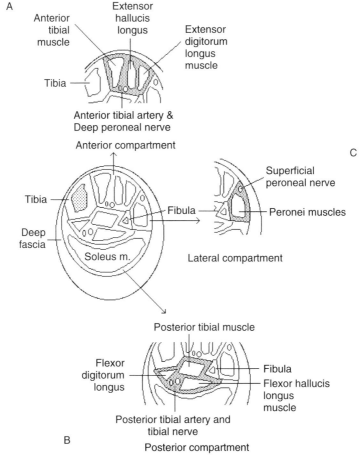

Fig. 10–3   Fibro-osseous compartments of the leg.

2. In crush syndrome, the **urine** may be markedly acidic with presence of casts and myoglobin. **Serum** potassium, blood urea nitrogen (BUN), and creatine kinase are elevated.

Course
Severe cases, if not treated as an emergency, may develop permanent damage to the affected muscles and nerves. Fibrosis of muscles and nerve palsies can give rise to severe deformities and loss of function. Pain subsides in a few days, and muscles become very hard. Contractures develop over a few weeks, and muscles become increasingly difficult to stretch. Very mild cases secondary to excessive activity usually recover completely.

Complications
Nerve palsies, muscle contractures and joint stiffness may develop over time.

Management

Early diagnosis is of paramount importance in preventing complications. Tight bandages and cast are cut down to the skin. If this does not improve symptoms and signs, they are completely removed. Appropriate treatment of shock and renal failure is undertaken. The next step is to incise the deep fascia and fascia of each individual muscle affected. If circulation to the muscle is still not restored, the proximal artery is explored for spasm or damage. When the compartment syndrome is precipitated by excessive activity, rest, elevation, and ice massage over the affected compartment should be tried. If these measures do not bring relief of signs and symptoms or intracompartmental pressure remains high, operation should be considered.

After the initial stage, the patient may require physical therapy to maintain joint mobility. In mild cases, this may be sufficient. When there is severe contracture and deformity, various surgical operations should be considered.

DIFFUSE IDIOPATHIC SKELETAL HYPEROSTOSIS

Diffuse idiopathic skeletal hyperostosis (DISH) is also known as **Forestier's disease**, **ankylosing vertebral hyperostosis**, and **ankylosing hyperostosis**. The presenting signs and symptoms are usually minimal. It is often seen as an incidental finding on chest or spine x-rays.

Etiology

The changes of DISH may occur in association with diabetes mellitus and degenerative joint disease because all these diseases are more common in the same age group. No definite causal relationship between DISH and other diseases or association with histocompatibility antigen has been established.

Pathology

There is an increased tendency to deposition of calcium in the ligaments, especially where they attach to the bone (**enthesopathy**). **Calcification** and/or **ossification** of the anterior and posterior longitudinal **ligaments** of the spine is commonly seen. The ligaments of the mid to lower thoracic and upper lumbar vertebrae are usually involved. Intervertebral discs and sacroiliac and apophyseal joints are not affected. These patients tend to form large osteophytes, develop soft tissue calcification after arthroplasty of the hip or knee, and develop calcium deposition in iliolumbar, sacrotuberous, and other ligaments. Large anterior osteophytes in the cervical region may cause dysphagia. The thickening and calcification of the posterior longitudinal ligament sometimes lead to cervical myelopathy.

History

DISH is fairly common in people over the age 60–65 years (5–10% of the population in that age group). Males are affected more often than females. The patient may complain of mild to moderate **back pain.** Occasionally, the patient may present with difficulty in walking or urinary incontinence due to cervical **myelopathy** secondary to ossification of the posterior longitudinal ligament. Difficulty in swallowing (**dysphagia**) may be secondary to a large osteophyte from the anterior cervical spine.

Physical Examination

There are no characteristic physical signs of this disease.

Range of motion of the spine may be limited.

Differential Diagnoses

Ankylosing spondylitis starts in a young adult with pain in the back. The pain is usually much more severe than in DISH. The patient experiences exacerbation and remissions of symptoms with increasing limitation of ROM of the spine and chest excursion. Plain x-rays should help in distinguishing between these two conditions. The sacroiliac joints are involved in almost all cases of ankylosing spondylitis but not in DISH.

Investigations

There are no blood tests that help in the diagnosis or management of this problem. Because nearly 40% of patients with DISH have diabetes mellitus, blood tests to rule out diabetes should be performed.

1. **Plain x-rays** of the thoracic or upper lumbar spine are useful. There is **calcification** of the anterior longitudinal ligament, especially over its anterolateral aspect (Fig. 10–4). The flowing calcified ligament may mimic "bamboo spine" of ankylosing spondylitis. The differentiation is usually easy. A radiolucent line between the calcified ligament and the vertebral body is characteristic of DISH, although it often is not present. Four contiguous vertebrae should be involved for a definite diagnosis of DISH. Unlike ankylosing spondylitis, there is no intra-articular bony ankylosis of the sacroiliac and apophyseal joints. Large osteophytes grow from the upper and lower ends of the vertebral bodies, the apophyseal joints of the vertebrae, and the sacroiliac joints. The disc spaces are usually well preserved.
2. **MRI** or **CT** scans of the cervical spine are requested when the patient presents with symptoms of cervical myelopathy.
3. **Barium swallow** studies may be necessary if the patient has dysphagia.

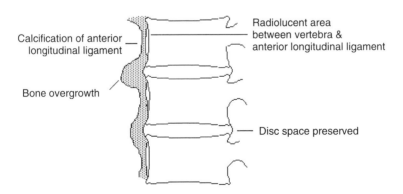

Fig. 10–4 Lateral view of the lumbar spine showing calcification of the anterior longitudinal ligament. The disc spaces are maintained. There are large bony outgrowths (hyperostosis) near the upper and lower borders of the vertebrae. A radiolucent area may be seen between the vertebra and the calcified anterior longitudinal ligament.

Course/Complications
The course is usually benign, and symptoms, if present, are usually mild. Soft tissue calcification after hip or knee arthroplasty may restrict ROM of that joint.

Management
1. **Medications.** Analgesics such as acetaminophen or an NSAID may be prescribed for pain.
2. **Ancillary.** Reassurance about the benign nature of the disease and exercises to maintain ROM are useful adjuncts in management.
3. **Surgical** treatment is necessary when there is spinal cord compression or dysphagia secondary to osteophytes.

AVASCULAR NECROSIS

Avascular necrosis is also known as **osteonecrosis**, **aseptic necrosis**, and **ischemic necrosis**. It is called **osteochondrosis** or **osteochondritis** when an epiphysis is affected. In this group of conditions, the blood supply to a part of bone and/or cartilage is cut off.

Anatomy
A **primary** center of ossification appears in cartilage which later forms the diaphysis of bone (Fig. 10–5). Secondary centers of ossification appear at the ends of the bone and form the epiphyses. The epiphysis that forms a joint is called a **pressure epiphysis** because of weight-bearing or other forces borne by it. The epiphysis to which a tendon is attached is called a **traction epiphysis** or **apophysis.**

Etiology
Many theories have been proposed to explain various causes of avascular necrosis. One frequent cause is a displaced **fracture** (e.g., fracture of the neck of the femur) or **dislocation.** Chronic, recurrent **injury** is blamed in osteochondrosis of the tibial tubercle (Osgood-Schlatter's disease) and calcaneal apophysis (Sever's disease). The other two common causes of avascular necrosis are ingestion of large doses of **steroids** and **alcohol** for a prolonged period. A **fat embolism** may occur in these two conditions. Sickle cell disease, renal transplantation, hyperlipidemia, and exposure to high altitude or high atmospheric pressure are some less common causes. When avascular necrosis of the epiphysis occurs without any apparent reason, it is termed **idiopathic.** In this group, most of the conditions are referred to by the names of people who described them, e.g., Perthes' disease for avascular necrosis of the epiphysis of the femoral head.

Pathology
The blood supply is cut off by disruption of the blood vessels in fractures and dislocations. In other cases, the insult to bone viability occurs due to intravascular blockage or extravascular pressure. Fat embolus from alcoholic fatty liver is an example of intravascular blockage. Increased intraosseous, extravascular, pressure is blamed for the idiopathic avascular necrosis of the femoral head in adults.

All cellular elements (osteocytes and marrow cells) die when the blood supply is cut off.

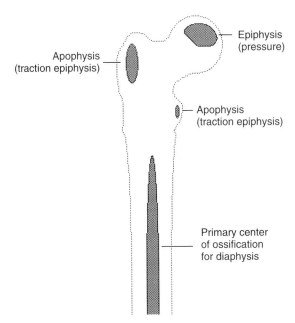

Apophysis (traction epiphysis)

Epiphysis (pressure)

Apophysis (traction epiphysis)

Primary center of ossification for diaphysis

Fig. 10–5   Centers of ossification in long bone.

The architecture of the bone (trabeculae and lamellae), however, remains intact. There is reactive hyperemia in the surrounding viable bone which leads to osteopenia (Fig. 10–6). The articular cartilage survives because it gets its nutrition from the synovial fluid. In children, the bone in the center of ossification of the epiphysis stops growing, but the epiphyseal cartilage continues to grow in thickness. On x-rays, this is seen as increased joint space and a smaller, more dense center of ossification on the affected side (Fig. 10–7). In adults, the joint space remains the same, and the necrotic area of bone looks denser than the surrounding viable bone.

New blood vessels slowly grow from the periphery and break the necrotic part into smaller areas (**fragmentation**). The dead tissue is removed and replaced by new cells, a process called **creeping substitution.** This newly formed tissue is more plastic and can be deformed by normal weight-bearing or muscle contraction. A fracture in the subchondral bone with collapse can also give rise to **deformity.** The deformed new bone is not congruous with the opposing articular surface and may lead to early **degenerative arthritis** of the involved joint.

History
Traumatic avascular necrosis can occur at any age. A history of other predisposing causes should be sought. Different sites affected often are referred to by special names:

Head of femur   Legg-Calvé-Perthes' disease
Lunate   Kienböck's disease
Head of metatarsal   Freiberg's infraction
Vertebrae   Scheuermann's disease

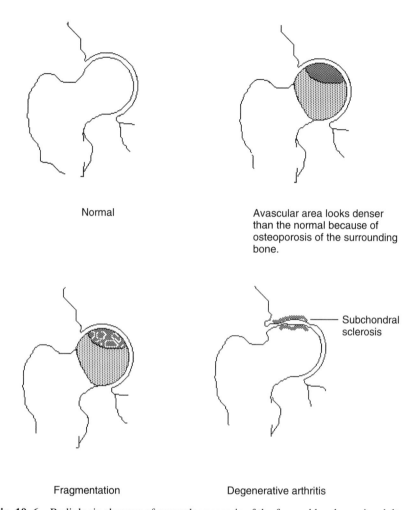

Normal

Avascular area looks denser than the normal because of osteoporosis of the surrounding bone.

Fragmentation

Degenerative arthritis

Subchondral sclerosis

Fig. 10–6 Radiologic changes of avascular necrosis of the femoral head seen in adults.

Osteochondrosis usually presents between the ages of 3 and 12 years. It may be **asymptomatic** during early stages of the disease. **Pain** in the affected part is the most common symptom. Parents may notice that the child is **limping** if a weight-bearing joint is involved.

Physical Examination
Physical examination is described in the separate chapters for each region.

Investigations
1. **X-rays** may be normal for a few weeks to a few months. Later, the necrotic area appears **denser** than the surrounding bone (Fig. 10–6). This part of the bone then undergoes **fragmentation,** and smaller islands of dense areas appear. The affected area may collapse and become **deformed.** Degenerative arthritis develops some years later.

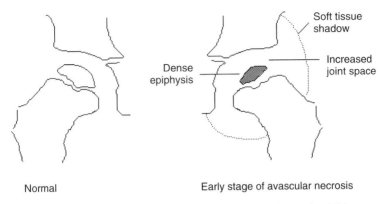

Fig. 10–7   Radiologic changes of avascular necrosis seen in children.

2. **MRI.** Avascular necrosis is seen earlier on MRI than on plain x-rays, and MRI is the preferred tool whenever this condition is suspected. It is especially useful in the early stages of the disease.
3. **Bone scan.** A bone scan is helpful only when the uptake is decreased. Increased uptake is too nonspecific to be useful.

Course/Complications

It takes about 2–3 years from the onset of avascular necrosis to fragmentation and final re-ossification. **Degenerative arthritis** develops in the involved joint if the epiphysis is deformed.

Management

Management of avascular necrosis for each joint is described in the separate chapters on individual joints. The outcome in the adult hip is not very satisfactory; only 15% or fewer improve spontaneously. Most develop significant impairment. The most important goal is to **prevent any deformity of the epiphysis** and hopefully prevent degenerative arthritis. This may be achieved by **non-weight-bearing** during the plastic stage of bone reformation. Many medications and orthopedic measures, such as core decompression, have been tried, but none have been universally accepted. Joint replacement **arthroplasty** offers the best relief after degenerative joint disease has developed.

OSTEITIS DEFORMANS

Osteitis deformans, or **Paget's disease,** is a slowly progressive disease of bone that gives rise to bony pain, deformities, and fractures.

Etiology

A genetic defect leading to an inborn error of metabolism of connective tissues and infection both have been implicated in the origin of this disease. Recent research has found inclusion bodies in the osteoclasts, and a slow virus is proposed as a cause.

Pathology

Any bone in the body may be affected, but the vertebrae, pelvis, femur, tibia, and skull are more commonly involved than other bones. There is increased activity of osteoclasts, leading to destruction of bone during the early stages. The bone is soft during this stage and can be deformed by normal stress of weight-bearing or muscle contraction. This leads to kyphosis and bowing of the femur and tibia (Fig. 10–8). An attempt to repair is made by formation of poorly organized bone. The early and late stages of the disease may be seen in the same bone at the same time. The cortex of the bone is thickened, and the trabeculae are coarse, though less in number.

History

The disease usually begins around age 50 years. The disease is **asymptomatic** in many and may be found incidentally on x-rays taken for some other problem. Increased vascularity gives rise to deep, boring **pain** in the affected bone. **Pathologic fractures** in the vertebrae, femur, or tibia can occur. A patient may present with **degenerative arthritis** of the hip due to deformity of the femur. Increasing circumference of the skull forces the patient to buy larger sized hats. He or she may also notice bowing of the femur or tibia.

Physical Examination

1. **Inspection.** The natural curvature of the tibia or femur is exaggerated. If the skull is involved, the top of the head looks larger (Fig.10–8).
2. **Palpation.** During the early stage, the temperature over a subcutaneous bone (e.g., tibia) may be increased.
3. **Range of motion** may be limited because of a fracture or degenerative arthritis.

Differential Diagnoses

Early osteolytic changes and increased density of bone in the late stages need to be distinguished from metastatic lesions of the bone. Plain x-rays in osteitis deformans show an increase in width of the bone which does not occur in metastasis. The uptake on gallium scan is increased in tumors but not in osteitis deformans.

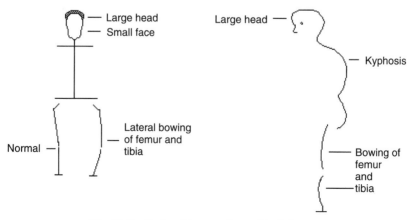

Fig. 10–8 Deformities seen in osteitis deformans.

Investigations

1. Serum **alkaline phosphatase** levels are markedly increased. Treatment is indicated if the level is more than double normal. **Urinary hydroxyproline** is also increased.
2. **Plain x-ray** findings vary with the stage of the disease. In the initial stage of osteolysis, a well-defined radiolucent area is seen (Fig. 10–9A). Later, small circumscribed areas of radiodensities ("cotton balls") appear. The cortex of the bone is thickened, and the size of the medullary cavity is reduced. The trabeculae are thicker and coarser than normal and reduced in number (Fig. 10–9B).
3. **Bone scan** (technetium) shows increased uptake.
4. **CT scan** may be indicated when spinal stenosis is suspected.
5. **Bone biopsy** is done if diagnosis is doubtful.

Course/Complications

The disease is usually very slowly progressive. Complications include:

1. **Fracture** occurs in the hard but brittle bone. They are common in the proximal femur and tibia.
2. **Degenerative arthritis** in the hip and knee is common.
3. **Sarcoma** in affected bone is an uncommon complication.

Management

Treatment is not necessary for patients who have no symptoms or when the alkaline phosphatase level is less than double the normal value. Bone pain or complications are the main indications for treatment.

1. **Medications.** Simple analgesics should be tried first. Calcitonin and diphosphonates (e.g., etidronate) have been tried to reduce the disease activity.
2. **Surgical.** Fracture of the femur or tibia requires internal fixation. Degenerative arthritis may need an arthroplasty.

NERVE COMPRESSION SYNDROMES

Peripheral nerves can be damaged by pressure which may be acute or chronic in nature. **Acute** pressure may develop within a fascial compartment of the forearm or leg due to hemorrhage or edema. **Long-standing** increased pressure within an osseofascial compartment occurs in the carpal tunnel syndrome involving the median nerve. The severity of pathologic changes in the nerve depend on the amount and duration of abnormal pressure. Severe pressure that occurs in acute compartment syndromes can damage a nerve within a few hours, whereas it may take much longer for carpal tunnel syndrome to develop. The nerve is vulnerable at locations where it can be compressed against a bone (e.g., radial nerve at midshaft of humerus) or where it passes through a unyielding fibro-osseous tunnel (e.g., carpal tunnel).

Pathology

Some damage to myelin sheath near nodes of Ranvier (**paranodal demyelination**) is seen in mild compression of a nerve. The process of demyelination extends in more severe compression and involves a few segments of the nerve (**segmental demyelination**). This leads to slowing of nerve conduction across the affected segment. **Wallerian degeneration** of

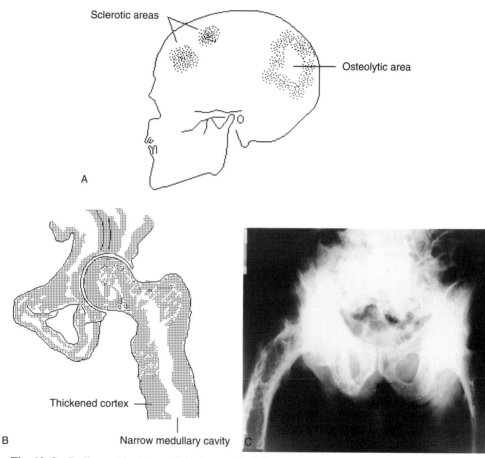

Fig. 10–9 Radiographic abnormalities in osteitis deformans. *A,* Well-defined osteolytic areas are seen during early stage. Sclerotic areas in skull are described as "cotton-wool" or "cotton ball" areas because of their fluffy appearance. *B,* Coarse trabeculae, diffuse sclerosis, thickened cortex, and narrow medullary cavity are seen in long bones. *C,* Osteitis deformans. X-ray of the pelvis and upper ends of femur shows diffuse osteosclerosis. The cortex of the bones is thickened with encroachment of medullary cavity. Bony trabeculae are thickened.

axons occurs in severe or long-standing compression neuropathy, which show up on elec-tromyography as fibrillations and positive sharp waves (Fig. 10–10). The peripheral nerves are more susceptible to compression neuropathies in patients with diabetes mellitus, alco-hol abuse, and other disorders causing peripheral neuropathy.

History

The patient usually complains of "pins and needles," hand or fingers "going off to sleep,"or "poor circulation" in the affected part. These symptoms (**paresthesias**) are restricted to the dermatomal distribution of the nerve. Some patients complain of **pain** in the distribution of the nerve or nerve root. It may extend proximal to the site of compression and may create difficulty in diagnosis. The symptoms may be aggravated at night (as in carpal tun-nel) or by certain activities or position of the extremity. **Weakness** of muscles may be re-ported by the patient as deterioration in handwriting or difficulty in holding a pen.

Physical Examination

1. **Special Tests. Neurologic** examination helps in confirming the diagnosis and in deter-mining the course of treatment. **Sensory exam** should include touch, two-point dis-crimination, and vibration tests. Muscle power is tested on both sides to look for any

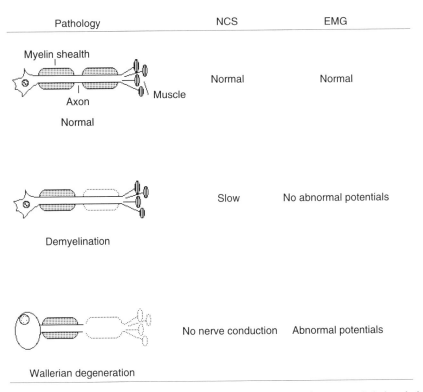

Fig. 10–10 Pathologic changes due to compression of a peripheral nerve and their relation to changes on nerve conduction studies (NCS) and electromyography (EMG).

weakness. **Atrophy** of muscles supplied by the affected nerve is usually a late finding. **Tendon reflexes** completes the neurologic exam. The whole course of the suspected nerve or nerve root is examined for any abnormality at the spine, bones, or joints.

Differential Diagnoses
Thorough neurologic exam, electromyography, and nerve conduction studies help to distinguish among conditions.
1. **Peripheral neuropathy** presents with tingling, numbness (usually of glove and stocking type), and muscle weakness. Initially, one nerve may be affected more than other nerves.
2. **Amyotrophic lateral sclerosis** (ALS) presents with muscle weakness, atrophy, and fasciculations. There are no sensory symptoms or signs in ALS.
3. **Mononeuritis** occurs in diabetes, connective tissue diseases with vasculitis, and other conditions. The onset is usually sudden with pain and weakness.
4. **Double crush syndrome** occurs when a nerve is compressed at two places along its course. This may make the diagnosis difficult, and often only one of the sites of compression is treated, with perseverance of symptoms.

Investigations
Electromyography and **nerve conduction studies** help to confirm the diagnosis and determine severity of involvement of the nerve.

Management
Management is considered separately under each individual compression neuropathy.

REFLEX SYMPATHETIC DYSTROPHY

Also known as Sudeck's atrophy, causalgia, algodystrophy, and shoulder-hand syndrome, reflex sympathetic dystrophy (RSD) is characterized by severe burning pain, hyperesthesia, hyperpathia, and vasomotor disturbances in the extremity. The upper extremity is affected more often than the lower. RSD of the hand is described in more detail in Chapter 17.

Etiology
Many hypotheses have been proposed to explain the signs and symptoms of RSD, but none can account for all of the related phenomena. Abnormal activity of the sympathetic nervous system is believed to be the final result that gives rise to the typical clinical picture. Local injury may lead to abnormal connections (artificial synapses) between sympathetic nerves and somatic sensory nerves. Somatic nerve impulses then cause hyper- or hypoactivity of the sympathetic nervous system, giving rise to pain, vasomotor instability, and trophic skin changes. Other hypotheses are based on some changes in the CNS pathways that perpetuate abnormal activity of the sympathetic nervous system.

Pathology
During initial stages of the disease, there is hyperemia and edema. Bones near the joints show osteopenia. The patient avoids all movements of the affected part, leading to **disuse**

atrophy of muscles. Soft tissue contractures develop, and the affected part becomes stiff and useless.

History

The onset usually follows minor trauma, operation on the extremity (e.g., to release carpal tunnel syndrome), myocardial infarction, or stroke. Constant, severe, burning **pain** develops immediately after the precipitating event or within a few weeks. In patients with degenerative disc disease or diabetic neuropathy, the onset may be very slow. The pain is aggravated by movements or touch.

The disease may be divided into three stages:

Stage I. There is severe burning pain with diffuse swelling of the hand or foot. The skin may be dry and warm or cold and sweaty. All movements are very painful. This stage may last up to 3 months.

Stage II. The pain spreads to involve a larger area and later subsides gradually. Muscle atrophy develops. This stage may last for another 3 months.

Stage III. The skin becomes thin and atrophic. Joint contractures produce deformities, and the hand cannot perform any function.

Physical Examination

1. **Inspection.** In the initial stage, the skin is edematous and hyperemic. Later, it may become thin, atrophic, and dry. In very late stage, the hand or foot may become shriveled with flexion contractures of fingers or toes.
2. **Palpation.** Even light touch is painful (**hyperesthesia** or allodynia) in the initial stage. The painful sensation persists after the stimulus is removed (**hyperpathia**).
3. **Range of motion.** The patient is reluctant to move the fingers or toes or let the examiner move them.

Differential Diagnoses

1. **Infection.** Pain is more localized, with systemic signs such as fever and high WBC count.
2. **Inflammatory arthritis.** The joints are swollen and tender. Other parts of the hand or foot are normal. The wrist, elbow, or knee may be involved in arthritis. ESR is elevated.
3. **Fracture.** Tenderness, swelling, and deformity are localized to the fracture site. X-rays will confirm the diagnosis.

Course/Complications

The **course** is variable. Milder cases with less than the full picture may be relieved of symptoms within a few weeks. A smaller percentage of patients go through all the stages and end up with a shriveled hand or foot with contractures, perhaps after months to a year.

Complications include:

1. **Chronic pain syndrome** and depression
2. **Contractures** may be very severe, and the patient may end up with a nonfunctional hand or foot.

Investigations

1. **Plain x-rays** may be completely normal during the first few weeks. Later, they may

show patchy osteoporosis, periarticular **osteoporosis,** or generalized osteoporosis of the involved part.

2. **Bone scan** (three phase) with technetium shows increased uptake. It may be abnormal before plain x-rays show any changes. There may be increased uptake in the opposite extremity, too.
3. **Thermography** shows increased vascularity and temperature during early stages.
4. **Sympathetic block** of appropriate sympathetic ganglia may stop the pain and vasomotor changes within minutes. This procedure is diagnostic as well as therapeutic.

Management

Prevention

Prevention of RSD should be attempted in patients who complain of undue pain and swelling after trauma, stroke, or myocardial infarction. These patients should be started on **ROM exercises** for the hand or foot as soon after the onset of symptoms as possible. It is better not to wait until the diagnosis is confirmed by x-rays or bone scan but to start when the diagnosis is suspected by severe, burning pain, hyperesthesia, hyperemia, and/or swelling of the hand or foot. **Analgesics,** elevation of the affected part, active **ROM exercises,** paraffin baths, and **transcutaneous electrical nerve stimulation** (TENS) are started initially. It is important to persevere with vigorous physical and occupational therapy and increase the time spent in therapies up to 4–6 hours/day. Any **associated conditions,** e.g., trigger points or cervical spondylosis, should be treated at the same time.

The patient may require treatments for many weeks to a few months. If the patient gets worse despite treatment or does not get better after 2–3 weeks, other differential diagnoses such as infection or fracture should be ruled out again. After that, the patient may be started on **prednisone,** 60–80 mg/day for 1–2 weeks, which is then gradually tapered. Prednisone may be started from the beginning if the symptoms are severe. Other treatments, including **sympathetic block** and **sympathectomy,** are considered after conservative measures fail.

Medications

1. **Analgesics.** Narcotics may be required for very severe pain. The dose and type of analgesic should be adjusted according to the patient's needs. Since the disease may linger for a long time, the possibility of addiction should be kept in mind.
2. **NSAIDs** help reduce pain, inflammation, and swelling.
3. **Steroids,** e.g., prednisone, have been found to be effective in some trials and are used extensively in practice.
4. **Sympathetic block** reduces overactivity of the sympathetic nervous system, and the effect on signs and symptoms of RSD is immediate. This can be used as a diagnostic test and therapeutic measure. It may be repeated three or four times. If the benefit is temporary, then sympathectomy may give more permenant relief.

Ancillary

Elevation, physical therapy, and occupational therapy are used as mentioned earlier. If pain becomes chronic, the help of a psychologist may become necessary to provide **relaxation, biofeedback,** meditation, imagery, and other techniques.

Surgical

Sympathectomy is carried out when sympathetic blocks have been partially effective or effective for short periods of time and other conservative measures have failed.

NEUROPATHIC JOINTS

Neuropathic joints are also known as **Charcot's joints**. When the CNS is deprived of sensory input from the joints, they become disorganized and deformed.

Etiology

Lack of pain sensation takes away protective mechanisms and predisposes joints to damage from minor trauma. The patient is able to carry on with activities without feeling any restraint imposed by pain. Another explanation for neuropathic joints is that reflex vasodilation leads to bone resorption. Fracture of bones and destruction of joints occur later. **Diabetes** is the leading cause of peripheral neuropathy and neuropathic joints in the United States. Other causes of peripheral neuropathy (e.g., alcohol abuse and leprosy), tabes dorsalis, and syringomyelia may also give rise to neuropathic joints. Occasionally, multiple intra-articular injections of steroids have resulted in this condition.

Pathology

Small joints of the foot, ankle, and knee are commonly affected. The spine and upper extremity joints are sometimes involved. There is marked destruction of articular cartilage and subchondral bone. The affected joints are swollen and subluxed or dislocated. New bone formation occurs at the margins of the bone. Severe deformity results (Fig. 10–11).

History

Patients usually present with swelling and deformity of the joints. There is no complaint of any significant pain despite severe deformity.

Physical Examination

1. **Inspection.** The involved joint is swollen. Deformity develops quickly (sometimes within a few weeks).
2. **Palpation.** There is very little tenderness. The skin may be slightly warmer over the joint. The small bones of the foot may feel like "a bag of bones" because of crepitus on squeezing the foot.
3. **Range of motion.** Abnormal mobility may be present because of lax ligaments.
4. **Special tests.** A complete neurologic exam is carried out to diagnose peripheral neuropathy, syringomyelia, leprosy, and other associated etiologies. **Absence of deep pain sensation** is the most important finding.

Differential Diagnoses

Infection should be ruled out. There is no pain or tenderness and the ESR and WBC counts are normal in neuropathic joint. However, differentiation from osteomyelitis in the diabetic foot may require aspiration and examination of joint fluid.

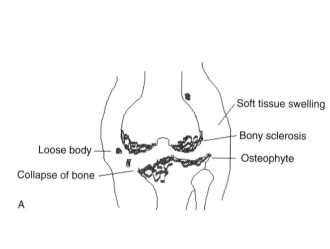
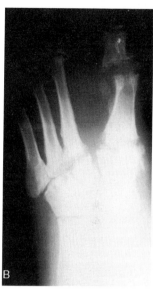

Fig. 10–11 X-ray abnormalities in neuropathic joint include soft tissue swelling, irregular patchy destruction of articular cartilage, subchondral sclerosis, collapse of bone, and loose bodies. There is gross disorganization of the joint with subluxation or dislocation, leading to deformity. *B,* X-ray of metatarsophalangeal joint of the big toe shows gross disorganization and subluxation. There is destruction of the head of first metatarsal and loose bodies in the joint space.

Investigations

1. **WBC** and **ESR** to rule out infection
2. **Blood sugar** to rule out diabetes
3. **VDRL** to rule out tabes dorsalis (tertiary syphilis)
4. **X-rays** show marked osteopenia with deformation of the bones. The articular cartilage is destroyed, and there may be subluxation or dislocation of joints. New bone formation occurs at the margins of the joint and in soft tissue around the joint (Fig. 10–11). The condition is sometimes described as "osteoarthritis with a vengeance."
5. **Joint fluid** aspiration and examination may be necessary to rule out infection.
6. **MRI** of the cervical region is ordered if syringomyelia is suspected.

Management

1. **Medications** are prescribed for any underlying disease, e.g., syphilis or diabetes.
2. **Ancillary.** The joints are protected by appropriate braces, and skin breakdown can be prevented by well-fitting shoes.
3. **Surgical** fusion of affected joints is not very successful because of the poor quality of bone.

Bibliography

1. Allman RM, Brower AC, Kotyarov EB: Neuropathic bone and joint disease. Radiol Clin North Am 26:1373–1381, 1988.

2. Bennett RM: Fibromyalgia and the facts. Rheum Dis Clin North Am 19:45–59, 1993.
3. Black KP: Compartment syndromes in athletes. Clin Sports Med 9:471–487, 1990.
4. Deese JM Jr, Baxter DE: Compressive neuropathies of the lower extremity. J Musculoskel Med 5:68–91, 1988.
5. Ellman MH: Neuropathic joint disease. In McCarty DJ (ed): Arthritis and Allied Conditions. Philadelphia, Lea & Febiger, 1989, pp 1255–1272.
6. Fan PT, Blanton ME: Clinical features and diagnosis of fibromyalgia. J Musculoskel Med 9:24–42, 1992.
7. Giurini JM, Chrzan JS, Gibbons GW, Habershaw GM: Charcot's disease in diabetic patients. Postgrad Med 89(4):163–169, 1991.
8. Gullough PG, DiCarlo EF: Subchondral avascular necrosis: A common cause of arthritis. Ann Rheum Dis 49:412–420, 1990.
9. Hamdy RC: Paget's disease of bone. Hosp Pract 25 (Oct):33–41, 1990.
10. Mandel S, Rothrock RW: Sympathetic dystrophy: Recognizing and managing a puzzling group of syndromes. Postgrad Med 87(8):213–218, 1990.
11. Matsen FA, Rorabeck CH: Compartment syndromes. Instr Course Lect 38:463–472, 1989.
12. Merkow RL, Lane JM: Paget's disease of bone. Endocrinol Metab Clin North Am 19:177–204, 1990.
13. Mirra JM: Pathogenesis of Paget's disease based on viral etiology. Clin Orthop 217:162–170, 1987.
14. Moore RE, and Friedman RJ: Current concepts in pathophysiology and diagnosis of compartment syndromes. J Emerg Med 7:657–662, 1989.
15. Nakano KK: Peripheral nerve entrapments, repetitive strain disorder, and occupation-related syndromes. Curr Opin Rheumatol 2:253–269, 1990.
16. Osterman AL: The double crush syndrome. Orthop Clin North Am 19:147–155, 1988.
17. Priebe MM, Werner RA, Davidoff GN: Diagnosis and treatment of the reflex sympathetic dystrophy syndrome of the upper extremity. J Back Musculoskel Rehabil 2(2):35–45, 1992.
18. Resnick D: Bone and Joint Imaging. Philadelphia, W.B. Saunders Co., 1989, pp 440–451.
19. Schwartzman RJ, McLellan TL: Reflex sympathetic dystrophy. Arch Neurol 44:555–559, 1987.
20. Travell JG, Simons DG: Myofascial Pain and Dysfunction: The Trigger Point Manual. Baltimore, Williams & Wilkins, 1983.
21. Weinstein SM, Herring SA: Nerve problems and compartment syndromes in the hand, wrist, and forearm. Clin Sports Med 11:161, 1992.
22. Wolf F: When to diagnose fibromyalgia? Rheum Dis Clin North Am 20:485–502, 1994.
23. Zizic TM: Osteonecrosis. Curr Opin Rheumatol 3:481–489, 1991.

11

Temporomandibular Joint

Steve M. Gnatz, M.D.

Pain or dysfunction of the temporomandibular joint (TMJ) is common and affects up to 20% of the population at least once in their life. It may be of acute onset, e.g., after biting on a hard item of food, or it may develop into a chronic pain syndrome. The chronic pain syndrome develops in about 1.6% of the population and can cause significant problems in eating and talking. The pain may be referred to other parts of the head and neck from the TMJ, or pain arising from other structures may be referred to this region, causing difficulty in diagnosis. The etiology of pain from the TMJ may be multifactorial, and for successful outcome, all factors need to be considered in the management of this syndrome. When the symptoms have been present for a long time, a complete "cure" may not be possible. In that case, treatment requires psychological counseling and adjustment of lifestyle.

Differential Diagnosis

Many conditions can give rise to pain in the TMJ and region. A detailed history and physical examination with proper investigations will help localize the problem.

1. **Myofascial pain dysfunction syndrome** is the most common (85–90% of all temporomandibular pain problems). The jaw movements are painful. There are palpable trigger points over the muscles of mastication. There is no tenderness over the TMJ. The trigger points may coexist with other pathology of the TMJ.
2. **Internal derangement** of the TMJ is due to problems with the intra-articular disc. The onset is likely to be acute after a traumatic event. A "pop" or click is felt on movements of the jaw. There may be some limitation of movements and pain. Arthrography or MRI may show the abnormal disc.
3. **Myofascial pain and internal derangement** are commonly seen together in the same patient. The clinical features of both are present.
4. **Degenerative joint disease** presents with insidious onset of pain, stiffness, and crepitus on movement. X-rays show an irregular joint surface, deformity of the head of the mandible, and osteophyte formation.
5. **Rheumatoid arthritis** affects the TMJ like any other synovial joint. There is morning stiffness and signs of inflammation around the joint. The joint may be involved in **juvenile rheumatoid arthritis** also.

Anatomy

The TMJ represents the only pair of joints in the body that are connected by a single bone (mandible). When the mandible moves, movement takes place at both joints. If one joint is affected by any pathology, the other becomes involved, too. Thus, both joints must be treated as a unit.

The head of the mandible articulates with the mandibular fossa and articular tubercle of the temporal bone (Fig. 11–1). An **intra-articular disc** separates these two bones and creates two compartments—an upper and a lower. The disc is made of fibrocartilaginous material. It glides forward and downward over the articular tubercle with the head of the mandible as the mouth opens. The mandible head can be palpated just in front of the tragus of the ear. Structural integrity of the disc is essential for smooth movements at the TMJ. The disc is supplied by blood vessels and has limited capacity for repair.

The fibrous capsule of the joint is lined by a synovial membrane. Generalized disorders of the synovial membrane, such as rheumatoid arthritis, also affect the TMJ. Muscles and ligaments maintain stability of the joint. Gravity facilitates opening of the jaw. Since active work of chewing is done by closing the jaw, the muscles that perform this movement are stronger than those that open the jaw. The temporalis, masseter, and medial pterygoid are the important muscles to close the mouth. The jaw is capable of side-to-side movements and protraction and retraction, too. The complex movement of grinding is a combination of different movements.

History
Details about the onset of **pain** and **difficulty in chewing** or speaking are requested. How did the symptoms start? Was there any trauma before the onset? Was the onset acute or insidious? Where is the pain? Is it brought on by any activity? Is it greater in the morning or evening? Has the patient had any previous treatment? Did it help?

Physical Examination
1. **Inspection** of the face from the front and side is done to look for any deformities and swelling. Is the lower jaw protruding in front of or too far behind the upper jaw and teeth?

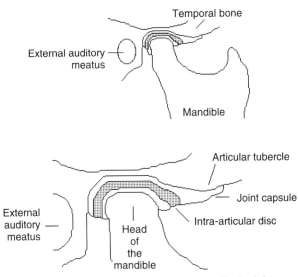

Fig. 11–1   Anatomy of the temporomandibular joint.

2. **Palpation.** The TMJ is in front of the external auditory meatus (Fig. 11–1). Its position can be confirmed by placing the finger in front of the tragus and asking the patient to open and close the mouth. Look for any warmth, **tenderness,** or swelling.
3. **Range of motion.** The movement of opening the mouth takes place at both TMJs. The range can be measured as the distance at midline between the medial incisors when the mouth is fully opened. It is called **interincisal distance** and is approximately 38–42 mm. The lower jaw can also be moved from side to side (lateral excursions) and protruded forward and retracted backward. It is important to listen or palpate for any pops, clicks, or crepitus during the movement. Auscultation with a stethoscope may be necessary to confirm crepitus.

Investigations

1. Examination for **alignment** of teeth (occlusion) is a specialized procedure carried out by a dentist.
2. **X-rays** are helpful in determining joint space and formation of osteophytes.
3. **MRI** is useful for internal derangements because it shows the position and condition of the intra-articular disc.
4. **Aspiration** can be done easily for joint fluid examination or arthrography. The joint is in front of the tragus and below the zygomatic arch. It can be located easily by asking the patient to open and close the mouth. The temporal artery runs in the vicinity, and damage to it should be carefully avoided. The needle should be inserted when mouth is fully open.
5. **Arthrography** is performed less frequently since the advent of MRI.

Management

Some general principles of treatment of painful TMJ are as follows:
1. **Rest** to the joints and muscles of mastication is provided by eating soft foods and taking small bites.
2. **NSAIDs** help reduce inflammation.
3. **Muscle relaxants** and **relaxation techniques** may assist in relieving painful muscle spasms.
4. A dentist can make a **splint** to take some of the stress off the TMJ.
6. ROM and stretching **exercises**

MYOFASCIAL PAIN DYSFUNCTION SYNDROME

This is the most common cause of pain in the TMJ region. The pain may radiate to the ear or neck and is aggravated by movements of the jaw. In a small percentage of patients, the pain may become chronic and recurrent.

Anatomy

One or more of the muscles of mastication are usually involved (Fig. 11–2). Temporalis, masseter, and medial pterygoid muscles close the mouth. Under normal conditions the

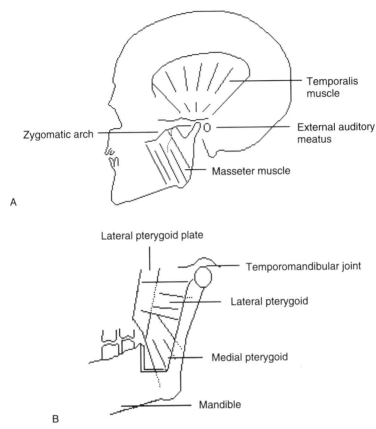

Fig. 11–2   Muscles of mastication involved in myofascial pain dysfunction syndrome. *A*, Superficial muscles. *B*, Part of the mandible is removed to show the deep muscles of mastication, the medial and lateral pterygoids.

mouth opens by gravity. **Temporalis** is a large and powerful muscle that arises from the temporal fossa. It is inserted into the coronoid process of the mandible. The muscle is palpable on the lateral side of the skull superior to the zygomatic arch. The **masseter** arises from the zygomatic arch and is inserted into the lateral aspect of the ramus of the mandible. It is palpable in front of the angle of the mandible. The pterygoid muscles (Fig. 11–2B) are deep to the mandible and are palpated by a finger in the mouth.

Etiology

The exact etiology of myofascial pain dysfunction syndrome is unknown. It is thought to be multifactorial. Some causes ascribed to this disorder are:

1. **Stress** can cause muscle spasm and **grinding of teeth** (bruxism). It becomes painful when trigger points develop.
2. **Malocclusion** of teeth can lead to abnormal stress on the muscles. This is commonly seen after some of the molars are removed.

3. It may coexist with **other pathology,** e.g., degenerative arthritis or rheumatoid arthritis of the TMJ.
4. **Trauma** of dental procedure, fracture or dislocation of the jaw, or cervical traction may precipitate this syndrome.
   Pain restricts mobility and may lead to development of contracture of the joint capsule and muscle. This may start a vicious cycle of pain, more restriction of movements, and tighter contractures.

Pathology
The histologic structure of the muscle is normal. There is some evidence now of a lack of some high-energy phosphates (ATP, etc.) in the involved muscle. It is thought to be a physiologic abnormality that leads to localized muscle spasm.

History
Myofascial pain dysfunction syndrome is common among young and middle-aged **females** (M:F ratio of 3:1 to 8:1). **Pain** is felt in the TMJ region or as a headache in the temporal or occipital area. A pain diagram is helpful in arriving at a correct diagnosis. Pain may radiate to the ear or neck. Chewing, yawning, or talking may aggravate the pain. A history of precipitating causes should be queried. Some patients may complain of fullness in the ear, hearing loss, or tinnitus. The TMJ dysfunction may be part of a **fibromyalgia** syndrome affecting other muscles. Abnormal sleep pattern and thyroid dysfunction may occur in generalized fibromyalgia.

Physical Examination
1. **Inspection** of teeth for **malocclusion** or missing teeth should be done.
2. **Palpation.** Muscles of mastication are palpated for muscle spasm and tender points. Palpation should be done from the outside and inside of the mouth. Localized tenderness over a muscle on firm palpation is an important sign. The pain, including its radiation, may be reproduced if the exact trigger point is palpated. In addition to the muscles of mastication, the sternocleidomastoid, cervical paraspinous, and trapezius muscles should be palpated for trigger points.
3. **Range of motion.** Opening of the jaw and its side-to-side movements are examined. The maximum distance between front incisors on full opening of the mouth is a useful measure of ROM of the TMJ. Active movement (especially against resistance) or passive stretching of the involved muscle is painful.
4. **Special tests**
   a. **Other joints** are examined for degenerative or rheumatoid arthritis, if these conditions are suspected.
   b. Examination of **cranial nerves** helps to rule out neurologic causes of pain.
   c. A **dental consultation** is necessary when malocclusion is suspected.

Differential Diagnoses
1. **Dental pathology** should be suspected if there is localized tenderness over a tooth.
2. **Otitis externa** or **otitis media** can give rise to severe throbbing pain. Examination with an otoscope may reveal the cause. Gentle pulling on the external ear is very painful in otitis externa.

3. **Sinusitis** usually starts after an upper respiratory tract infection with pain and tenderness over the maxillary sinus.

Investigations
There are no diagnostic tests for fibromyalgia or temporomandibular myofascial pain dysfunction syndrome. It is usually recommended to rule out anemia and abnormal thyroid function. Other tests depend on precipitating factors, such as malocclusion or degenerative arthritis.

Course/Complications
The course of this disease is marked by exacerbations and remissions. It may go on for years without diagnosis, and the patient may go to many different health professionals and try many different treatments. The patient may become **depressed** because of different diagnoses given by the health professionals and lack of relief from chronic pain.

Management
The patient should be **reassured** that the condition is benign and not crippling. Addictive narcotic pain killers should be avoided. **NSAIDs** and **physical therapy** measures should be tried first. Well-localized trigger points are **injected** with local anesthetic. A **tricyclic antidepressant** is added if necessary.

Medications
1. NSAID
2. Tricyclic antidepressant
3. Injection of local anesthetic

Ancillary
1. **Physical therapy** modalities may help:
   a. **Local heat** in the form of a hot pack or ultrasound helps relieve pain. A cold pack can be used in a similar fashion.
   b. **ROM exercises** for muscle spasm and for improving contracted soft tissues.
   c. General **stretching and flexibility exercises** prevent muscle spasm and tightness in other muscles.
   d. **Aerobic exercises** and/or swimming
2. **Soft diet** helps in reducing stress on muscles of mastication.
3. A **splint** made by a dentist can be used at night.

INTERNAL DERANGEMENT OF THE TEMPOROMANDIBULAR JOINT

The abnormal intra-articular disc causes **pain** on movements of the jaw. There is **popping** or **clicking** because of abnormal mobility of the disc.

Anatomy
The intra-articular disc separates the head (condyle) of the mandible from the temporal bone and creates two separate joint spaces. At the periphery, it is attached to the capsule of

the joint. The disc is made up of fibrocartilaginous material and supplied by blood vessels from its posterior end. The head of the mandible rotates during opening of the mouth and then slides forward and downward over the tubercle on the undersurface of the temporal bone (Fig. 11–3).

Etiology
Internal derangement is often due to an acute trauma to the jaw. However, chronic biomechanical stress on the joint may damage the disc, too.

Pathology
The disc is displaced from its normal position and is **subluxated** or **dislocated**. The capsule of the joint and the disc may be torn. The condyle of the mandible may come in direct contact with the mandibular fossa, giving rise to pain on movements. Abnormal movements of the disc can cause clicks and pops. **Degenerative arthritis** may follow. Fibrosis and scarring of the capsule can limit the ROM.

History
Patients with internal derangement complain of **painful** limitation of movements of the jaw similar to myofascial pain dysfunction syndrome. However, it is more likely to be accompanied by **clicking, popping,** or grinding noise or sensation. The jaw may **lock** in the open or closed position and require manipulation by the patient to bring it back in alignment. History of significant trauma to the jaw is common but not invariable. The patient may have difficulty in speaking.

Physical Examination
1. **Inspection.** Look for any facial asymmetry or swelling. Erythema around the joint indicates inflammation.
2. **Palpation.** The TMJ is palpated in front of the external auditory meatus for increased warmth and tenderness.
3. **Range of motion.** The interincisal distance (normal, 38–42 mm) is a good indicator of limitation in the ROM. The TMJ should be palpated during movement for clicks or

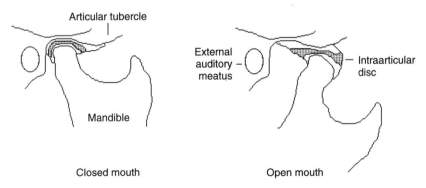

Fig. 11–3 Relation of the head of the mandible to the articular tubercle of the temporal bone in the closed and open mouth.

crepitus. Auscultation by a stethoscope over the joint is more sensitive than palpation. Both sides should move equally and smoothly. If the disc has dislocated anterolaterally, the jaw will deviate toward the affected side when the mouth is opened.

Investigations

1. **Plain x-rays.** A transcranial view shows any narrowing of joint space and osteophyte formation. The joint space is narrowed if the intra-articular disc is degenerated or displaced.
2. **MRI** is useful in detecting disc abnormalities, such as tears and displacements. It has reduced the need for invasive procedures like arthrography.

Management

Conservative measures should be tried first. After an acute injury, **rest,** local **cold** pack, and **NSAIDs** are given until pain, swelling, and tenderness subside. Gentle **ROM exercises** are started as tolerated. A **splint** is useful in reducing stress on the joint. **Ultrasound** is prescribed for chronic disorders.

Surgery is considered only after a good trial of conservative treatment has failed to relieve symptoms. **Discoplasty** (repair of the disc), discectomy (removal of the disc), or silicone implant arthroplasty are some of the surgical procedures that can be done.

INFLAMMATORY ARTHRITIS OF THE TEMPOROMANDIBULAR JOINT

The TMJ is involved in various inflammatory arthritides, including rheumatoid arthritis, gout, calcium pyrophosphate deposition disease, and systemic lupus erythematosus. The diagnosis and management of TMJ disorders is part of the whole picture.

Pathology

In rheumatoid arthritis, both TMJs are usually affected late in the course of disease. Erosions start in the neck of the condyle. There is uniform narrowing of the joint space. The TMJ may be the first joint involved in systemic lupus erythematosus.

History

Pain and **stiffness** in the region of the TMJ are common. These symptoms are more severe in the morning and after overuse. Pain is usually progressive and unrelenting. Systemic symptoms of fatigue, loss of appetite, and fever may also be present.

Physical Examination

1. **Inspection.** Slight, diffuse, swelling in front of the tragus may be visible.
2. **Palpation.** Increased temperature and tenderness are present during exacerbation of the disease.
3. **Range of motion.** Active and passive ROMs are restricted and painful.
4. **Special tests.** Other joints and systems are examined, depending on the suspected diagnosis.

Investigations

Additional testing will depend on the clinical diagnosis.
1. **ESR** is high in inflammatory diseases.
2. **Serum antinuclear antibody** titer is >1:40 in some inflammatory joint diseases.
3. **Muscle creatine kinase** may be elevated in polymyositis or dermatomyositis.
4. **Plain x-rays** may show erosions near the synovial attachment in rheumatoid arthritis. Destruction of articular cartilage is seen as joint space narrowing. The intra-articular disc may be seen on plain x-rays because of calcium deposition in calcium pyrophosphate deposition disease.
5. **MRI** is useful in detecting a mass due to infection or malignancy.

Management is similar to that for the inflammatory arthritides.

DEGENERATIVE JOINT DISEASE OF THE TEMPOROMANDIBULAR JOINT

Degenerative joint disease (DJD) of the TMJ may be part of the primary (idiopathic) process or secondary to trauma or disc disease. Pain in the TMJ area and difficulty with chewing are the main symptoms.

Etiology

The primary disease is idiopathic. Secondary DJD can occur after fractures of the mandible, dislocation of the TMJ, displaced or damaged intra-articular disc, or long-standing malocclusion.

Pathology

The joint space is irregularly narrowed because of destruction of the cartilage. Osteophytes are seen in the late stage of the disease.

History

Pain in the region of the TMJ is a common presenting symptom. It is usually of insidious onset and long duration. It is aggravated by **chewing,** especially hard substances. There may be some stiffness around the joint in the morning for 15–30 minutes. In primary disease, other joints including the distal interphalangeal joints, knees, or hips may be symptomatic. Other symptoms such as clicking and popping may be present in DJD secondary to intra-articular disc problems. The **course** is slowly progressive.

Physical Examination

1. **Inspection** may not show any abnormality.
2. **Palpation.** Tenderness over the joint is common. There may be palpable crepitus on movement of the jaw.
3. **Range of motion.** All movements are painful. There may be some restriction of movements in the late stage of disease.

Investigations

1. **X-rays** show irregular narrowing of the joint space and osteophytes. The condyle of the mandible may be flattened.
2. **MRI** is not necessary unless intra-articular disc pathology is suspected.

Management

The treatment is similar to that for DJD of any other joint. **NSAIDs** are given for relief of pain and inflammation. Local **heat** over the joint helps in relieving symptoms. If DJD is secondary to internal derangement, the primary disease should be treated.

Bibliography

1. Block SL: Differential diagnosis of masticatory muscle pain and dysfunction. Oral Maxillofac Surg Clin North Am 7:29–49, 1995.
2. Gnatz SM: Physiatric management of temporomandibular joint syndrome and myofascial pain of the craniomandibular apparatus. Curr Concepts Rehabil Med 5:7–18, 1989.

12

Neck and Cervical Spine

Andrew Fischer, M.D., Ph.D., and Aerie Rim, M.D.

The neck connects the head to the trunk. The spinal cord, food and air passages, and major blood vessels, to and from the head, are contained within the neck. There are many lymph nodes in the neck that may become enlarged because of infection or malignancy. Many of these structures do not belong to the musculoskeletal system, but diseases of these structures can present as a differential diagnosis and need to be considered in the diagnostic workup.

Clinical Manifestations and Differential Diagnosis

1. **Pain** is the most frequent presenting complaint of patients with neck disorders. It is important to concentrate on common causes of neck pain, such as myofascial **trigger points,** degenerative arthritis of the cervical spine, and degenerative disc disease. The pain may **radiate** down one of the upper extremities, or it may be felt in the interscapular region. It is always better to keep diagnoses of infection and tumor in the back of your mind, because the result of missing these conditions in any patient may be disastrous. The pain may sometimes be **referred** to the neck from the heart, lungs, or muscles of the chest wall.
2. **Swelling** in the neck is usually in connection with a **lymph node** or thyroid gland.
3. **Deformity. Torticollis** or wryneck may be due to painful spasm or contracture of the neck muscles.
4. **Tingling and numbness** in the upper extremity. Upper extremities are innervated by cervical 5 to 8 nerve roots. Impingement of any of these nerve roots or pathology of the brachial plexus in the neck can give rise to sensory changes in the upper extremity.
5. **Weakness** in the upper extremity may be due to lesions of the nerve roots, brachial plexus, or primary muscle disease, e.g., myopathy.
6. **Difficulty in walking** is sometimes the presenting symptom of **cervical myelopathy.** It may also cause frequency and dribbling incontinence of urine.

Anatomy

The primary function of the cervical spine is to **support** the head and to allow it to **move** in different directions. It also **protects** the spinal cord and vertebral artery. There are seven cervical vertebrae. The first vertebra articulates with the occiput above and second vertebra below. There are no intervertebral discs between the occiput and first vertebra and between the first and second cervical vertebrae. One intervertebral disc is present between each of the subsequent vertebrae.

The first and second cervical **vertebrae** are very different from the rest. The first is like

139

a ring and is called the **atlas** (Fig. 12–1A). It has an anterior and posterior arch and two lateral masses. The lateral masses articulate with the occiput above and with the second vertebra below. **Atlanto-occipital joints** are lined by synovial membrane. Flexion and extension movements (nodding) occur at these joints. The second vertebra, named **axis,** has an odontoid process that forms a pivot around which the atlas and head rotate (Fig. 12–1B). This gives the head its ability to turn from side to side—lateral rotations. The C3 to C7 vertebrae are small irregular bones that are held together by intervertebral discs, ligaments, and articular processes. The body of the vertebra is anterior and the arch is posterior (Fig. 12–2). Between the body and the arch is the vertebral foramen, within which lies the spinal cord and its meninges. The intervertebral disc lies between the bodies of two adjacent vertebrae.

The **intervertebral discs** have two parts, a central soft nucleus pulposus and a surrounding annulus fibrosus. The disc acts as a shock absorber and allows movements between two vertebrae. The blood supply to the disc is cut off by the second decade, and the disc becomes the largest avascular structure in the body. It receives nutrition by diffusion, a process which is facilitated by intermittent compression and decompression.

The neck **muscles** are divided into flexors and extensors according to their function. Sternocleidomastoid muscles acting together **flex** the neck. Acting individually, they rotate the head to the opposite side and pull the occiput toward the sternoclavicular joint. Other anterior muscles, i.e., longus capitis, longus colli, scalenus, infrahyoid, and anterior rectus capitis, are secondary flexors. The **extensors** of the neck are the upper part of the trapezius, semispinalis capitis, erector spinae, and semispinalis cervicis. Lateral flexion is performed by three scalene muscles.

The cervical spinal cord is protected by the vertebrae and surrounding tissues. Eight pairs of spinal roots emerge from the spinal cord and form cervical and brachial plexuses. These nerves supply the neck and both upper extremities. The first cervical nerve comes out between the occiput and C1, and the eighth comes out between C7 and T1.

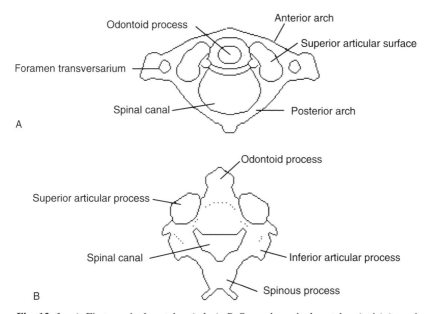

Fig. 12–1 *A,* First cervical vertebra (atlas). *B,* Second cervical vertebra (axis) (top view).

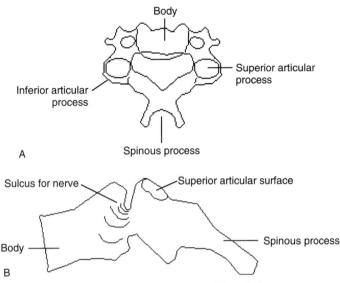

Fig. 12–2 A cervical vertebra. Top and lateral views.

History

The onset, duration, and progress are considered for each symptom. Some of the painful conditions are brought on by injury, e.g., a fall or rear-end collision, and certain movements of the neck or activities may aggravate pain and stiffness. Reading or working at a computer terminal with bifocal lenses requires the neck to be in an extended position for a prolonged time. Symptoms of nerve root entrapment can be made worse by these activities.

Physical Examination

1. **Inspection. Posture** of the head is observed as soon as the patient walks into the office. Is it held to one side? Are the eyes level? When the patient is slouched forward and has sagging shoulders, it puts strain on the muscles of neck. Are the shoulders level? Is there any difficulty in walking? Does he or she keep the head very stiff? The patient is asked to undress down to the waist. Look for any deformity, swelling, or scars of operations in the back, sides, or front of the neck.
2. **Palpation** can be carried out with the patient sitting or lying. The muscles may be more relaxed when the patient is lying on an examination couch. As with inspection, the posterior aspect, sides, and anterior part of the neck are systematically palpated for local warmth, tenderness, muscle spasm, and swelling.
   a. **Posterior aspect** is palpated from the occiput to base of the neck. In the occipital region, the occipital bone, muscles, and mastoid process are examined for tenderness and muscle spasm. Trigger points in muscles here can give rise to occipital headache. Sometimes, the occipital nerves are palpable and tender. In the midline, spinous processes are covered by ligamentum nuchae. The spinous process of C7 is the most prominent one and is easily palpable. The trapezius and paraspinous muscles are examined for spasm and trigger points.
   b. The **space between the trapezius and sternomastoid muscles** is palpated for swellings. Normal lymph nodes are not palpable. The superior border of the trapezius

is a very frequent site for trigger points. The sternomastoid muscle is also palpated from its insertion in the mastoid to the sternoclavicular joint.

    c. The **anterior region** is examined from the submandibular area to the suprasternal notch. The submandibular lymph nodes and salivary gland may be palpable. The thyroid cartilage, thyroid gland, and carotid pulsations are palpated for any abnormalities.

3. **Range of motion** is not examined if there is any doubt about the stability of the spine. Flexion, extension, right and left lateral flexions, and right and left lateral rotations are tested. These movements occur at multiple intervertebral levels and cannot be measured very accurately. Limitation of movements may be due to spasm of cervical muscles, inelastic intervertebral ligaments, or fusion between two vertebrae. The extent of limitation in ROM may correlate with severity of functional deficit. The patient is asked to touch his or her chin to the chest to examine the range of flexion. For extension, the patient bends the head backward to look up to the ceiling. A major portion of flexion-extension takes place at the atlanto-occipital joint. Some flexion-extension also takes place at other intervertebral levels. There is more movement at the lower cervical level (i.e., C5–6 and C6–7) than upper (C2–4). Rotation of the head in relation to the shoulders (lateral rotation) occurs largely at the atlanto-axial joint and to lesser extent at other levels. To test this, have the patient look to his or her sides without moving the shoulders. Lateral flexion occurs at multiple levels when the patient bends his head to his side to touch his ear to his shoulder without lifting up the shoulder.

    The normal range of motion in the cervical spine is 60° of lateral rotation and 45° of flexion, extension, and lateral flexion (Fig. 12–3).

    a. **Active** and passive ROMs are always restricted when there is pain, muscle spasm, shortening of ligaments, or fusion between vertebrae. While the patient is performing ROM, observe whether the movement is smooth or guarded and jerky.

    b. **Passive.** In some patients with polymyositis, the passive movements are normal but active movements, such as lifting the head off the bed, are not possible.

4. **Special tests**

    a. **Compression tests** should *not* be done if fracture, dislocation, or metastatic disease of the cervical spine is suspected. While the patient is sitting, the examiner puts his or her hands on the top of patient's head and pushes down. The test is positive when the patient experiences pain in the neck or pain radiating down one of the upper extremities. Pressure is transmitted to the intervertebral discs and facet joints. It is positive in degenerative disease of the discs or facet joints or in cervical radiculopathy and myelopathy.

    b. **Neurologic examination** is performed when there is history of radiating pain or sensory disturbance, weakness, and difficulty in walking.

    c. **Radial pulses** are palpated in different positions of the upper extremity and neck when thoracic outlet syndrome is suspected.

    d. **Heart** and **lungs** are examined when myocardial infarction or pneumonia is suspected.

    e. **Shoulder** pathology may sometimes give rise to neck pain.

Investigations

1. **Plain x-rays** tell us about the vertebrae, intervertebral discs, and facet joints. Anteroposterior, lateral, and oblique views are usually done. The **oblique views** are useful in showing the condition of the intervertebral foramina, which are commonly narrowed in degenerative disease of the cervical spine (*see* Fig. 12–10). **Open-mouth view** gives information about the odontoid process of C2 and the atlanto-axial and atlanto-occipital joints. Degenerative disc and joint disease, fractures, and tumors of bone are visualized on plain x-rays.

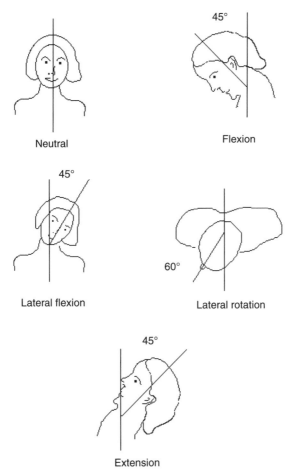

Fig. 12–3 Normal range of motion in the cervical spine.

2. **Blood tests,** such as the WBC count and ESR, are useful when infection or inflammatory arthritis is suspected.
3. **CT** is useful for a more detailed look at fractures of the spine.
4. **MRI** is helpful in prolapsed discs, syringomyelia, or spinal cord tumors.
5. **Electromyography** is positive when nerve root, brachial plexus, or nerve compression syndrome is present.

TORTICOLLIS

There are many causes of torticollis or **wryneck.** The head is tilted (lateral flexion) to one side and turned (lateral rotation) toward the opposite side. The most common cause of this deformity is contracture of the sternomastoid muscle.

Anatomy

The sternomastoid or sternocleidomastoid muscle arises from the manubrium sterni and medial one-third of the clavicle. It goes obliquely upward and backward to insert in the mastoid process (Fig. 12–4). When sternomastoid muscles on both sides of the neck contract together, they flex the head forward. If only one muscle contracts, it pulls the mastoid process toward the medial end of the clavicle, tilts the head to the same side, and rotates it toward the opposite side.

Etiology

Fibrosis of the sternomastoid muscle may occur as a result of **injury** or ischemia during the intrauterine period or childbirth. Bleeding inside the muscle results in fibrosis. Contracture of this fibrous tissue leads to shortening of the muscle. Alternatively, the muscle may be irritated by **infection** of one of the cervical lymph nodes or inflammation in some other structure. This may lead to muscle spasm and wryneck. Lymphadenitis may be due to pyogenic infection or tuberculosis.

Pathology

A swelling consisting of fibrous tissue may form within the sternomastoid muscle during early infancy. Contracture of the muscle may take some years to develop, and deformity becomes apparent around the second or third year of life. If the deformity is not corrected, the face on the affected side does not develop and remains smaller than the other side (Fig. 12–4).

History

Parents notice that the child's head is turned to one side and cannot look straight. This deformity gradually worsens. If it is due to acute infection, the child may have fever, chills, pain, and dysphagia.

Physical Examination

1. **Inspection.** A localized swelling in the sternomastoid muscle can be seen sometimes in early infancy. In the older child, the head is tilted to one side, and the chin is turned to the opposite side. The whole length of the sternomastoid muscle may be visible.

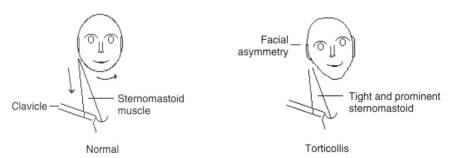

Fig. 12–4 In torticollis, the sternomastoid muscle pulls the mastoid process down and turns the head toward the opposite side. The face on the affected side remains smaller than on the unaffected side.

2. **Palpation.** The findings of inspection can be confirmed by palpation.
3. **Range of motion.** Lateral rotation toward the same side and lateral flexion to the opposite side are limited.

Differential Diagnoses
If torticollis is secondary to infection, the primary cause of infection should be looked for and treated.

Complications
Permanent changes in bones of the face and cervical vertebrae may occur if the deformity is not corrected early.

Management
1. **Ancillary.** Initial treatment of idiopathic torticollis consists of gentle stretching of the sternomastoid muscle. This can be taught to the parents and carried out many times during a day.
2. **Surgical.** If conservative treatment fails, release of the muscle near its origin or a Z-plasty is carried out to correct the deformity.

CERVICAL FLEXION-EXTENSION INJURY

In flexion-extension injury (**whiplash**), the head is forced into flexion and/or extension in relation to the trunk, often during a rear-end or head-on collision of motor vehicles. The soft tissues of the neck are injured, and the patient presents with pain and muscle spasm. This is the most common traumatic condition of the cervical spine.

Etiology
Automobile accidents are the most frequent cause of this injury. The incidence of this injury is increasing because of increasing numbers of car accidents. This type of injury occurs as a result of sudden acceleration or deceleration of the body.

Pathology
Soft tissues of the neck (muscles and ligaments) are stretched when there is movement beyond extremes of normal range. Some fibers may tear, with bleeding within the tissues. Usually, there are no fractures and the spine is stable. The interspinous ligaments, capsule of the facet joints, anterior and posterior longitudinal ligaments, cervical disc, and various muscles of the neck may be affected. Rear-end collisions lead to **hyperextension** injury with overstretching of the anterior muscles and ligaments. Head-on collisions cause **hyperflexion** and damage to the posterior muscles and ligaments, such as the ligamentum nuchae and interspinous ligaments. Muscles are overstretched in the mild form of injury, but in more severe injuries ligaments are also damaged. In very severe injuries, there may be fracture of the articular processes and subluxation or dislocation of the facet joint. Concussion of the brain may be associated with severe "whiplash."

Clinical Features

Evaluation of these patients is difficult because there is great disparity between abundant symptoms and very few objective signs.

History

Details about the accident give useful information about the forces involved and extent of injuries sustained. The patient may be confused after the accident. Severe **pain** starts about 24–48 hours after the injury. The pain may radiate to the shoulders, interscapular region, or head. It is aggravated by any movement of the head. The pain may be referred to the occipital region or shoulder. The patient frequently complains of headache. After a severe injury, there may be nausea, blurred vision, or vertigo. The symptoms last for a few days if the injury was minor but may last for months after a severe accident.

Physical Examination

1. **Inspection.** Cervical lordosis may be lost as a result of muscle spasm.
2. **Palpation.** The muscles and other soft tissues are markedly tender. Initially, the **tenderness** is diffuse. After a few weeks, the patient may develop localized tenderness with **trigger points.** The sternomastoid and/or paraspinal muscles may be firm because of **muscle spasm.**
3. **Range of motion.** All active and passive movements are markedly restricted because of pain and muscle spasm.
4. **Special tests.** Neurologic exam is normal.

Differential Diagnoses

1. **Fractures** and **dislocations** of the spine should be ruled out by appropriate x-rays.
2. **Cerebral concussion** should be ruled out if the patient has severe headache.

Investigations

X-rays should be normal in flexion-extension injury. Cervical lordosis may be lost because of muscle spasm.

Course

Pain, muscle spasm, and limitation of movements usually subside gradually over a period of weeks. They may last for a few months if injuries are severe.

Management

Bed rest for a few days may be necessary after a severe injury. Local rest is provided by a soft **cervical collar. Ice packs** are prescribed for a couple of days after the accident. After that, **local heat** helps relieve some of the pain and muscle spasm. **Analgesics** or NSAIDs are prescribed to relieve pain, and **muscle relaxants** are used if there is muscle spasm. Gentle **exercises** to increase ROM of the cervical spine are started as soon as the patient can tolerate. Cervical traction with light weight may also help in overcoming muscle spasm. It may, however, aggravate pain and spasm if the weight is too much. Other modalities, including transcutaneous electrical nerve stimulation and spray-and-stretch therapy, are also used. Later, when definite trigger points are present, they are treated by local injections and stretching exercises.

FRACTURES, FRACTURE-DISLOCATIONS, AND DISLOCATIONS

Fractures and dislocations of the cervical spine are very serious injuries and should be managed by specially trained professionals. Traffic accidents account for more than half of serious cervical spine injuries. The mechanism of injuries are varied. Correlation between vertebral displacement and neurologic damage remains elusive; however, certain types of injury are known to be commonly associated with recognizable patterns of neurologic damage. For example, bilateral facet joint dislocation is commonly associated with a complete cord lesion, whereas nerve root injury is accompanied by unilateral facet joint dislocation. Burst fracture of the vertebral body usually leads to anterior cord syndrome.

The vascular gray matter in the central part of the spinal cord suffers more severe injury than the peripheral part. In some instances, the lesion is virtually restricted to the anterior and posterior gray matter (**central cord syndrome**). It affects motor function in the upper extremities more than in the lower extremities. Urinary retention occurs in some patients. Sensory deficit is minimal. Hyperextension injury is the one most often associated with central cord syndrome.

Physical Examination
When a patient complains of pain in the neck after an accident, the neck should be immobilized until fracture/dislocation of the cervical spine is ruled out. The spine should be examined very carefully. Open wounds, bruises, swelling, and deformity of head and neck are noted without moving the patient. Air in the subcutaneous tissue gives a peculiar crepitus and indicates rupture of the air passage or esophagus.

Range of motion. Do not test ROM if a fracture/dislocation is suspected.

Neurologic examination is done to determine the level and type of spinal cord injury and level of consciousness.

Management
If fracture or dislocation of the cervical spine or spinal cord injury is suspected, the patient should be transported to a specialized trauma center. Details of management are beyond the scope of this book.

RHEUMATOID ARTHRITIS

Anatomy
The facet joints, atlanto-occipital, atlanto-axial, and posterolateral intervertebral joints are lined with synovial membrane. There is a synovium-lined cavity between the odontoid process and the transverse ligament (Fig. 12–5). During flexion of the cervical spine, the transverse ligament holds the odontoid process close to the anterior arch of the atlas.

Pathology
All synovial joints in the neck can be involved by the rheumatoid process. The inflammatory changes damage the articular cartilage and ligaments. The transverse ligament of the

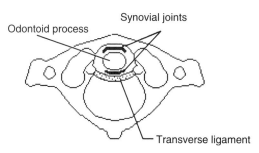

Fig. 12–5 There are synovial joints between the odontoid process and the anterior arch of atlas and another one between the odontoid process and the transverse ligament.

atlas is no exception and may be damaged or destroyed in rheumatoid arthritis. Then, the odontoid process can move independently to the atlas and compress the spinal cord (Fig. 12–6). The upper cervical vertebrae (C1–4) are more frequently involved in rheumatoid arthritis than the lower vertebrae. Degenerative joint disease develops in facet joints later as secondary changes.

Clinical Features
The severity of clinical features is variable in different patients and even in the same patient over time.

Ill-defined aching **pain** is felt in the upper part of the neck. This pain may be referred to the occipital region. It is aggravated by movements. Neck symptoms may be exacerbated during flareup of the disease.

Physical Examination
1. **Inspection.** Cervical lordosis may be lost during acute exacerbation.
2. **Palpation.** Diffuse tenderness and muscle spasm may be palpable during an exacerbation. Localized tenderness due to trigger points should be looked for along the paraspinals, trapezius, and suboccipital muscles.
3. **Range of motion.** During an exacerbation, all active and passive movements are restricted due to muscle spasm. If the patient complains of tingling of both hands or other neurologic symptoms when he or she flexes the neck, atlanto-axial subluxation (*see* Complications) should be suspected and appropriate x-rays ordered.
4. **Special tests.** A neurologic exam is carried out if the patient complains of any paresthesias, weakness, or difficulty in using the hands.

Investigations
Plain x-rays. Rheumatoid arthritis affects the upper cervical spine more often than the lower (unlike degenerative arthritis). Narrowing of disc spaces between C2–3 and C3–4 is more likely due to rheumatoid involvement than degenerative disc disease. Generalized **osteoporosis** of the cervical vertebrae is a common finding in long-standing rheumatoid arthritis. **Erosions** are seen near facet joints. Subluxation of a vertebra may occur due to laxity of ligaments (Fig. 12–6B).

If **atlanto-axial subluxation** and spinal cord compression are suspected, flexion-extension and open-mouth views are requested. The distance between the posterior aspect of the

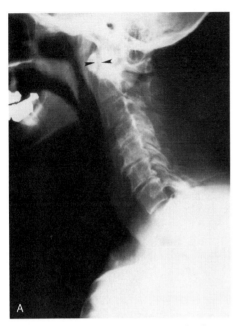 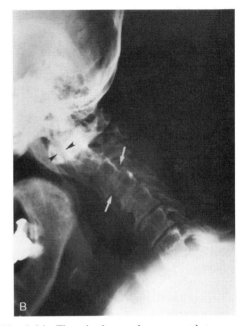

Fig. 12–6 Subluxation of vertebrae in rheumatoid arthritis. There is abnormal movement between vertebrae because of laxity of ligaments. This becomes more apparent in flexion of the cervical spine. Lateral flexion-extension views are requested if subluxation of cervical vertebrae is suspected. The x-ray in *A* is taken in the neutral position, and the one in *B* is taken in flexion. The black arrow heads mark the distance between the anterior surface of odontoid process and the posterior surface of the arch of atlas. This space is increased in flexion because of subluxation of the arch of atlas on the second vertebra. The white arrows show anterior slippage of the third cervical vertebra on fourth. In a normal cervical spine, the posterior surface of vertebral bodies forms a smooth curve that is convex anteriorly (lordosis). This curve is disturbed and a step-like deformity is seen (white arrows) at the posteroinferior angle of upper vertebra and posterosuperior angle of lower vertebra in subluxation.

anterior arch of the atlas and the anterior surface of the odontoid process is measured in the flexed position. This distance should not exceed 2.5 mm in women and 3 mm in men. Abnormal separation indicates laxity of the transverse ligament and subluxation of the atlanto-axial joint (Fig. 12–6). Erosions may be seen over the odontoid process, or it may be completely destroyed in the very late stages of disease.

Complications
1. **Atlanto-axial subluxation** is the most serious complication of rheumatoid arthritis in the cervical spine. It may give rise to minor neurologic symptoms, such as tingling and numbness in hands, to quadriplegia and sudden death. Paresthesias are intermittent initially and are brought on by flexion of the neck. A rear-end collision or less severe injury may lead to quadriplegia in a patient with preexisting subluxation.
2. **Occipital neuralgia** from compression of the occipital nerve
3. **Vertebral artery compression** due to subluxation may manifest by sudden loss of balance and fall.

Management

Management of rheumatoid arthritis is described in Chapter 4. Local **heat** and support by a soft **cervical collar** help in relieving pain during acute exacerbation of neck symptoms. Gentle **ROM exercises** are added as tolerated by the patient. Atlanto-axial subluxation may require a hard cervical collar or surgical fusion.

ANKYLOSING SPONDYLITIS

Ankylosing spondylitis is a chronic inflammatory disease of the axial skeleton occurring in late adolescence and early adulthood. The sacroiliac joints are involved in all patients. Inflammatory arthritis occurs in hips, shoulders, and knee joints in some patients. Males are affected 7 times more often than females. Almost 90% of the patients with ankylosing spondylitis have HLA-B27, but this antigen is present in only 8% of the general population. (*See also* Chapter 4.)

Pathology

The anterior longitudinal ligament is especially affected in this disease. Calcification of this and other ligaments gives rise to "bamboo spine." (*see* Fig. 4–4).

History

Pain and stiffness usually start in the low back during adolescence or young adulthood. It gradually migrates upward to affect the thoracic and then the cervical spine. The cervical spine may not be involved in all cases. The course of the disease is marked by exacerbations and remissions.

Physical Examination

1. **Inspection.** Flexion deformity of the whole spine can develop. In severe cases, the patient is bent over and unable to look forward when standing.
2. **Palpation.** During acute exacerbation, there may be tenderness and muscle spasm palpable over paraspinal muscles.
3. **Range of motion.** There is marked limitation of active and passive movements of the involved spine in all directions, especially extension.

Complications

The spine becomes very rigid after the ligaments are calcified, and the spine is likely to fracture after relatively minor trauma. **Spinal cord injury** is also more frequent after fractures of the ankylosed spine.

Management

Prevention of deformity and **relief** of pain are the main goals of treatment. These are achieved by NSAIDs, local heat, proper posture, ROM exercises, and stretching exercises.

INFECTIONS

Infections of the musculoskeletal tissues of the neck occur in children, the aged, debilitated, and drug addicts. Infection spreads to the bones and joints via the bloodstream. The cervical spine is not as frequently affected as the lumbar or lower thoracic spine. *Staphylococcus, Pseudomonas,* and *Klebsiella* are commonly found in infectious lesions. The incidence of spinal tuberculosis is increasing.

Clinical presentation is usually insidious, with progressive **pain** and little systemic reaction. Pain is made worse by movement. Later, it becomes constant and unremitting, even on bedrest. A history of diabetes, chronic renal failure, recent urinary tract or pulmonary infection, and intravenous drug abuse may be present. Typically, there is tenderness over spinous processes of the affected vertebrae and muscle spasm.

Plain **x-rays** do not show any changes in the involved vertebrae for several weeks. Radionuclide bone scan may show increased uptake earlier than plain x-rays. Increase in soft tissue shadow is the first sign on x-rays. Later, destruction of bone or disc may be seen. **Aspiration,** culture, and sensitivity testing help in selection of proper antibiotics. A **brace** or **cast** may be required to provide rest and support to the spine.

Lymphadenopathy. Palpable and painful lymph nodes may give rise to neck pain. Groups of lymph nodes are located along the external and internal jugular veins. Normal lymph nodes are not palpable but become enlarged because of infection or malignancy in the head or neck. Metastasis from carcinoma of the breast, lung, or even stomach can occur in nodes in the lower cervical region. Enlarged lymph nodes may be the first sign of a malignant tumor in these regions.

CERVICAL SPONDYLOSIS

Degenerative disease of the disc and facet joints is included under this title because they occur simultaneously and may be difficult to distinguish clinically. Cervical spondylosis is also known as **degenerative disc disease,** degenerative joint disease, **osteoarthritis,** and osteoarthrosis. It is a very common condition encountered in people over 45 years of age.

Anatomy

There are two synovial joints, one in front and one behind each intervertebral foramen (Fig. 12–7). Osteophytes growing from these joints can compress nerve roots to produce radiculopathy (Fig. 12–8). There are seven cervical vertebrae and eight cervical nerve roots. The first nerve root comes out between the occiput and C1, and the eighth comes out between C7 and T1. The third to eighth roots pass through the intervertebral foramina. The dimensions of the intervertebral foramina are reduced on both sides when the neck is extended and reduced on the same side when it is bent or rotated to one side (Fig. 12–9).

Etiology

The prevalence of degenerative changes increases with age. Nearly half of the population around 60 years of age shows changes of degenerative disc disease or degenerative arthritis of facet joints on x-rays.

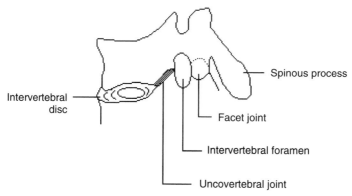

Fig. 12–7 Nerve roots emerge through intervertebral foramina. These foramina are seen on oblique views of cervical spine. The uncovertebral joint (of Luschka) is anterior to, and the facet joint is posterior to, the intervertebral foramen. Extension of the neck, lateral flexion to the same side, and lateral rotation toward the same side reduce the dimensions of the foramen.

Pathology

Blood supply to the intervertebral disc is cut off by the late second decade or early third decade of life. The disc begins to lose its water content, and fibrillations appear within the fibers of the annulus fibrosus. X-ray changes of degeneration are seen in the fifth decade. The disc loses some of its height, subchondral sclerosis develops under the cartilage plate, and osteophytes start appearing near the margins of the annulus fibrosus. Similar changes are seen in facet joints. Degenerative changes in the disc and facet joints occur most frequently at cervical 5, 6, and 7 vertebral levels, where much of flexion-extension movement occurs. The osteophytes growing from the facet joint and uncovertebral joint (posterolateral intervertebral joints of Luschka) compress the nerve root in the intervertebral foramen (Fig. 12–8). Nerve roots supplying the upper extremity (C5–8) are larger and are more likely to be compressed and become symptomatic. The diameter of the spinal cord is relatively large at this level, and it can be compressed by thickened posterior longitudinal ligament, posterior osteophytes, or a protruded disc. The spinal cord is especially vulnerable

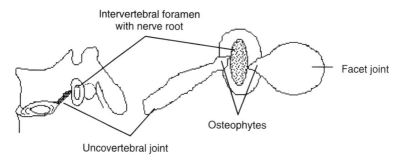

Fig. 12–8 In cervical spondylosis, osteophytes grow from the facet joint and uncovertebral joint into the intervertebral foramen. This diminishes the dimensions of the foramen and may cause nerve root impingement.

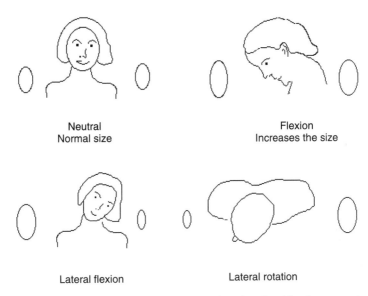

Neutral
Normal size

Flexion
Increases the size

Lateral flexion

Lateral rotation

The size of the intervertebral foramina is reduced on the side of movement

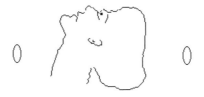

Extension reduces the size of intervertebral foramina on both sides

Fig. 12–9   Extension of the cervical spine narrows the intervertebral foramina on both sides of the neck. Lateral rotation and lateral flexion of the neck reduce the size only on the side toward which the head moves.

if there is congenital narrowing of the spinal canal. The symptoms of nerve root and spinal cord compression may be brought on and exacerbated by inflammation of the soft tissue around the osteophytes.

History
Onset of symptoms is usually insidious but may be acute with exacerbations and remissions. Acute exacerbations may be brought on by excessive activity such as reading (especially with bifocals) or painting a ceiling with the neck in extension. Trauma, e.g., a fall or rear-end collision, may precipitate an acute exacerbation, too. There may be dull aching **pain** in base of the neck or interscapular region. It may radiate to the shoulder or arm on one side. Pain is aggravated by movements and may be worse after activities. The pain is relieved by lying down and avoiding certain activities. There may be some difficulty moving the neck during exacerbation.

Physical Examination

1. **Inspection.** During an acute exacerbation, the patient avoids all movements of the neck and holds it **stiff** and straight. Normal lordosis of the cervical spine is lost.
2. **Palpation.** Paraspinal muscles may be **tender** and firm because of **muscle spasm.** Special effort should be made to look for coexisting **trigger points.**
3. **Range of motion.** All movements may be restricted during an acute exacerbation. If there is narrowing of the intervertebral foramen and pressure on the nerve root, then extension and lateral flexion toward the affected side are especially limited and may reproduce the pain.
4. **Special tests**
   a. **Compression test.** While the patient is in a sitting position, downward pressure is exerted by the palms of the examiner's hands placed on the patient's head. This may reproduce the pain if there is narrowing of the intervertebral foramen and pressure on the nerve root. If there is no pain, the patient is asked to bend the neck to the affected side and similar pressure is exerted. This test should not be performed if instability of the cervical spine is suspected.
   b. **Neurologic exam** is done to rule out nerve entrapment at the intervertebral foramen or compression of the cervical spinal cord (*see* Complications).

Differential Diagnoses

1. **Trigger points** in the paraspinal muscles can give rise to pain in the neck that sometimes radiates to the shoulder and arm. Careful palpation of the paraspinal muscles, suboccipital region, and upper border of the trapezius for trigger points should always be carried out when a patient complains of neck or arm pain. Lateral flexion of the neck toward the opposite side reproduces pain in a trigger point as opposed to flexion toward the same side for root impingement.
2. **Carpal tunnel syndrome.** Symptoms of tingling and numbness are confined to the radial 3½ fingers. Sometimes, patients have pain in the forearm or arm. If the diagnosis is in doubt, nerve conduction and electromyography can help localize the problem.
3. **Peripheral neuropathy.** Tingling and numbness of the feet and depressed deep tendon reflexes in lower extremities suggest diffuse peripheral neuropathy.
4. **Prolapsed intervertebral disc** is not as common in the cervical region as in the lumbar spine. Radicular symptoms due to a prolapsed disc in the cervical region can be treated successfully by conservative measures in the vast majority of patients.
5. **Thoracic outlet syndrome** usually causes symptoms in young females in the distribution of the eighth cervical nerve root and not in the cervical fifth or sixth nerve root. The eighth nerve root is not commonly involved in cervical spondylosis. Vascular symptoms due to microemboli should be looked for in thoracic outlet syndrome.

Investigations

1. **Plain x-rays** for cervical spondylosis should include anteroposterior, lateral, and oblique views. The posterolateral intervertebral joints may show degenerative arthritis with irregular narrowing of the joint space, subchondral sclerosis, and osteophytes. Cervical lordosis, facet joints, and disc spaces are seen well on lateral views. Narrowing of disc space and osteophyte formation should be observed. Minor degrees of subluxation can also occur in cervical spondylosis. Narrowing of the intervertebral foramen is seen on oblique views (Fig. 12–10). These changes are very common after age 50 years, even in patients who do not have any symptoms, and x-ray changes do not always correlate well with clinical findings.

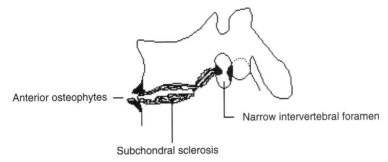

Anterior osteophytes —

Narrow intervertebral foramen

Subchondral sclerosis

Fig. 12–10 In cervical spondylosis, the disc space is narrowed and there is subchondral sclerosis. Osteophytes from uncovertebral joints and facet joints reduce the dimensions of the intervertebral foramen.

2. **Electromyography** is useful in confirming the diagnosis of radiculopathy and in ruling out carpal tunnel or cubital tunnel syndrome.
3. **MRI** is requested when spinal cord compression by a prolapsed intervertebral disc is suspected.
4. **CT** is useful in fractures of the cervical spine.
5. **Myelography** is not being done as often because MRI can give information about spinal cord pathology. Myelography may be combined with CT to show any obstruction to the flow of cerebrospinal fluid by a prolapsed disc or intraspinal tumor.

Course/Complications

The vast majority of patients have exacerbations and remissions. Complications include:
1. **Radiculopathy.** When a nerve root is compressed at the intervertebral foramen, radiating pain is felt along the affected nerve root. This compression is usually caused by osteophytes, but sometimes disc herniation may be the cause. The patient complains of pain and stiffness in the neck. Pain may radiate down the arm and forearm. Pain is aggravated by extension, lateral flexion, and lateral rotation toward the affected side (Fig. 12–9). The patient may complain of some paresthesias in one or two digits innervated by the nerve root or slight clumsiness or weakness of the hand. There may be sensory, motor, and reflex changes in the distribution of that nerve root. Sixth and seventh cervical nerve roots are most commonly involved. When the sixth cervical nerve root is affected, the pain radiates from the arm to forearm. The patient may complain of paresthesias in the thumb. Biceps and brachioradialis reflexes may be depressed or absent. Cervical seventh radiculopathy is by far the most frequent, seen in 60–70% of all patients with cervical radiculopathy. The triceps reflex may be absent or depressed. Sensation over the middle finger may be impaired.
2. **Cervical myelopathy.** Patients usually present with difficulty in walking, with slight unsteadiness and weakness of one or both legs. The leg feels stiff and heavy and gives out quickly on activity or exercise. The patient may complain of tingling and numbness of the feet. The symptoms begin insidiously and progress slowly. Fine hand movements may be impaired. There is usually no pain. Increased frequency of micturition or dribbling incontinence indicate involvement of bladder function.

On examination there is increased muscle tone in the lower extremities, with exaggerated deep tendon reflexes and extensor plantar responses. The vibratory and tactile sensation may be impaired from the hip down, and joint position sense in the toes may be diminished. Flexion of the neck may induce an electric-like sensation down the spine (Lhermitte's sign) which is characteristic of cervical myelopathy. Later, the patient may develop hesitancy of micturition. Cervical myelopathy may have to be distinguished from multiple sclerosis with spasticity of both lower extremities. In multiple sclerosis, there may be spasticity of both upper extremities, visual symptoms, and signs of involvement of other parts of the CNS. Amyotrophic lateral sclerosis, subacute combined degeneration of the spinal cord due to vitamin B12 deficiency, and spinal cord tumor are other conditions that may need to be ruled out.

Management

Conservative treatment helps in relieving symptoms in most patients, and surgical intervention is rarely required. Local heat, cervical traction, gentle ROM exercises, and NSAIDs are tried first. If there is muscle spasm, muscle relaxants and cervical collar are also prescribed. A cervical pillow may help in maintaining proper posture. Surgical intervention is considered for progressive spinal cord compression.

1. **Medications.** NSAIDs and analgesics help relieve pain. Injection of trigger points with local anesthetic gives immediate relief of pain.
2. **Ancillary.** Physical therapy, cervical pillow, and cervical collar are useful measures.
3. **Surgical.** Spinal fusion by an anterior approach will maintain space between the vertebrae and prevent any movement at the offending level. A laminectomy with posterior decompression is performed for spinal stenosis and progressive symptoms and signs of cervical myelopathy.

TRIGGER POINTS

Trigger point is a frequent cause of pain in the neck, shoulder, and head. The pain may be referred to a distant part of the body or described as radiating down the arm. It is likely to be confused with many other conditions. No definite pathology has been shown to cause this condition and its existence and management are controversial.

The patient may complain of referred pain in a different area depending on the site of the trigger point. The upper border of the trapezius, cervical paraspinal muscles, small muscles in the suboccipital region, supra- and infraspinatus muscles, and sternomastoid muscle are common sites in the neck and shoulder regions. The **onset** may be spontaneous, with pain that is aggravated by activity. Deep **palpation** over the trigger point reproduces the pain. Passive stretching or active contraction of the affected muscle is also very painful.

There may be more than one trigger point in the same patient. Trigger points may be the only cause of pain, or they may coexist with other conditions such as flexion-extension injury, degenerative disease of the cervical spine, or rheumatoid arthritis. The pain from trigger points in the upper border of the trapezius, supraspinatus, and infraspinatus may be referred to the shoulder, arm, or forearm, whereas that from suboccipital muscles may be referred to the occipital region.

The most effective **treatment** consists of injection with a local **anesthetic** in the tender area. This may be combined with a steroid preparation or needling technique and is followed by local heat and stretching exercises for the specific muscles involved. The injections may be repeated. It is very important for the patient to continue a home program of stretching and aerobic exercises for a prolonged period of time.

TUMORS OF THE SPINE

Primary tumors of the cervical spine are rare. The bone tissue is composed of osteogenic, chondrogenic, and fibrous tissue cells as well as vascular, neural, lipomatous, hematopoietic, and undifferentiated mesenchymal elements. Any of these components may give rise to benign or malignant tumors. Metastatic tumors of bone are much more common than primary tumors. The tumor tissue replaces or displaces normal bone and surrounding soft tissues, inducing pain and possibly neurologic symptoms. Pathologic fracture may occur in the weakened bone.

The most common symptom of a tumor is **pain.** Unfortunately, pain is also the most common symptom of many other nonneoplastic diseases of the spine. However, pain caused by neoplasia is persistent and not relieved by rest. It may be worse at night. Age at onset of symptoms helps in distinguishing possible cause. Tenderness over the spinous process of the involved vertebra, muscle spasm, limitation of ROM, or deformity should be looked for on physical examination. Detailed neurologic examination may also help in localizing the problem.

THORACIC OUTLET SYNDROME

Thoracic outlet syndrome is also called cervical rib syndrome, costoclavicular syndrome, scalenus anticus syndrome, and hyperabduction syndrome. The clinical presentation of all these syndromes is very similar, even though their pathology may differ. The complex of symptoms and signs is caused by compression of the neurovascular bundle at the outlet of the thoracic cage. The entire bundle containing the subclavian artery, vein, and the lower trunk of the brachial plexus or its individual components may be involved.

Anatomy

The brachial plexus descends from the cervical vertebrae as nerve roots. They merge into trunks and cords and ultimately form peripheral nerves. The neurovascular bundle emerges through a triangle formed by the scalenus anterior muscle, scalenus medius muscle, and first rib (Fig. 12–11). It passes behind the scalenus anterior muscle and over the first rib. A cervical rib is an extra rib arising from the seventh cervical vertebra. Sometimes, instead of a rib, there may be a fibrous ligament extending from the transverse process of C7 to the first rib. Presence of a cervical rib pushes the neurovascular bundle upward and increases the chances of symptoms due to compression (Fig. 12–12). Further down the course, the axillary artery surrounded by medial, lateral, and posterior cords of brachial plexus passes behind the pectoralis minor muscle and below the coracoid process of the scapula.

Pathology

The lower trunk of the brachial plexus is usually affected. Because compression is intermittent, there may be no neurologic deficit on physical examination. Symptoms are limited to the seventh and eighth cervical nerve root distribution. The subclavian artery may show a poststenotic dilatation or aneurysm formation distal to the site of compression. Small blood clots may form in the dilated portion of the artery, leading to embolic phenomena in the fingertips.

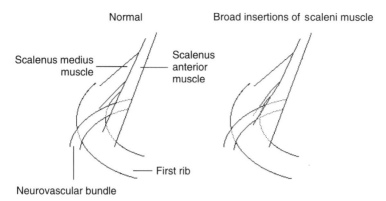

Fig. 12–11   The subclavian artery, subclavian vein, and brachial plexus are within a triangle formed by the first rib, scalenus anterior muscle, and scalenus medius muscle. If the insertions of these muscles are broad, the triangular space is narrowed, and the neurovascular bundle may be compressed.

Different mechanisms may compress the lower trunk of the brachial plexus and/or the subclavian artery. Drooping of the shoulders in middle-aged females because of poor posture pulls the neurovascular structures down against the cervical or first rib (Fig. 12–13). Abnormal configuration of the scalenus medius or anticus muscle near their insertion in the first rib may narrow the triangle through which these structures pass (Fig. 12–11). Carcinoma of the upper lobe of lung can involve the same structures and cause similar symptoms (Pancoast's tumor). Full abduction of the upper extremity may cause compression of the neurovascular structures here (Fig. 12–14), which is called the pectoralis minor syndrome or hyperabduction syndrome.

History

Thoracic outlet syndrome is more common in young and middle-aged women. The onset is usually very gradual. Symptoms depend on whether the nerves or blood vessels are compressed. Nerve compression symptoms are more common and include tingling and numbness of the little finger, medial aspect of the hand, and forearm that may wake the patient from sleep. Occasionally, the symptoms are brought on by carrying something or maintaining certain positions of the arm for prolonged times. The paresthesias are worse at night. Weakness of the small muscles of the hand may be seen in more severe cases. Vascular symptoms include coldness and discoloration of fingertips or Raynaud's phenomena.

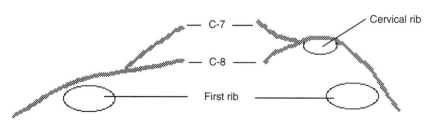

Fig. 12–12   Presence of a cervical rib may stretch the lower trunk of the brachial plexus and lead to thoracic outlet syndrome.

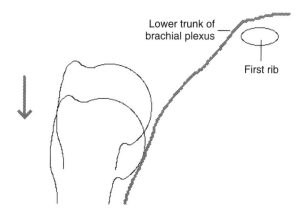

Fig. 12–13 Drooping shoulder because of poor posture may stretch the lower trunk of the brachial plexus over the first rib.

Physical Examination

1. **Inspection.** The patient may present with drooping shoulders. Atrophy of the small muscles of the hand or gangrene of fingertips may be seen in late cases.
2. **Palpation.** A cervical rib may be rarely palpated in the lower anterior part of the neck. Poststenotic dilatation of the subclavian artery, if large enough, may be palpable.
3. **Special tests**
   a. On auscultation, a **bruit** may be heard over the subclavian artery.
   b. **Adson maneuver** tests for arterial occlusion by the scalenus anterior muscle. The patient hyperextends the neck, turns the head to the side of the paresthesia, takes a deep breath, and holds it. The arm is held at the patient's side, and the radial pulse is palpated bilaterally. The radial pulse is occluded on the side toward which the head is turned. This maneuver may reproduce paresthesias in the hand.
4. **Intermittent claudication test.** The patient is asked to raise her arms above the head and flex and extend her fingers quickly. A patient with thoracic outlet syndrome is not able to continue this activity for a minute.

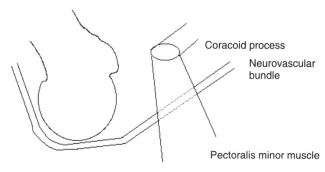

Fig. 12–14 Abduction of shoulder may stretch the brachial plexus and cause thoracic outlet syndrome.

Differential Diagnoses

1. **Ulnar neuropathy** at the elbow may present with tingling and numbness of the little finger and weakness of interossei and lumbrical muscles. These may be worse at night. Ulnar neuropathy is much more common than thoracic outlet syndrome and should be ruled out by electromyography and nerve conduction tests.
2. **Cervical eighth radiculopathy** usually starts with pain and paresthesias in the medial forearm and hand. There may be some pain and stiffness of the neck. Movements of the neck may aggravate pain. Electromyography and nerve conduction tests help in localizing this problem.

Investigations

1. **Plain x-rays** may show a cervical rib or a large transverse process of the seventh cervical vertebra. An old fracture of the clavicle with large callus or malunion can also cause thoracic outlet syndrome.
2. **Electromyography** and **nerve conduction test** are useful in localizing ulnar neuropathy and cervical radiculopathy.
3. **MRI** can help in confirming cervical rib, fibrous band, and other anomalies in the region.

Management

Most patients get better with **conservative treatment.** The patient should be given instructions in how to improve sitting, standing, and walking posture and how to correct drooping shoulders. Many patients with thoracic outlet syndrome are middle-aged with dorsal kyphosis and weak shoulder girdle muscles. Exercises to strengthen these muscles and patient education may be all that is necessary. Patients whose symptoms are brought on by abduction of arms should be asked to avoid those activities. **Surgical treatment** is considered when conservative measures fail or when the patient has evidence of embolic phenomena.

Bibliography

1. Bland JH: Disorders of the Cervical Spine. Philadelphia, W.B. Saunders Co., 1987.
2. Carroll C, MacAfee PC, Riley LH: "Whiplash" injuries and how to treat them. J Musculoskel Med 9(6):97–114, 1992.
3. Fischer AA: Diagnosis and management of chronic pain in physical medicine and rehabilitation. In Ruskin AP (ed): Current Therapy in Physiatry. Philadelphia, W.B. Saunders Co., 1984, pp 123–145.
4. Fischer AA: Local injections in pain management. Phys Med Rehabil Clin North AM 6:851–870, 1995.
5. Goodman BW: Neck pain. Prim Care 15:689–708, 1988.
6. Hardin JG: Complications of cervical arthritis. Postgrad Med 91(4):309–318, 1992.
7. Herkowitz HN: The surgical management of cervical radiculopathy and myelopathy. Clin Orthop 239:94–108, 1989.
8. Lipson SJ: Rheumatoid arthritis in the cervical spine. Clin Orthop 239:121–127, 1989.
9. MacDonald D: Sternomastoid tumor and muscular torticollis. J Bone Joint Surg 51-B:432–443, 1969.
10. Maricic MJ, Gall EP: Cervical arthritis: Which therapy for your patient. J Musculoskel Med 6(10):66–77, 1989.
11. Pedowitz RA, Garfin SR, Roberts WA, White AA: Evaluating the causes of neck, shoulder, and arm pain. J Musculoskel Med 5(6):61–74, 1988.
12. Sartoris DJ, Resnik D: What radiology reveals about painful neck. J Musculoskel Med 5(10):52–71, 1988.
13. Teasell RW, Shapiro AP (eds): Cervical flexion-extension/whiplash injuries. Spine State Art Rev 7:329–570, 1993.
14. Thorne RP, Curd JG: A systematic approach to disorders of cervical spine. Hosp Pract 28(6):49–58, 15, 1993.

13

Thoracic Spine and Chest Wall

Arun J. Mehta, M.B., F.R.C.P.C.

Pain in the chest immediately brings to mind cardiac and pulmonary causes, such as myocardial infarction or pneumonia. However, in > 10% of patients, it is due to musculoskeletal problems. Sometimes, it may be due to more than one condition. Since cardiac and pulmonary causes can be life-threatening, they need to be ruled out. Pain also may be referred from the shoulder or cervical or thoracic spine.

Differential Diagnosis

Spine
1. **Osteoporosis.** Compression fracture usually affects the lower thoracic and upper lumbar vertebrae. The patient gives a history of a fall with sudden onset of severe pain.
2. **Metastasis** to the spine can give rise to severe pain, which may be worse at night.
3. **Ankylosing spondylitis** occurs in young adults and starts as low back pain. It involves the thoracic spine later.
4. **Infection. Osteomyelitis** of the spine should be suspected in intravenous drug users.

Spinal nerves
1. **Herpes zoster** can give rise to pain and skin eruption along the affected nerve root.
2. **Radiculopathy** is not very common in the thoracic region but may occur as a result of metastatic lesions of the spine.

Ribs
1. **Fracture** of the ribs is common in the elderly, and injury due to falls is the common cause of it.
2. **Metastasis** from breast or lung carcinoma may involve the ribs.

Myofascial pain syndromes
1. **Fibromyalgia.** The patient presents with pain over the anterior aspect of the chest wall. A tender point may be palpable in the pectoral muscle near the costochondral junction. It may or may not be associated with other tender points.
2. **Overuse syndromes** of pectoral muscles can cause chest pain.
3. **Precordial catch syndrome** is characterized by sudden, sharp, severe pain in the precordial region. It is aggravated by deep breathing.

Costal cartilage

1. **Costochondritis** is also known as anterior chest wall syndrome, parasternal costodynia, and costosternal syndrome. The patient complains of pain over the costal cartilage, and the whole cartilage is tender. However, unlike Tietze's syndrome, there is no swelling. Costochondritis may be associated with coronary artery disease.
2. **Tietze's syndrome** is a rare disease of the costochondral junction. The patient presents with a painful swelling in this region. It usually affects the second or third costochondral junction, which is tender. There are exacerbations and remissions of signs and symptoms. Treatment of this self-limiting disease is symptomatic with NSAIDs and local heat.

Sternoclavicular joint

1. **Degenerative joint disease** may cause localized pain, tenderness, and swelling over the joint.
2. **Infection** may be due to gonococci or pseudomonas.
3. **Inflammatory arthritis. Rheumatoid arthritis** or ankylosing spondylitis can affect this joint.

Other

1. **Referred pain.** Pain due to cervical spondylosis of the lower cervical vertebrae is usually felt in the interscapular region.

Anatomy

The thoracic cage is formed by 12 thoracic vertebrae, 12 pairs of ribs, and the sternum. These bones protect important organs such as the heart and lungs in the thorax and liver and spleen in the abdomen. They also provide attachment for the muscles involved in respiration. The spinous process of the seventh cervical vertebra is the most prominent one at the base of the neck. The medial end of the spine of the scapula is at the same level as the tip of the spinous process of the third thoracic vertebra (Fig. 13–1). These two landmarks help in localizing different thoracic vertebrae.

The head of each rib articulates with the vertebral body by a synovial joint. There is another synovial joint between the tubercle of the rib and the transverse process of the corresponding vertebra (Fig. 13–2). These joints can be involved in ankylosing spondylitis,

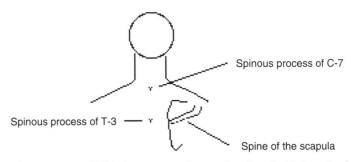

Spinous process of C-7

Spinous process of T-3

Spine of the scapula

Fig. 13–1   The spinous process of C7 is the most prominent and easily palpable bony landmark. The tip of the spinous process of T3 is at the level of the medial end of the scapular spine.

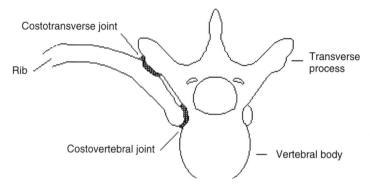

Costotransverse joint

Rib

Transverse process

Costovertebral joint

Vertebral body

Fig. 13–2   There are two synovial joints between each rib and thoracic vertebra.

which restricts chest expansion. The ribs 1 through 7 articulate with the sternum through costal cartilages. The second costal cartilage articulates with the sternum at the manubriosternal angle. Since this is palpable as a subcutaneous ridge, it is easy to identify the second costal cartilage. The costal cartilages of the 8th, 9th, and 10th ribs join the cartilage of the rib above. The ends of the 11th and 12th ribs are free (floating ribs).

The medial end of the clavicle articulates with the sternum at the sternoclavicular joint. This joint is a synovial joint with an intra-articular disc. The pectoralis major muscle arises from the medial end of the clavicle, sternum, and upper six costal cartilages. It is a large flat muscle that covers the upper part of the front of the chest. It is deep to the breast and is not easily palpable in females. It inserts into the proximal humerus and adducts the arm.

History
If pain started after an injury, details of "how, when, and where" about the injury should be elicited. Pain related to overuse syndromes develop over a period of time. Pain arising from the chest wall muscles, ribs, or pleura is aggravated by deep breathing. If it is due to cervical spine or shoulder pathology, then it is aggravated by movements of the involved structures.

Physical Examination
The cervical and thoracic spine, rib cage, costal cartilages, muscles covering the chest wall, clavicle, sternoclavicular joint, and neck should be examined for the cause of pain. Routine examination of the heart and lungs is carried out *without exception*.
1. **Inspection.** The **spine** is observed from the back and sides for any **deformity** or swelling. Rib hump of structural scoliosis becomes prominent when the patient bends forward. Any swelling or deformity in connection with the sternoclavicular joint or sternum is seen from the front.
2. **Palpation.** Localized tenderness is the most helpful sign in diagnosing musculoskeletal problems.
3. **Range of motion.** Tests for ROM of the thoracic spine, cervical spine, and shoulder and chest expansion are performed. Pain on movements or limitation of ROM is noted.
4. **Special Tests.** Percussion over the spinous processes is tender when there is vertebral pathology.

Investigations
X-rays of the chest may not show abnormalities of the thoracic spine, ribs, or sternum. Special views of these structures may be necessary.

FRACTURE OF THE RIBS

Rib fracture is a common painful condition of the chest wall. Most patients do not need any special treatment, except for those who have associated injury to an internal organ.

Mechanism of Injury
Direct trauma to the chest wall fractures the rib at the site of injury. **Indirect injury,** e.g., crush injuries, give rise to fractures near the angle of the rib. This can happen during cardiopulmonary resuscitation or in major car accidents. Pathologic fractures can occur in metastatic disease, osteoporosis, or Paget's disease.

History
The patient complains of pain at the fracture site. It is aggravated by breathing and movements.

Physical Examination
1. **Palpation.** There is localized **tenderness** at the site of the fracture. **Surgical emphysema** is a typical crepitus felt due to air in the subcutaneous tissue. It indicates leakage of air from the lung and needs special attention.
2. **Special tests** are carried out to check for injury to internal organs, such as the heart, lungs, liver, or spleen. Ribs in children are very resilient and do not break easily. Children may have an internal organ injury without a rib fracture.

Investigations
Fractures of ribs may be missed on plain chest x-rays. A special view for the ribs may be necessary.

Course
Rib fractures heal without any immobilization in 6–8 weeks. The muscles attached to the ribs usually anchor them well. However, when there is a loose segment of chest wall because of fractures at two sites or on both sides (**flail chest**), it needs to be immobilized by external fixation.

Complications
Pneumothorax, hemothorax, and rupture of the liver or spleen can occur due to fracture of the ribs.

Management
Uncomplicated fractures of the ribs are treated with **analgesics.** If pain is very severe, local injection of long-acting local anesthetic is given to the intercostal nerve. Breathing exercises are started to prevent pneumonia as soon as the patient can tolerate them.

FRACTURES OF THE VERTEBRAE

Vertebral fractures are common in the lower thoracic and upper lumbar regions. Upper and mid-thoracic regions are more stable and less prone to fractures because of the ribs, shape of the articular processes, and direction of facets.

Anatomy

The thoracic spine is much more stable and less mobile than the cervical or lumbar spine. The rib cage and articular processes provide this additional stability. Articular facets in the thoracic spine are in the coronal plane and restrict rotational movements. Ribs restrict flexion and extension. Fracture-dislocations in the upper and mid-thoracic region therefore are rare. The supraspinous and interspinous ligaments, articular capsule of the facet joints, intervertebral discs, and other ligaments help in maintaining stability in all the regions of the spine.

Mechanism of Injury

A fall from height with landing on the feet or buttocks flexes the spine. The force compresses the anterior part of the vertebra and leads to **compression fracture** (Fig. 13–3). This fracture can occur after minimal trauma in the osteoporotic spine. Sometimes, the anterior and posterior surfaces of a vertebra are compressed to the same extent, especially in metastatic disease of the spine. (Fig. 13–4) In a third type of injury, the spine remains straight, instead of flexing, and pushes the disc into the body of the vertebra above or below; the vertebral body explodes into small fragments that get displaced in all directions.

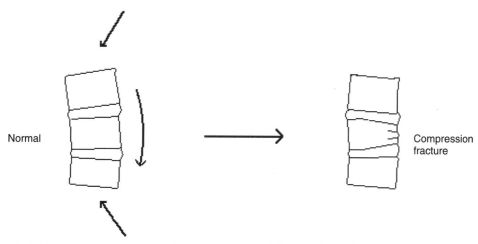

Normal

Compression fracture

Fig. 13–3 Compression fracture. After a fall from a height, the spine is forcefully flexed when we land on our feet or buttocks. The anterior part of the vertebral body is crushed, resulting in a compression fracture.

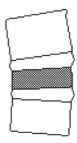

Fig. 13–4 When the whole vertebral body is compressed, it looks denser than the normal vertebra. This type of compression fracture is sometimes seen in metastatic disease of the spine.

This is called the **burst fracture** (Fig. 13–5). More violent injuries, as in a car accident, tear ligaments and fracture parts of vertebrae, resulting in **fracture-dislocation.** The mechanism of injury is a combination of flexion and rotation of the spine.

Classification of Fractures
1. **Compression fracture.** Height of the anterior part of the vertebral body is reduced in comparison with the posterior. This fracture frequently happens in the osteoporotic spine. The posterior ligaments and articular processes remain intact. Compression fractures are **usually stable** and can be treated conservatively in most patients. Sometimes, the whole body is compressed equally, as occurs in metastatic disease.
2. **Burst fracture** is not very common. One or more fragments may compress the spinal cord or cauda equina causing neurologic deficit. This type of fracture **may be unstable.**
3. **Fracture-dislocations** are **unstable** and should be treated by a specialist. There is displacement of the body and, at times, articular processes. Rarely, the displacement may not show up on the x-rays because it is reduced without any treatment. Fracture-dislocation may require open reduction and internal fixation with fusion of the spine.

History
The mechanism of injury gives an important clue as to the type of fracture that is sustained. There is severe pain in the region of the fracture, although fracture of an osteoporotic spine sometimes may give rise to very little pain. The patient is unable to sit or walk. It is very important to know if the patient has tingling, numbness, difficulty in moving any of the extremities, or loss of control of the bladder or bowel.

Physical Examination
1. **Inspection.** Abrasions and bruises indicate the direction and severity of forces involved. Visible deformity suggests a displaced, unstable fracture.
2. **Palpation.** Tenderness over the spinous processes helps localize the fracture. Normally, the interspinous ligament feels firm on palpation. When this ligament is torn, the interspinous space feels softer. This suggests that stability of the spine may be compromised.
3. **Range of motion** tests are **not** done when a fracture is suspected, for fear of damaging the spinal cord or cauda equina.
4. **Special tests.** A detailed neurologic exam is carried out.

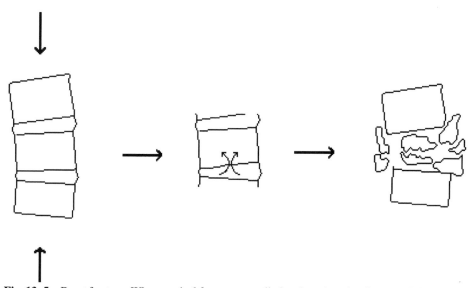

Fig. 13–5 Burst fracture. When vertical forces are applied to the spine, the disc material is pushed into the vertebral body. The vertebral body may burst into multiple fragments.

Investigations

1. **Plain x-rays** confirm the diagnosis of fracture, identify the type of fracture, and help in determining the course of treatment.
2. **CT scan** gives more detailed information about displaced bone fragments. This knowledge is very helpful in burst fractures and fracture-dislocations before deciding on surgical intervention to relieve pressure on neurologic structures.

Complications

The most dreaded complication of fracture of the spine is injury to the spinal cord or cauda equina.

Management

Prevention of neurologic complications is the most important goal, and **determination of spinal stability** is the first step in the management process. Treatment of stable fractures is simple—bedrest and analgesics. The patient's activities are increased as tolerated. He or she is allowed to sit up, transfer from bed to chair, and start ambulating with a therapist. If pain and muscle spasms are very severe, a brace to support the spine may be ordered. Unstable fractures require the immediate attention of a specialist team.

HERPES ZOSTER

Herpes zoster (**shingles**) is an acute viral infection of the dorsal root ganglion, with pain and skin vesicles in the distribution of a cutaneous nerve. Thoracic nerves are most commonly affected.

Etiology

The virus that causes chickenpox (**varicella**) also causes herpes zoster—hence the name varicella-zoster virus.

Pathology

The affected nerve cells in the dorsal root ganglion and dorsal horn of the spinal cord undergo necrosis. Some of the sensory nerves show demyelination. There may be partial recovery later. No unique pathologic features are seen in patients with postherpetic neuralgia to explain their chronic pain.

History

People over age 50 years are commonly affected. There may be some prodromal symptoms, like fever and malaise for a few days before the pain starts. **Pain** is constant, severe, and burning and is felt along the affected nerve root. It is aggravated by light touch, and the patient may not be able to tolerate any clothes over that area.

Physical Examination

1. **Inspection.** Typical rash (**vesicles**) appears 4 or 5 days after the onset of pain. It is restricted to the skin supplied by the involved nerve root. A scab forms over the vesicles in 4–7 days.
2. **Palpation.** The affected area is painful even to light touch (**hyperesthesia**).

Differential Diagnoses

It may be difficult to rule out cardiac, pulmonary, or abdominal causes of pain before the rash appears. Sometimes, herpes simplex infection may give similar rash. Cultures for viral studies help to distinguish the two.

Course/Complications

The pain usually subsides without any specific treatment. In about 10% of the patients, especially the elderly, pain persists after the rash disappears, resulting in **postherpetic neuralgia.**

Management

Treatment is symptomatic. Antiviral agents are being studied to see if they can reduce the pain and prevent complications. **Prednisone,** 50–60 mg/day, may be given. It should be tapered off in 2–3 weeks. **Analgesics** and a cold, moist pack over the painful area as well as **transcutaneous electrical stimulation** (TENS) may partially relieve pain. The affected nerve may be injected with a long-acting local anesthetic to relieve pain.

COSTOCHONDRITIS

Costochondritis and Tietze's syndrome are often confused. Some even use these terms to mean the same condition. Costochondritis, however, produces no swelling and is more common than Tietze's syndrome. Costochondritis is also known as costosternal syndrome, anterior chest wall syndrome, or parasternal chondrodynia. Its exact etiology is not known. The patient complains of pain in the region of the costochondral junction. The pain may become severe and more diffuse. The disorder may develop following some injury to the chest wall, or it may be associated with other rheumatic disease. The affected costal cartilage is tender to palpation. In Tietze's syndrome, a tender swelling of the costal cartilage is palpable. The pain may be aggravated by deep breathing or coughing.

Conservative treatment with **NSAIDs** and local **heat** usually relieves the symptoms. The course of these diseases is without any complications, and they are self-limiting.

KYPHOSIS

Increased anteroposterior curvature of the spine with posterior convexity is a common deformity. It may be due to:
1. Poor posture
2. Senile osteoporosis
3. Compression fractures of the vertebral bodies
4. Idiopathic origin (e.g., adolescent kyphosis)
5. Metastasis
6. Tuberculosis of the spine

Only adolescent kyphosis will be covered here because compression fracture is described on page 165 and osteoporosis is dealt with in Chapter 6. Tuberculosis of the spine is uncommon in the United States.

Adolescent Kyphosis
A kyphotic deformity may develop during adolescence. It is also known as Scheuermann's disease, epiphysitis of the spine, adolescent vertebral osteochondritis, and juvenile round back. The symptoms are minimal with x-ray changes in the epiphyseal plate of the vertebrae. The etiology is unknown.

Anatomy
The vertebral body develops by three ossification centers—one in the center of the vertebral body and two at either end. The ossification centers at the superior and inferior ends of the vertebral body are called annular or ring epiphyses.

Pathology
There is damage to the ring epiphysis of the vertebral body, which is more marked anteriorly than posteriorly. This damage interferes with growth of the anterior part of the vertebral body, leading to wedging of the vertebral body and exaggeration of normal kyphosis (anterior concavity) in the thoracic region. Thoracic vertebrae are most commonly involved. The intervertebral disc protrudes into the vertebral bodies through the vertebral endplates. There is reactive sclerosis around the protruded disc material. These changes are described as **Schmorl's nodes** on x-rays.

History
A 12- to 16-year-old adolescent may present with **pain** in the thoracic region of the back. Later, the pain subsides and the patient may only have **deformity.**

Physical Examination
1. **Inspection** reveals increased backward convexity in the thoracic region. The curvature is smooth and rounded and not angular.
2. **Range of motion.** The deformity is fixed and not corrected by movements.

Differential Diagnoses
1. **Postural kyphosis** can be corrected by voluntary effort, whereas adolescent kyphosis is a fixed deformity.
2. **Compression fracture** occurs in older individuals and is usually secondary to osteoporosis.

Investigations
Plain lateral **x-rays** of the thoracic spine show missing anterior angles of the vertebral bodies. Osteophytes are seen at a later stage.

Management
Rest is recommended during the painful stage of the disease. **Analgesics** and **extension exercises** help relieve pain. A body cast in extension or Milwaukee-type brace may be necessary for severe deformity. Surgical correction is rarely required for very severe and progressive deformity, pain secondary to deformity, or spinal cord involvement.

SCOLIOSIS

The normal spine does not have any lateral curvature (scoliosis).

Etiology
Patients with scoliosis can be divided into two major groups:
1. **Structural scoliosis**—when the shape of the vertebrae is altered. A rib hump becomes prominent on forward flexion in patients with structural scoliosis.
2. **Nonstructural scoliosis**—when the structure of the vertebrae is normal. The scoliosis disappears on forward flexion of the spine.

The vast majority (80–85%) of patients with structural scoliosis have no definite cause (**idiopathic**). Secondary causes, including congenital disease and infection, can be identified to explain the structural scoliosis in a minority of patients, as listed in Table 13–1. Causes of nonstructural scoliosis include poor posture, painful muscle spasm on one side, and leg-length discrepancy.

Pathology
The main curve is described as the **primary curve,** and the curves proximal and distal to it are called **secondary curves.** Sometimes, there are two primary curves. In structural sco-

Table 13–1 Causes of Secondary Structural Scoliosis

Bone	Muscle disease
Congenital hemivertebra	Muscular dystrophy
Vertebral fracture	Arthrogryposis multiplex
Tuberculosis of the spine	Thorax
Neurologic disease	Post pneumonectomy
Cerebral palsy	Miscellaneous
Syringomyelia	Neurofibromatosis
Poliomyelitis	Marfan's syndrome
Spina bifida	

liosis, the vertebral body rotates toward the convexity of the curve. The ribs rotate and are distorted to produce the **rib hump.** Degenerative changes develop early in the disc and facet joints and may give rise to pain.

History
The age at onset of idiopathic adolescent scoliosis is usually around 10–12 years, though it may be seen at any age from early childhood to late adolescence. It is five times more common in females. There is no pain to start with, and the deformity may be noticed by the parents or a health professional on routine physical examination.

Physical Examination
1. **Inspection.** Scoliosis is described by the location of the primary curve as thoracic, thoracolumbar, or lumbar. If the primary thoracolumbar curve is convex toward right side, it is called right thoracolumbar scoliosis. Rib hump becomes more prominent on forward flexion and is seen on the convex side. The levels of shoulders, nipples, and iliac crests are noted on both sides.
2. **Special tests.** Lengths of both lower extremities are measured for any difference. Neurologic exam is done to rule out neuromuscular diseases.

Investigations
Plain x-rays are done to measure the angle of the curvature. Sequential measurements help in determining if the curvature is worsening and will need surgical treatment.

Course
Structural scoliosis tends to get worse as long as the individual is growing. Skeletal growth stops when the epiphysis of the iliac crest unites with the ilium. If scoliosis develops in early childhood, then the deformity has a much longer time to progress and get worse. The later in life the scoliosis appears, the better is the prognosis.

Complications
Severe deformity may lead to respiratory embarrassment. Degenerative arthritis and back pain develop at an earlier age than usual.

Management
Scoliosis is managed by a specialist, usually an orthopedic surgeon. Mild curves ($> 25°$) are followed closely to see if they are worsening. If the curve is worsening, it is treated by a **brace,** e.g., Milwaukee brace. Special exercises are prescribed. Some patients need **spinal fusion** with Harrington rods.

MISCELLANEOUS DISORDERS

Muscles of the chest wall can become painful due to overuse or disease. These and other miscellaneous conditions are included in this chapter.

Overuse Syndromes

Unaccustomed use of muscles of the chest wall, as in weight-lifting or repetitive work such as painting a ceiling, can result in pain. The pain is aggravated by active contraction of the muscle and passive stretching. It is treated with NSAIDs, rest, and local heat.

Fibromyalgia

Fibromyalgia (also known as fibrositis or myofascial pain syndrome) results in chronic recurrent pain in various muscles of the body, including those of the chest wall. The trigger points in the chest wall are found in pectoralis major muscle near the sternum. Fibromyalgia may be precipitated by trauma to the chest wall (e.g., car accident or thoracotomy), cervical spondylosis, or rotator cuff problems. It is treated like any other trigger point. (*See also* Chapter 10.)

Precordial Catch Syndrome

This condition, also known as chest wall twinge syndrome, occurs in healthy young individuals. They experience sudden sharp pain in the precordial region which is aggravated by deep breathing. This condition is of unknown etiology but is self-limiting.

Epidemic Myalgia

Also known as epidemic pleurodynia or Bornholm disease, this disease is due to group B coxsackievirus. The patient experiences sharp lateral chest wall pain which is aggravated by deep breathing and movements. There also is fever, headache, and pharyngitis. Viral cultures from the throat and feces may clinch the diagnosis. Treatment is symptomatic.

Bibliography

1. Calabro JJ, Jeghers H, Miller KA: Classification of anterior chest wall syndromes. JAMA 243:1420–1421, 1980.
2. Keim HA: Spinal deformities: Scoliosis and kyphosis. Clin Symp 41(4):3–32, 1989.
3. Lonstein JE: Adolescent idiopathic scoliosis: Screening and diagnosis. Instructional Course Lect 38:105–113; 1989
4. Sima MA: Evaluation of chest pain. Postgrad Med 91(8):155–164, 1992.
5. Song K, Herring JA: Early recognition and assessment of idiopathic scoliosis. J Musculoskel Med 10(4):63–76, 1993.

14

Lumbosacral Spine

Arun J. Mehta, M.B., F.R.C.P.C.

Pain in the low back is a very frequent complaint. Even though most patients with back pain do get better without active medical intervention, a sympathetic and intelligent approach to the problem may reduce their suffering.

Differential Diagnosis
The following is a classification of causes of pain in the low back:
A. **Soft tissue** (muscles and ligaments)
    1. Trauma
        a. Acute soft tissue strain
        b. Chronic strain
        c. Overuse syndromes
    2. Trigger points
    3. Generalized inflammatory joint disease
        a. Ankylosing spondylitis
        b. Psoriatic and other spondyloarthropathies
B. **Disc**
    1. Degenerative disc disease
    2. Prolapsed disc
C. **Facet joints**
    1. Degenerative joint disease
D. **Spinal canal**
    1. Spinal stenosis
E. **Vertebra**
    1. Osteoporosis
        a. Generalized
        b. Compression fracture
    2. Infection
    3. Metastasis
    4. Spondylolisthesis
F. **Adjacent structures**
    1. Aneurysm of abdominal aorta
    2. Hips (degenerative joint disease)
    3. Pelvic organs

Anatomy

Injury or disease of a range of anatomical structures may give rise to pain (Fig. 14–1).

1. **Ligaments**
   a. Anterior and posterior longitudinal ligaments
   b. Interspinous and supraspinous ligaments
   c. Ligamentum flavum
2. **Muscles.** Injury or spasm secondary to other pathology
3. **Facet joints.** Degenerative joint disease or stretching of the capsule of facet joint due to effusion
4. **Anterior dura mater**
5. **Nerves.** Traction or compression of a nerve is very painful. A nerve root stretched over a protruded intervertebral disc is a good example of this mechanism. Nerves are also very susceptible to ischemia.
6. **Periosteum of the vertebra**

It may be difficult to localize the lesion to any particular anatomical structure. However, every attempt should be made to come to as exact an anatomical and pathologic diagnosis as possible, because certain conditions have definite treatment, e.g., metastatic disease of the spine. As mentioned, there are many structures besides the intervertebral disc that can give rise to back pain. Lesions of the spinal cord do not give rise to pain as a general rule.

Pathology

Prof. Kellgren injected hypertonic saline solution in normal volunteers to determine which structures in the back can give rise to pain. He found that when saline was injected in the superficial tissues, the subject was able to localize the site of injection very well. The deeper the source of pain, the more difficult it became for the subject to pinpoint the involved structure. The pain was felt as a dull, diffuse pain at a distance from the source, but it occurred in the same segmental distribution as the structure injected. Severity of pain determined size of the painful area—the more severe the pain, the wider the distribution. These experiments have shown that radiating pain is not necessarily due to nerve root pathology. When a nerve trunk was injected; intense burning pain was felt in the skin throughout the territory of that nerve.

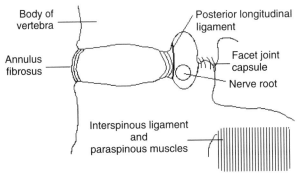

Fig. 14–1 Anatomical structures that may give rise to pain in the back.

History

How did the pain start (**onset**)? Was there any history of injury, overuse, or activity involving bending or twisting of the back? When did the pain start (**duration**)? Were there similar episodes in past? What was the frequency and duration of a typical episode? What is the location of pain? The **site** of maximum pain and the entire area of pain can be marked out in a pain diagram. Does the pain **radiate** to the hip or down the leg? The path of pain and how far down the leg it radiates are noted. Are there any activities or movements that make the pain worse (**aggravating factors**)? Usually, pain due to a herniated disc is made worse by bending forward, sneezing, or sitting and is relieved by rest in bed. Has the patient received any **treatments** for back pain? What was the result of these treatments?

1. **Past illnesses.** Is there any history of malignant tumor, intravenous drug abuse, or major trauma?
2. **Review of systems.** Involvement of other joints may suggest ankylosing spondylitis or rheumatoid arthritis. Chronic back pain may affect vocational and avocational activities. Has the pain affected his or her work or ability to enjoy life or hobbies?

Physical Examination

1. **Inspection.** Observe the patient as he or she walks into the office—the gait, how he or she sits, any expressions, and, if possible, how he or she undresses. Is the spine kept rigid, or are certain movements avoided? How does he untie his shoe laces? Is color of the skin normal? Is there any swelling or a tuft of hair over the lumbosacral region (suggestive of spina bifida occulta)?

    a. **From behind**—Alignment of the spine (abnormal lateral curvature) is observed from behind. Are the shoulders and scapulae level (Fig. 14–2)? Is there a rib hump? The relation of spine with head, neck, iliac crests, dimples of Venus, gluteal folds, and greater trochanters is observed.

    b. **From sides**—Normal spine has a cervical and lumbar lordosis (convex toward front) and dorsal kyphosis (convex posteriorly). These curvatures are observed from the sides.

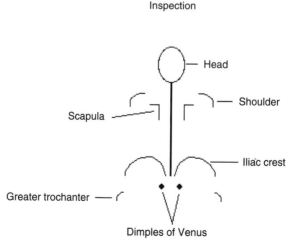

Fig. 14–2 Anatomical landmarks to observe during back examination.

c. **From front**—Head and neck, level of shoulders, anterior superior iliac spines, and relation of the trunk to lower extremities (lateral list) can be seen from the front.
2. **Palpation.** Try to visualize the structures you are palpating, including the spinous processes, supraspinous ligaments, and paraspinous muscles. Is one of the superficial structures **tender,** or is it a deep one? Renal angles, sacroiliac joints, coccyx, and greater trochanters are palpated. Deep palpation over a trigger point may reproduce a patient's pain. The paraspinous muscles feel more firm than usual when there is **muscle spasm.** **Spinous processes** are palpated for alignment and their relation to iliac crests and rib cage.

Facet joints between L4–5 can be palpated at the level of iliac crests about 1 inch lateral to the midline, whereas those between L5–S1 are about 1 inch lower and those at L3–4 are 1 inch above that level (Fig. 14–3). Deep palpation at these levels may reveal tenderness due to degenerative facet joint disease.

The **sciatic nerve** runs down between the ischial tuberosity and the greater trochanter. It can be palpated there. Tenderness over the sciatic nerve indicates irritation of one of the nerve roots forming the nerve.
3. **Range of motion**
   a. **Flexion** or forward bending is tested with the knees straight. Most of this complex movement takes place at the hips. Maximum flexion in the spine takes place at the lumbosacral junction (L5–S1) and (L4–5) levels. The range can be measured approximately by the distance from the fingertips to the floor or, more accurately, by inclinometer held over the sacrum and L1 in upright and bent positions.
   b. **Extension**—The patient is asked to bend backward while the pelvis is supported.
   c. **Lateral flexions**–Right and left lateral flexion is tested by stabilizing the pelvis and asking the patient to bend sideways. The distance between the fingertips and floor is measured. There is always an element of rotation involved in lateral flexion.
   d. **Rotation**—Right and left lateral rotation is measured after fixing the pelvis so that anterior superior iliac spines are facing straight ahead and then asking the patient to twist to the left or right side. Rotation is measured by the angle the plane of the shoulders make with the plane of the anterior superior iliac spines.
4. **Special tests**
   a. **Lower extremity**
      i. **Straight leg raising test**—With the patient supine, one leg is raised from the hor-

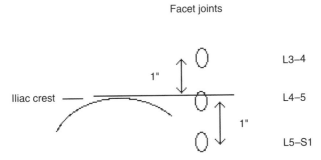

Facet joints

Fig. 14–3   The facet joints between L4–5 are at the level of highest point of the iliac crest, about 1 inch lateral to the midline. The facet joints between L3–4 are 1 inch proximal to this level, and facet joints between L5–S1 are 1 inch distal.

izontal position by the examiner. The heel is supported and the knee is kept straight. The angle between the leg and the horizontal is measured when the patient begins to complain of pain. Normally, one is able to raise the leg up to 70°–80°. The location and radiation of pain are also noted. Pain in back of the knee is usually due to tight hamstrings. With the leg in the raised position, the patient's foot is dorsiflexed to put more stretch on the sciatic nerve. Pain radiating along the sciatic nerve indicates irritation of one of its nerve roots.

ii. **Cross leg (or well leg) straight leg raising test**—The asymptomatic lower extremity is raised in the same manner as in straight leg raising test. The test is positive if the patient complains of pain in the back or in the involved extremity (opposite to the one being raised). Sometimes, in a central disc protrusion, raising the affected side gives rise to pain in the unaffected leg.

iii. **Leg lengths** are measured to rule out significant discrepancies between the lower extremities.

b. **Sacroiliac joints.** The sacroiliac region is palpated for tenderness. The examiner's hands are placed on the outer aspect of the patient's anterior superior iliac spines, and pressure is exerted to bring them together. Pain in the sacroiliac region indicates pathology in the sacroiliac joint.

c. **Neurologic exam.** Appropriate sensory, motor, and reflex examination is carried out depending on the differential diagnoses being considered.

d. **Hip joints.** Osteoarthritis of the hip or trochanteric bursitis may give rise to pain in the back or knee or radiating pain in the lower extremity. Tenderness just posterior to the greater trochanter suggests trochanteric bursitis. ROM of the hips should be tested for any limitations.

e. The **abdomen** is palpated for any intra-abdominal pathology, such as aneurysm of the aorta or tumor of an intra-abdominal organ.

f. **Rectal exam** for enlarged prostate or rectal carcinoma may suggest a cause for back pain.

Investigations

The diagnosis of a herniated disc can be arrived at in most patients on the basis of a good history and physical examination.

1. **Plain x-rays** of the lumbosacral spine are done for most back pain patients. However, they are useful in relatively few conditions, such as bony metastasis, osteoporosis, compression fracture of a vertebral body, ankylosing spondylitis and spondylolisthesis. Plain x-rays do show changes of degenerative disc and facet joint disease, but these conditions are so common after the fifth decade that x-rays are not very useful in confirming the structure giving rise to pain in a patient.

2. **Blood tests** are done if there is need to rule out rheumatoid arthritis, ankylosing spondylitis, or infection of the spine.

3. **Electromyography** is carried out if nerve root compression is suspected. It is a relatively innocuous investigation that helps confirm and localize the lesion. It does not help in determining whether it is a disc that is pressing on the nerve root or which disc is protruding.

4. **CT scan** is useful in confirming the diagnosis of spinal stenosis and narrowing of the lateral recess. It shows the architecture of bone well and helps in difficult cases of spinal fracture.

5. **MRI** shows soft tissue pathology very well and is useful in disc herniations and neoplastic and infectious diseases of the spine. Like CT, it also shows changes in the spinal canal dimensions.

6. **Myelogram** helps in anatomical localization of herniated discs before operation. It may be ordered when conservative measures have failed to relieve pain, and operative treatment is being considered or a tumor is suspected. Many specialists now rely on MRI more than myelography because it is noninvasive.
7. **Bone scan** is ordered to rule out metastasis or infection. However, it may be positive in degenerative disc or joint diseases or in inflammatory spondyloarthropathies.

Management
General principles of management of back pain are discussed here. Treatment of specific problems is dealt with in appropriate chapters. **Conservative treatment** should be the main emphasis in the management of any patient with back pain, because it helps relieve the pain in 70% of the patients within 3 weeks and in 90% within 2 months.

   Goals of conservative treatment are to:
   1. Relieve pain
   2. Improve mobility
   3. Prevent recurrence
1. **Bedrest.** There is debate about the role of bedrest in the treatment of back pain. It should be prescribed for patients with severe pain and muscle spasm. The patient lies in the most comfortable position, which is usually with hips and knees flexed, on a firm mattress. Pillows can be used to support the knees. Rest must be continuous with bathroom privileges. The length of bedrest depends on the severity of the symptoms and signs. Other measures, such as analgesics, muscle relaxants, local heat, and traction, may be used with bedrest. Gradually increasing activities are permitted as muscle spasm and pain begin to subside. If these symptoms recur with resumption of activities or if bedrest fails to relieve symptoms within a reasonable time, the diagnosis and management plan should be reconsidered.
2. **Analgesics.** An **NSAID** is selected to help control pain and inflammation. Preparations with codeine may be added for severe pain during initial stages. Uncontrolled severe pain may require a parenteral analgesic. Analgesics are more effective if given on a regular basis rather than as needed (prn).
3. **Muscle relaxants.** Skeletal muscle relaxants on their own or combined with an analgesic help overcome muscle spasm in the initial stages.
4. **Massage** with or without salicylic acid derivatives also helps relieve pain.
5. **Corticosteroids.** A short course with tapering dose is used by some physicians to reduce inflammation.
6. **Local heat** in the form of a heating pad or moist hot packs 3 or 4 times a day for 20–30 minutes at a time relieves pain temporarily and reduces muscle spasm. Putting hot packs on a patient in the prone position may aggravate pain because of increased lordosis. Other forms of heat, e.g., shortwave diathermy or ultrasound, can also be used.
8. **Traction** helps by:
   a. Reducing load on the discs
   b. Overcoming muscle spasm
   c. Stretching ligaments and joint capsule
   Indications
   a. Acute low back pain with or without radiculopathy
   b. Chronic recurrent low back pain
   Contraindications
   a. Large central disc herniation with cauda equina or cord lesion
   b. Metastatic disease of the spine

   c. Infection of the disc or vertebral body

   d. Severe osteoporosis

   e. Recent fracture of the spine

   f. Pregnancy, especially last trimester

   g. Aortic aneurysm or abdominal tumor

    Traction is discontinued if the pain gets worse or new neurologic deficits appear. It may be used up to 2–3 weeks or until the pain is reduced to a reasonable level. Improvements in straight leg raising test or muscle spasm are other indicators.

9. **Exercises** to increase mobility are prescribed initially and are followed by exercises to increase strength and improve posture. They are prescribed after the acute stage of severe pain and muscle spasm is over or for milder attacks. During the acute stage, symptoms may be aggravated by exercises. Exercises should be continued for maintenance of benefits.

10. **Local injections.** Trigger points may coexist with other pathology or may be the main reason for back pain. Treatment of this condition is dealt with elsewhere (*see* Chapter 10). Local injection of an anesthetic should be tried to rule out a trigger point.

11. **Epidural injection** of local anesthetic and steroid may be given when bedrest and analgesics have failed to relieve back pain within a reasonable time or if there is recurrence of pain after laminectomy. It is contraindicated if the patient is allergic or when there is skin infection in the low back.

12. **Intradiscal injection of chymopapain** is a very specialized procedure. Because of serious potential complications, such as anaphylactic shock and paraplegia, very few centers provide this treatment.

13. **Patient education** regarding back protection and pain management forms a very important part in returning to work and improving quality of life. This education may be provided by the physician, physical or occupational therapist, nurse, or other suitable person. Commercially available programs come in various formats, e.g., reading materials, slides and tapes, and video cassettes. The patient is advised to use a firm mattress. Good lumbar support while sitting for prolonged periods (e.g., while driving or typing) and increasing the inclination of the chair backrest by 10°–20° beyond the vertical reduces strain on the back muscles. An armrest is used when getting up from a chair. Movements requiring flexion and rotation of the spine frequently precipitate acute back pain because of high loads on the lower lumbar discs. The patient is advised to avoid these movements, especially while lifting. He is taught proper lifting techniques with legs bent and load as close to the body as possible. Exercises to maintain strength and flexibility of the back and strength of the abdominal muscles are very important to the program.

14. **Corsets and braces** help by controlling the range of movements of the back and by taking some of the load off the spine. Many different types of braces are available. They should be considered for following conditions:

   a. Postoperative period—After laminectomy, when the patient is beginning to increase activities.

   b. Degenerative disc disease—When other conservative measures have failed to control the pain.

   c. After an acute episode of low back pain—During the recovery phase, when the patient is beginning to increase activities.

   d. Compression fracture of the spine

   e. Malignant disease of the spine

15. **Surgical.** Removal of the offending disc is considered when:

   a. Conservative treatment fails to relieve severe pain.

   b. Bladder and/or bowel function is affected (surgical emergency).
   c. Worsening of neurologic status, e.g., acute paresis of toe extensors
   d. Recurrent attacks of back pain which interferes with work

Best results are obtained if a herniated disc is found at the time of operation and if surgery is performed within 3 months of onset of sciatica. Chances of surgery failing to relieve pain are 80% if no protruded disc is found. A second operation at the same level may relieve pain in only in 25% of cases.

Referral

The patient is referred to a specialist when:
1. **Very severe pain** not relieved by ordinary analgesics within a reasonable time. Depending upon the severity, refer immediately or in a few days.
2. **Pain worse at night** or on lying down, when infection or malignancy is suspected.
3. Failure of conservative treatment

INTERVERTEBRAL DISC DISEASE

The disc begins to degenerate early in life. Degenerative disc disease and prolapsed intervertebral discs are common causes of low back pain. All low back pains are not due to prolapsed disc, and not all prolapsed discs need to be removed by operation. Most patients with back pain due to prolapsed intervertebral discs can be treated successfully by conservative means.

Anatomy

The intervertebral disc consists of two parts (Fig. 14–4):
1. **Annulus fibrosus** is the thick ring of fibrous tissue surrounding the nucleus pulposus.
2. **Nucleus pulposus** is the inner gelatinous center.

   The cartilaginous endplates of vertebrae above and below the disc form its upper and lower boundaries. Very few nerve terminals are found in the disc. However, the peripheral part of the annulus and surrounding ligaments are well supplied by nerves and probably play an important role in the pain sensation.

Pathology

Nutrition of the disc depends on diffusion. This diffusion is facilitated by movements of the spine and alternate loading and unloading of the disc. Fluids and metabolites are pushed out when pressure on the disc increases, whereas the reverse process takes place when the

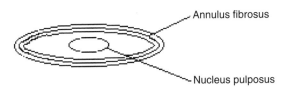

Fig. 14–4 The intervertebral disc is made up of two parts, the outer annulus fibrosus and an inner nucleus pulposus.

load on the disc is reduced (Fig. 14–5). Spinal fusion may have an adverse influence on nutrition of the disc because of immobility. Maximum mechanical stress occurs at the lumbosacral junction (L5–S1) and at the disc between L4–5, and these discs are the ones most likely to degenerate, bulge, and prolapse.

Intradiscal pressure was measured by Nachemson by inserting a needle in the nucleus pulposus of the disc. The results of this study have very important bearing on understanding and treatment of disc diseases. The intradiscal pressure is least when the subject is lying down, flat on his or her back, and this is the basis for conservative treatment of protruded intervertebral disc. Pelvic traction further reduces this pressure. There is nearly 1.5 times more pressure on the disc in the unsupported sitting posture than when standing upright. Patients with pain due to a prolapsed intervertebral disc prefer to stand rather than sit because it is less painful.

The exercise commonly recommended to increase abdominal muscle strength (sit-ups) also increases the pressure considerably and should be avoided when a protruded intervertebral disc is suspected. During patient health education on lifting techniques, the patient is instructed to bend from the knees and to keep the object as close to the body as possible. Keeping the inclination of backrest of a carseat to 110° (slightly beyond the vertical) and using a lumbar support can reduce electrical activity in the back muscles considerably and intradiscal pressure.

Degenerative changes in the intervertebral discs are very common. The intervertebral disc loses its blood supply after the second decade and becomes the largest avascular structure in the human body. The water content of the nucleus pulposus diminishes as we advance in age, and the annulus develops tears. These changes predispose the disc to prolapse.

History

Onset. There may or may not be any history of trauma, such as lifting a heavy object while bending and twisting, falling on the buttocks, or an activity to which the patient is not accustomed. The **duration** of symptoms is very variable. Patients with chronic pain (>6 months in duration) may need a special treatment program. The **course** is usually marked with episodes of exacerbations and remissions. The **pain** is usually located in the low back or gluteal region on one or both sides. It may **radiate** down the thigh and leg to the foot depending on severity of the nerve root involvement. In milder involvements, the pain may be felt only in the gluteal region. In more severe cases, the pain may radiate to the toes.

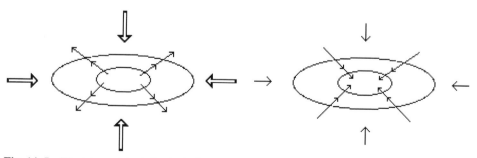

Fig. 14–5 The intervertebral disc is the largest avascular structure in the body. Nutrients enter the disc by diffusion. Fluids are pushed out of the disc when it is compressed, and they enter the disc substance when pressure is reduced.

Forward bending, coughing, sneezing, prolonged sitting (e.g., while driving), and lifting may aggravate the pain. Bedrest, local heat, and analgesics usually provide some relief.

It is very important to inquire about **neurologic symptoms,** including tingling, numbness, or weakness in the lower extremities. The patient may present with **foot drop** due to weakness of dorsiflexors of the foot. Recent onset of incontinence of bladder or bowel is a good reason for emergency referral to a surgeon. History of **previous treatments** helps in determining further management. It is useful to know what kinds of treatments were found to be effective or which treatment modalities made the pain worse. Inquiry about involvement of other joints and systems (**review of systems**) helps to rule out systemic diseases, e.g., ankylosing spondylitis or malignancy.

Physical Examination

1. **Inspection.** The patient's **gait** is observed as he or she walks in. There may be foot drop, limp, or guarding due to pain. If at all possible, see how the patient undresses or unties shoelaces, which may give a better idea of ROM of the spine. The back is examined from behind for any prominence of paraspinous muscles due to **muscle spasm.** Scoliosis or lateral list is commonly seen due to unequal muscle spasm on two sides. **Scars** of previous operations may suggest a different approach in management. A tuft of hair in the midline over the low back indicates congenital anomaly of the spine such as spina bifida. Lumbar lordosis may be obliterated because of muscle spasm. **Abdominal obesity** puts strain on the lumbar discs and muscles of the back and requires consideration in the treatment program.
2. **Palpation.** Localized tenderness may help in pinpointing the structure involved. Muscle spasm is felt as a firm muscle mass, usually on one side more than the other. Spinous processes are palpated to confirm any scoliosis.
3. **Range of motion.** During the acute stage, all movements may be restricted because of pain. Forward flexion is especially restricted in disc disease, whereas extension is painful in facet joint disease or spinal stenosis.
4. **Special tests**
   a. **Straight leg raising test** is positive when one of the nerve roots forming the sciatic nerve is compressed. Patients with severe nerve root compression complain of pain immediately on lifting the leg. In milder cases, pain starts after the leg is raised beyond 40°–50°. This test also helps in following the patient's progress.
   b. **Neurologic exam** helps in localizing the nerve root involved. Sensation, muscle strength, and reflexes are tested. Lumbar fifth and sacral first nerve roots are commonly affected.
   Fifth lumbar nerve root affects:
      i. Sensation over the dorsal aspect of the base of the big and second toe
      ii. Dorsiflexion of the big toe and foot
   First sacral nerve root affects:
      i. Sensation over the lateral aspect of the foot and little toe
      ii. Plantar flexors of the foot
      iii. Achilles tendon reflex
   c. **Hip joint** and **abdomen** are examined to rule out any referred pain from the hip or intra-abdominal pathology.

Differential Diagnoses

1. **Soft tissue problems.** Ligament or muscle strain are very common and may mimic disc disease. There may be a history of overuse with localized tenderness in the back, negative straight leg raising test, and normal neurologic exam in soft tissue problems.

2. **Trigger points** are common in the iliolumbar ligament in the angle between the iliac crest and fifth lumbar vertebra. Localized tenderness in this area with pain radiating to the gluteal region is a common finding in trigger point.

Other possible conditions are listed at the beginning of this chapter.

Investigations

1. **ESR** and **WBC count** are normal in disc disease.
2. **Bence-Jones protein** in urine is sought if multiple myeloma is suspected.
3. **Plain x-rays** of the lumbosacral spine are done mainly to rule out infection and metastatic or inflammatory disease. Because a large proportion of patients after age 45–50 will have degenerative changes in the spine, plain x-rays may help in a very small percentage of them. In degenerative disc disease, the **disc space** is narrowed, there are horizontally directed osteophytes, and there is reactive sclerosis of vertebral endplates. Vacuum phenomenon is the description for a dark line seen in the intervertebral space and is considered a definite sign of disc degeneration. Scoliosis may be secondary to degenerative disc disease, or degeneration may be secondary to primary scoliosis. Sometimes, a vertebral body slides posteriorly (**retrolisthesis**) in relation to the one below it. This may be secondary to disc space narrowing. There is increased load on the facet joints when the disc degenerates, which leads to degenerative changes in the facet joint with **osteophyte** formation and encroachment of intervertebral foramen.
4. **Electromyography** may help in confirming nerve root involvement.
5. **MRI** has become a very useful, noninvasive procedure for determining the severity of disc disease and is fast replacing myelography, discography, and CT.

Management

Management is described on page 178.

DEGENERATIVE DISEASE OF THE FACET JOINT

The facet joints (apophyseal joints) are synovial joints between the superior and inferior articular processes of the vertebrae. They undergo degenerative changes as any other joint and are also involved in diseases such as ankylosing spondylitis.

Etiology

The articular cartilage of the joint degenerates with age. These changes may occur at an earlier age if there is hereditary tendency, degenerated intervertebral disc, or deformity of the spine. Occupations requiring the lifting of heavy loads and frequent bending or poor posture may also predispose facet joints to degenerative changes.

Pathology

The articular cartilage develops fibrillations and loses superficial layers. The surface of the cartilage becomes irregular, and bone underneath becomes sclerosed. Osteophytes develop from joint borders, encroach upon the lateral recess of the spinal canal, and may press on the intervertebral nerve. Injection of hypertonic saline solution into facet joints of normal volunteers produced low back pain with radiation into the lower extremity, even to the foot. It may also affect the straight leg raising test and deep tendon reflexes in lower extremities.

History

Onset of the disease may be early if there are any predisposing factors. Otherwise, degenerative disease of the facet joint may become symptomatic after the fifth decade. The patient complains of **low back pain** which is usually worse in the morning after getting up from sleep. This may be accompanied by **stiffness.** These symptoms are relieved by activity but may return after a full day's work. Pain and stiffness are usually aggravated during cold and damp weather and are relieved by local heat and analgesics. The low back pain may or may not radiate down the lower extremities. The clinical picture may sometimes be confused with a prolapsed intervertebral disc with radiculopathy.

Physical Examination

1. **Inspection.** Increased dorsal kyphosis, scoliosis, or poor posture (**deformity**) may be present. The lumbar spine may lose its lordosis and become straight because of muscle spasm.
2. **Palpation.** Paraspinous **muscle spasm** may be palpable as firm muscle mass on one or both sides of the spine. There may be focal paraspinal tenderness.
3. **Range of motion. Extension** of the lumbar spine is painful in degenerative disease of the facet joints. All movements may be restricted if there is muscle spasm.
4. **Special tests. Neurologic exam** is carried out if entrapment of a spinal nerve or spinal stenosis is suspected.

Differential Diagnoses

Patients with disc disease have more pain on flexion, whereas in facet joint disease, there is pain on extension of the spine. Facet joint disease does not give rise to dermatomal sensory loss or specific motor weakness of a particular nerve root distribution. Degenerative disc disease, spinal stenosis, or tender points may coexist with degenerative facet joint disease. It may be difficult to determine which disease is causing the symptoms.

Investigations

Irregular narrowing of the joint space, subchondral sclerosis, and osteophyte formation are seen in affected facet joints on x-rays. Plain x-rays may not be very useful, because after age 50 years, degenerative changes are seen in 70–80% of people. CT or MRI give more information regarding narrowing of lateral recess and spinal canal stenosis.

Management

Rest, local heat, and NSAIDs are tried. If the pain and muscle spasm are severe, bedrest until the acute stage subsides may be necessary. General principles used in the management of disc disease are followed. Activities are increased gradually. A lumbosacral corset may help during this phase of mobilization. Exercises to increase ROM after local heat helps to stretch tight muscles and ligaments. Later, exercises to increase the strength of paraspinous and abdominal muscles are added. If conservative measures fail to relieve pain, surgical fusion of the spine may be considered.

SPINAL STENOSIS

Patients with narrowing of the spinal canal in the lumbar region usually present with pain or weakness in the lower extremities on walking. This sensation may be mistaken for intermittent claudication due to vascular disease. An estimated 10% of patients attending vascular clinics have spinal stenosis.

Anatomy
The spinal canal is formed anteriorly by the posterior surface of the vertebral body and the posterior longitudinal ligament. The pedicles and laminae form the sides and posterior boundaries of the canal (Fig. 14–6). The facet joint is at the junction of the pedicle and lamina. In the lower lumbar region, the canal is triangular in shape. The spinal nerve root comes out from the lateral recess.

Etiology
The size of the canal may be small since birth due to some congenital or developmental factors in certain individuals. Later in life when degenerative changes occur, the canal is further narrowed by osteophytes from facet joints and the vertebral body, thickening of the posterior longitudinal ligament or ligamentum flavum, or retrolisthesis of the vertebral body secondary to narrowing of the disc space (Fig. 14–7).

Pathology
The intermittent nature of symptoms may be due to increased venous congestion within the confined space of the spinal canal. Lower extremity activities such as walking bring on the symptoms. The diameter of the canal is narrowed by extension of the spine, and thus, any activity carried out with the spine in extension, e.g., going down a hill, brings on the symptoms. The symptoms are relieved by flexion of the spine, which increases the spinal canal dimensions and reduces congestion and pressure on the cauda equina.

History
The symptoms start gradually and usually occur in males over age 45–50 years. The history may be vague, and he may complain of weakness, pain, tingling, or numbness of one or both legs after walking. His legs feel "heavy" or "rubbery." There may be some pain in

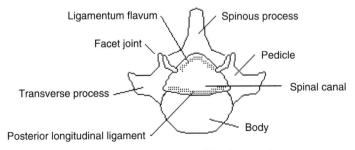

Fig. 14–6   Parts of a normal lumbar vertebra.

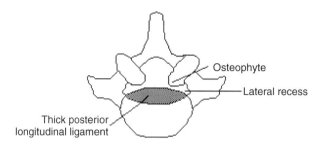

Osteophyte

Lateral recess

Thick posterior longitudinal ligament

Fig. 14–7 The spinal canal may be narrow from birth, or it may become narrow due to ingrowth of osteophytes, protrusion of disc material, or thickening of the posterior longitudinal ligament.

the gluteal region or legs, and he has to sit down or stand with the spine flexed to relieve symptoms. It usually takes much longer to resume walking for someone with spinal stenosis than with vascular disease. Some patients may complain of pain radiating down the sciatic nerve.

Physical Examination

Usually, there are very few physical signs on examination. The neurologic deficits may be brought on by asking the patient to walk until symptoms develop and then examining him while he is symptomatic.

1. **Inspection.** Observe the patient after a long walk, and see how he relieves his symptoms.
2. **Range of motion.** Spinal movements may be restricted because of associated degenerative changes in the disc and facet joints.
3. **Special tests.** Peripheral arterial pulses are examined to rule out vascular disease.

Differential Diagnoses

Peripheral vascular disease occurs in the same age group and is more common than spinal stenosis. Pain due to intermittent vascular claudication occurs after walking the same distance every time and is relieved by standing in one place for a few minutes. The pain is felt in calf muscles or buttocks, and there are no neurologic symptoms or signs (tingling, numbness, weakness, absent reflexes). Arterial pulses in the lower extremities may be absent.

Investigations

1. **X-rays** of the lumbar spine may show narrowing of disc spaces, osteophyte formation, narrowing of intervertebral foramina, and retrolisthesis of vertebrae. The anteroposterior dimension of the spinal canal is not visualized on plain x-rays.
2. **Doppler studies** are done to evaluate peripheral circulation in the legs.
3. **CT** and **MRI** can show the narrowing of the spinal canal or lateral recess. The extent of pathology in the vertical axis can be determined by MRI or myelography.

Course

The course is variable in each patient. The disease may progress and then stop deteriorating, or it may gradually worsen.

Management

Conservative measures, including **NSAIDs, exercises** to strengthen abdominal muscles, and a **corset** to keep the lumbar spine in slight flexion, are tried initially. Epidural injection of **steroids** may reduce some soft tissue inflammation and swelling in the canal. If all these measures fail and symptoms progress or markedly curtail the patient's activities, then **surgical decompression** may be advisable.

SPONDYLOLYSIS AND SPONDYLOLISTHESIS

A defect of the pars interarticularis of a lumbar vertebra (**spondylolysis**) usually does not give rise to symptoms. When a vertebra slips forward from its position, it is called **spondylolisthesis.** This condition may give rise to low back pain and/or radiculopathy.

Anatomy

The vertebral arch is formed by two pedicles and two laminae (*see* Fig. 14–6). They protect the spinal cord and cauda equina. Two articular processes attach on either side and are called the superior and inferior articular processes. They articulate with the upper and lower vertebrae. The bony part between the superior and inferior articular processes is called the **pars interarticularis** (Fig. 14–8A).

Etiology

The following factors contribute to spondylolysis and spondylolisthesis:

1. **Traumatic.** A defect in the pars interarticularis may be due to some injury, especially in childhood.
2. **Congenital malformation.** Instead of bone, fibrous tissue forms the pars.
3. **Degenerative disc disease.** The height of an intervertebral disc decreases, giving rise to laxity of ligaments. The upper vertebra slides forward or, sometimes, backward (**retrolisthesis**) because ligaments are not able withstand shearing forces. In degenerative disc disease, spondylolisthesis develops without spondylolysis.

Pathology

In spondylolysis, the part of the vertebra between the superior and inferior articular processes is not ossified (Fig. 14–8B) and remains fibrous. Stability of the spine depends on an intact vertebral arch and strength of muscles and ligaments. The defect in the arch (spondylolysis) may put undue stress on the soft tissues, giving rise to pain or slippage of a vertebra (spondylolisthesis). Spondylolysis occurs most often in the fifth lumbar vertebra. An estimated 5% of the population has this defect.

History

Spondylolysis and spondylolisthesis are usually asymptomatic. **Low back pain** due to spondylolysis is usually dull and aching in character. It is made worse by standing or walking for long periods and is relieved by rest. The pain may radiate to the buttocks and thigh. Accidental injury may mark the onset of pain in childhood or adolescence. Another period in life when pain due to spondylolysis may start is pregnancy. Spondylolisthesis secondary to degenerative changes presents in fifth or sixth decade.

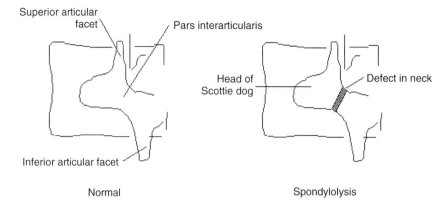

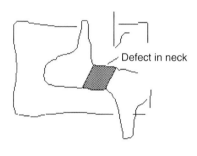

Spondylolisthesis

Fig. 14–8   The part of the vertebra between the superior and inferior articular processes is called the pars interarticularis. *A,* Normally, it looks like the neck of a Scottish terrier dog on oblique views of the lumbar spine. *B,* In spondylolysis, there is a defect in the pars which looks like a collar around the dog's neck. *C,* In spondylolisthesis, there is separation of the head from the dog's body.

Physical Examination

1. **Inspection.** No abnormalities are seen on physical examination in spondylolysis. However, in spondylolisthesis (forward slippage of the vertebra), the distance between the lower rib and iliac crest is reduced. There may be an increased hollow in the midline and a transverse skin crease in the lumbar region.
2. **Palpation.** Localized midline tenderness is present when pain is due to spondylolysis. A step-like defect may be palpable between the spinous processes in severe cases of spondylolisthesis.
3. **Range of motion.** Forward flexion is usually normal. At times, the patient is more supple and is able to touch the floor easily. Extension of the spine may be limited.
4. **Special tests.** Straight leg raising test is negative in most patients. It may become positive when nerve roots are compressed in severe spondylolisthesis.

Course/Complications

A small percentage of patients progress from spondylolysis to spondylolisthesis. Compression of nerve roots is uncommon because the diameter of the spinal canal increases in spondylolisthesis. The posterior elements of the neural arch remain in their place, whereas anterior elements slide forward. In very severe cases of spondylolisthesis, one or more nerve roots may be compressed.

Differential Diagnosis

All other common causes of low back pain, such as degenerative disc disease, prolapsed intervertebral disc, or facet joint arthritis, should be ruled out.

Investigations

Plain x-rays of the lumbosacral spine with AP, lateral, and oblique views are usually sufficient for diagnosis. The oblique views show the defect in pars, and lateral views are useful for determining the extent of slippage in spondylolisthesis. The bony portion between the superior and inferior articular processes looks like the head of a Scottish terrier dog on oblique views (Fig. 14–8B). The defect in the pars is described as a collar on the dog's neck. In spondylolisthesis, the "head" separates from the front feet (inferior articular process), and the dog is decapitated (Fig. 14–8C). **CT scan** or **MRI** may be ordered if surgical treatment is considered.

Management

No treatment is necessary for asymptomatic patients. Most patients with symptoms due to spondylolysis and mild spondylolisthesis can be treated conservatively. The treatment of spondylolysis is very similar to treatment of idiopathic back pain.
1. **Medications.** Analgesics or **NSAIDs** can be prescribed for pain.
2. **Ancillary.** A program of isometric **exercises** to strengthen the abdominal and back muscles may be helpful. A **corset** to support the lumbosacral spine is prescribed for symptomatic patients.
3. **Surgical** treatment should be considered when:
   a. Conservative treatment fails to relieve symptoms, and pain interferes with daily activities.
   b. Single or multiple nerve root involvement causes radiating pain, positive neurologic signs, and abnormal electromyographic findings.
   c. Grade III and IV slippage with symptoms

Bibliography

1. Boachie-Adjei O: Conservative management of low back pain: A evaluation of current methods. Postgrad Med 84(3):127–133, 1988.
2. Ciricillo SF, Weinstein PR: Lumbar spinal stenosis. West J Med 158:171–177, 1993.
3. Daum WJ: The sacroiliac joint: An underappreciated pain generator. Am J Orthop 24:475–478, 1995.
4. Davids JR, Wenger DR: Back pain in children and adolescents: An algorithmic approach. J Musculoskel Med 11(3):19–32, 1994.
5. Eisenstein SM: The lumbar facet arthrosis syndrome: Clinical presentation and articular surface changes. J Bone Joint Surg 69-B:3, 1987.
6. Hensinger RN: Spondylolysis and spondylolisthesis in children and adolescents. J Bone Joint Surg 71-A:1098–1107, 1989.
7. Katz JN, Dalgas M, Stucki G, Lipson SJ: Diagnosis of lumbar spinal stenosis. Rheum Dis Clin North Am 20:471–484, 1994.

8. Kellgren JH: The anatomical source of back pain. Rheumatol Rehabil 16:3–12, 1977.
9. Kirkaldy-Willis WH (ed): Managing Low Back Pain, 2nd ed. New York, Churchill Livingstone, 1988.
10. McCowin PR, Borenstein D, Wiesel SW: The current approach to medical diagnosis of low back pain. Orthop Clin North Am 22:315–325, 1991.
11. Modic MT, Ross JS: Magnetic resonance imaging in the evaluation of low back pain. Orthop Clin North Am 22:283–301, 1991.
12. Mooney V, Robertson J: The facet syndrome. Clin Orthop 115:149–156, 1976.
13. Nachemson AL: The lumbar spine: An orthopedic challenge. Spine 1:59–71, 1976.
14. Portenoy RK: Back pain in the elderly patient. Hosp Pract 28(4):81–98, 1993.
15. Porter R: Management of Back Pain. Edinburgh, Churchill Livingstone, 1986.
16. Strausbaugh LJ: Vertebral osteomyelitis: How to differentiate it from other causes of back and neck pain. Postgrad Med 97(6):147–154, 1995.
17. Spengler DM: Degenerative stenosis of the lumbar spine. J Bone Joint Surg 69-A:305–308, 1987.
18. Weinstein JN, Wiesel SW (eds): The Lumbar Spine. Philadelphia, W.B. Saunders, 1990.
19. Wiesel SW, Cuckler JM, Deluca F, et al: Acute low back pain: An objective analysis of conservative therapy. Spine 5:324–330, 1980.

15

Shoulder

Arun J. Mehta, M.B., F.R.C.P.C.

Musculoskeletal problems in the shoulder region are common. Movement of this joint is very important for placing the hand in space where it can function. Pain or limitation of movement of the shoulder makes it difficult for the hand to perform its function.

Anatomy
The shoulder complex consists of:
Three **synovial joints**
1. Glenohumeral joint. Formed by the head of the humerus and glenoid of the scapula (Fig. 15–1A)
2. Acromioclavicular joint. Between the acromion and lateral end of the clavicle
3. Sternoclavicular joint. Medial end of the clavicle and sternum
Two **sliding surfaces**
4. Scapulothoracic. Scapula glides over the posterior thoracic wall.
5. Acromiohumeral. The head of the humerus moves under the coracoacromial arch formed by the acromion, coracoid process, and coracoacromial ligament (Fig. 15–1B). It is separated from the coracoacromial arch by the subacromial bursa.
The last two structures are not real joints, but a lot of movement takes place between these adjoining surfaces.

Differential Diagnosis
Pain in the shoulder region may be due to pathology in that area, or it may be referred from another structure at some distance from the joint.
Shoulder problems may be due to:
1. **Subacromial bursitis** may present with pain on abduction of the shoulder and tenderness over the subacromial region.
2. **Adhesive capsulitis.** All movements of the shoulder are painful and limited.
3. **Rotator cuff injuries.** The patient has difficulty maintaining abduction of the shoulder against gravity and initiating abduction of the shoulder.
4. **Bicipital tendinitis.** Tendon sheath surrounding the biceps tendon is inflamed, and there is tenderness over the front of the shoulder joint.
5. **Dislocation** of the shoulder joint is common because of a lax capsule. If not treated properly, the patient may end up with recurrent dislocation.
6. **Fractures** of the surgical neck of the humerus are common in the elderly.
7. **Degenerative arthritis** of the acromioclavicular joint causes pain on movements of the

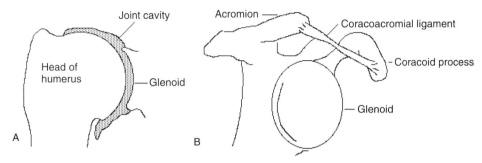

Fig. 15–1 Anatomy of the shoulder. *A*, Glenohumeral joint. *B*, Glenoid and coracoacromial arch (lateral view).

shoulder and tenderness over this joint. Degenerative arthritis does not commonly affect the glenohumeral joint.
8. **Shoulder-hand syndrome.** Shoulder may be painful with some limitation of movements in reflex sympathetic dystrophy of the hand.
   Referred pain may be from:
1. **Cervical radiculopathy.** Entrapment of the fifth cervical nerve may present with shoulder and arm pain.
2. **Trigger points** over the upper border of the trapezius or supraspinatus muscles may cause pain the shoulder.
3. **Cardiac** problems. Pain of myocardial infarction is well known to be felt in the left shoulder region.
4. **Liver** and **gallbladder** diseases, such as cholecystitis, may produce pain in the right shoulder.
5. **Diaphragmatic pleura** (e.g., basal **pneumonia**) causes pain in the shoulder region on the same side.
6. **Subdiaphragmatic** conditions (e.g., liver abscess)
   Shoulder conditions also commonly differ in prevalence in the different age groups (Table 15–1).

Table 15–1 Shoulder Conditions Common in Different Age Groups

Children
   Shoulder conditions uncommon
Young adults
   Overuse syndromes (e.g., subacromial bursitis)
   Trigger points
   Dislocation
Middle life
   Rotator cuff injuries
   Bicipital tendinitis
   Cardiac
   Trigger points
Elderly
   Fractures
   Cervical radiculopathy
   Adhesive capsulitis
   Rupture of biceps tendon
   Metastasis to head of humerus

History
Pain originating in structures around the shoulder may be dull aching or severe and felt deep inside the joint. It may radiate down from the tip of the acromion over the lateral aspect of the arm to its middle near the insertion of the deltoid muscle. Pain from the acromioclavicular and sternoclavicular joints is felt right over those joints. The pain is aggravated by movements or lying on the affected shoulder. It is important to find out which movements aggravate the pain. Restriction of movements is expressed by the patient as limitation in performance of function (e.g., difficulty in reaching the hip pocket). Symptoms related to cardiac, pulmonary, or gallbladder disease may need to be specifically elicited.

Physical Examination
1. **Inspection.** The shoulder region is observed from the front, side, and back. Look for symmetry and **contour** on both sides. The normal shoulder is nicely rounded. It becomes flat when the shoulder joint is dislocated or deltoid muscle is atrophied. Color of the skin, scars, and swelling are noted. **Atrophy** of deltoid, trapezius, supraspinatus, and infraspinatus muscles may be due to disuse or to nerve or muscle pathology. Patients with shoulder problems have difficulty removing their shirts. Look for exaggerated kyphosis of the thoracic spine or scoliosis. Is one scapula higher or more prominent than the other?
    Observe:
    a. Suprasternal notch and sternocleidomastoid muscle
    b. Sternoclavicular joint
    c. Clavicle, supra- and infraclavicular fossae
    d. Acromioclavicular joint
    e. Rounded contour of the shoulder
    f. Upper border of the trapezius muscle
    g. Spine of the scapula, supra- and infraspinatus muscles, and medial or vertebral border of scapula
    h. Position of the scapula in relation to the thorax and spine
    i. Spinal curvature
2. **Palpation.** Palpate the shoulder structures listed above and look for increased temperature, tenderness, and swelling. Additional structures that need to be palpated are:
    a. **Long head of biceps** is palpated between the greater and lesser tuberosities of the humerus. It is felt over the anterior aspect of shoulder 1–1.5 inches distal to the acromioclavicular joint. Palpation of the long head of biceps will be facilitated by keeping your palpating fingers over the anterior aspect of the shoulder and rotating the humerus with the elbow flexed to 90°. There is tenderness in this area in bicipital tendinitis.
    b. **Subacromial region** is just distal to the lateral border of the acromion. Tenderness indicates subacromial bursitis, supraspinatus tendinitis, or rotator cuff tear. In subluxation of the shoulder, there is diminished resistance to a palpating finger in the subacromial region.
    c. Palpate for **trigger points** along the superior border of the trapezius muscle, paraspinous muscles, and supra- and infraspinatus muscles.
    d. Axilla is palpated for enlarged or tender lymph nodes.
3. **Range of Motion.** ROM of the shoulder is measured from the neutral position with the arm by the side of the body. Various motions taking place at the shoulder joint complex are:
    a. Flexion. The arm is moved anteriorly from the neutral position. Normal range is 0° (neutral) to 180° (arm straight up).

b. Extension. The arm is moved posteriorly. Normal range is 0° to 45°–50°.
c. Abduction. The arm is moved sideways and outward in the coronal plane. Normal range is 0° to 180° (arm straight up). The first 20°–30° of motion takes place at the glenohumeral joint. After that, abduction takes place at the glenohumeral joint and the scapulothoracic surface. For every 3° of abduction, 2° take place at the glenohumeral joint and 1° at the scapulothoracic surface.
d. **Adduction.** The arm is moved toward the opposite arm, either in front of or behind the body. Normal range is up to 45°–50°.
e. **Rotations.** Internal and external rotation can be measured in two different positions:
  i.   Arm in neutral position by the side of the body and elbow flexed to 90°. The forearm is then moved outward (external rotation) or inward (medial rotation); *or*
  ii. Arm is abducted to 90° at the shoulder and elbow is flexed to 90°. The forearm is moved upward (external rotation) from the horizontal position or downward (internal rotation). **Normal range** is up to 90° for both.
f. **Functional.** Functional movements are a combination of two or more of the aforementioned movements. These movements are performed actively by the patient.
  i.   Ask the patient to touch the inferior angle of the opposite scapula. This will test internal rotation and adduction. This movement is necessary in hooking a bra.
  ii. Ask the patient to touch the back of the head or medial angle of the opposite scapula. This movement is required for doing the hair and tests abduction and external rotation.
g. **Elevation.** Whole shoulder girdle is moved upward.
h. **Depression.** Opposite of previous movement.
i. **Retraction.** Scapula and shoulder are pushed backward.
j. **Protraction.** Opposite of previous movement.

Active ROM tests are performed by the patient and are examined first. If the patient is able to do full range of active movements, then passive ROM tests need not be done. A patient may not be able to perform full ROM in all directions because of:
  a. Pain
  b. Soft tissue contracture
  c. Bony restriction
  d. Muscle weakness

Passive ROM tests are performed by the examiner and may be the same as the active ROM in soft tissue contracture and bony restrictions. If active ROM is restricted and not the passive, it is very likely due to muscle weakness or ruptured tendon. Pain, under certain circumstances, may restrict active movements more than passive (e.g., painful arc syndrome).

Active movements against resistance, e.g., abduction against resistance offered by the examiner, are painful in inflammation or partial rupture of the supraspinatus tendon.

4. **Special Tests. Neurologic examination** is carried out when the shoulder involvement may be secondary to a neurologic condition such as a stroke, or when shoulder pain may be a presenting symptom of a neurologic condition such as cervical radiculopathy. Appropriate neurologic tests are essential for diagnosis and management.

Investigations

1. **Plain x-rays** are useful in diagnosis of fractures, dislocations, calcific tendinitis, and metastatic diseases.
2. **MRI** is useful in rotator cuff tears and recurrent dislocations.
3. **Arthrography** may be indicated in adhesive capsulitis to delineate the synovial cavity, and it may help in breaking adhesions and improving ROM.

4. **Arthroscopy** helps in diagnosing rotator cuff tears and determining pathology in recurrent dislocations. Some surgical procedures can be done through an arthroscope.

FRACTURE OF THE CLAVICLE

Fracture of the clavicle is very common, especially among children and young adults.

Anatomy
The clavicle is a horizontally located bone articulating with the sternum medially and the acromion of the scapula laterally. It helps in transmitting the weight of the upper extremity to the axial skeleton. Its contours are easily visible and palpable because it lies subcutaneously. Some very important structures, including the brachial plexus, subclavian artery, and apex of the lung, lie deeper to it and may be injured at the time the clavicle is fractured.

Pathology
The weakest part of the clavicle is at the junction of the lateral with the middle third, and most fractures occur there. A fall on an outstretched hand is the most common mechanism of injury. Pain is localized over the fracture site.

Physical Examination
1. **Inspection.** The patient walks around supporting the injured arm with the opposite hand. Deformity due to a complete fracture is easily visible. The lateral end is depressed because of the weight of the upper extremity. Later, discoloration of skin due to hematoma becomes apparent.
2. **Palpation** elicits localized tenderness and a gap in the continuity of the clavicle.
3. **Range of Motion.** All active and passive movements of the shoulder are painfully restricted.
4. **Special Tests**
   a. Neurologic exam of the upper extremity is necessary to rule out **brachial plexus injury.**
   b. **Pulsations** of ulnar and radial arteries are checked.
   c. Auscultation of **lungs** is carried out to rule out pneumothorax.

Investigations
X-rays are taken to confirm the diagnosis, determine the type of the fracture, and rule out pneumothorax. If injury to the subclavian artery or vein is suspected, **angiography** may be necessary.

Management
1. **Ancillary.** Most fractures can be treated by a figure-of-eight bandage. This can be removed after 3 weeks in children and young adults. Stiffness of the fingers and shoulder should be prevented by active ROM exercises as soon as allowed by pain.
2. **Surgical.** Open reduction and internal fixation are needed only rarely.

FRACTURES OF THE PROXIMAL END OF HUMERUS

Anatomy
The constriction around the articular surface of the proximal end of the humerus is called the **anatomical neck** of the humerus (Fig. 15–2). The **surgical neck** is the region where the expanded proximal end meets the shaft of the humerus. Fractures commonly occur at the surgical neck.

Pathology
Fracture of the proximal end of the humerus is commonly seen in the elderly with osteoporosis. If the bone is severely osteoporotic, it takes minimal trauma to cause the fracture. In younger individuals with strong bones, it takes much greater force to Łfracture the humerus. In the very young, epiphyseal separation occurs instead of a fracture.

Types of fractures (Fig. 15–3) include:
1. **Surgical neck** of humerus. The fracture line is transverse at the junction of the proximal expanded end and shaft of the humerus.
   a. **Impacted**—Both fragments are driven into each other, and the fracture is stable.
   b. **Displaced**
2. **Greater tubercle**
   a. **Undisplaced**—Crack fracture without any displacement of the fragment.
   b. **Displaced**—The fragment of the greater tubercle is pulled away by supraspinatus.

History
The patient usually presents with **pain** in the shoulder region after a **fall.** Severity of pain depends on the severity of trauma, and in the elderly osteoporotic with an impacted fracture, there may not be much pain.

Physical Examination
1. **Inspection.** The injured arm is supported by the other hand. Visible swelling is seen in the upper arm. Later, ecchymosis appears which may track down to the elbow or forearm.

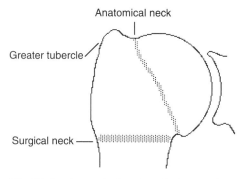

Fig. 15–2   Anatomical and surgical neck of humerus.

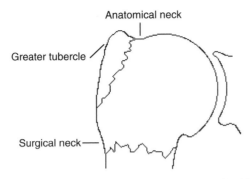

Fig. 15-3   Common sites of fracture in the proximal humerus.

2. **Palpation.** There is localized tenderness at the fracture site. In case of fracture of the neck, tenderness is palpated over the medial aspect of the upper arm in the axilla as well as over the lateral aspect.
3. **Range of motion.** All active and passive movements are painful. In patients with impacted fracture, pain and discomfort may be minimal, and the patient may be able to actively move the arm.
4. **Special tests**
   a. **Neurologic**—The involved upper extremity is examined for axillary nerve or brachial plexus injury.
   b. Radial and ulnar artery **pulsations** are checked to rule out axillary artery injury.

Investigations
Plain **x-rays** of the shoulder confirm the diagnosis of fracture and type of fracture.

Management
1. **Medications.** Analgesics are prescribed to control pain.
2. **Ancillary.** Treatment depends on the type of fracture. For impacted fracture of surgical neck and undisplaced fracture of the greater tuberosity in an elderly patient, support in a **sling** until pain subsides is prescribed. Gentle passive ROM exercises are started as soon as pain permits. Later, pendulum exercises and active exercises against gravity are started. The main goal in this group of patients is to **prevent a stiff shoulder.**
   Details of other forms of treatments are beyond the scope of this book.
3. **Surgical.** Open reduction and internal fixation may be necessary in some cases.

Complications
1. **Stiffness** of the shoulder is the most common problem in elderly patients. It is easier to prevent than to cure. **ROM exercises** are started in these patients as soon as possible.
2. **Axillary nerve palsy.** This nerve supplies the deltoid muscle, and muscle atrophy and weakness are seen when the axillary nerve is damaged.
3. Brachial plexus injury
4. Injury to axillary artery

DISLOCATION OF THE SHOULDER

Anatomy
The shoulder is the most mobile joint and also the most vulnerable joint as far as dislocation is concerned. Half of all dislocations of any major joint occur in the shoulder. The stability of this joint is maintained not by bony configuration but by muscles and ligaments. The glenoid is very shallow and covers only part of the head of the humerus. The joint capsule is very lax to allow extensive ROM.

Pathology
Shoulder dislocations are described by the position the head of humerus takes in relation to the glenoid (Fig. 15–4):
1. **Anterior dislocation**—The head of the humerus is under the coracoid process. It is also called **subcoracoid** dislocation. This is the most common variety of dislocation, comprising >90% of all shoulder dislocations. Forceful abduction, external rotation, and extension may cause the shoulder to dislocate. Pathologic features seen in this variety may include one, two, or all of the following:
    a. The joint capsule, which is continuous with the periosteum over the scapula, is lifted off the bone, and the head of the humerus comes to lie between these two structures.
    b. The glenoidal labrum, the cartilaginous rim around the glenoid, is detached from the bone.
    c. A defect in the posterolateral aspect of the head of the humerus (Hill-Sachs) is due to compression fracture that develops as the head slides over the rim of the glenoid.
2. **Inferior dislocation**—The head of the humerus is displaced inferiorly, in the subglenoid region.
3. **Posterior dislocation**—This variety may be seen after an epileptic seizure.
   The following injuries may be associated with dislocation of the shoulder joint:
1. Fracture of the greater tuberosity
2. Rupture of the rotator cuff
3. Fracture of the neck of the humerus

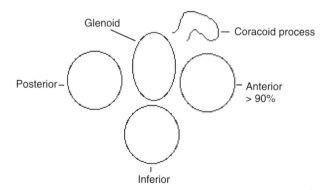

Fig. 15–4 Dislocations of the shoulder joint are described by the position of the head of the humerus in relation to the glenoid. If the head is anterior to the glenoid and under the coracoid process, it is called an anterior dislocation. The other two positions are inferior and posterior to glenoid.

4. Axillary nerve palsy leading to paralysis of the deltoid muscle
5. Damage to the axillary artery
6. Brachial plexus injury

History
Sudden, severe pain develops in the shoulder region after a fall or some other form of trauma. The patient tends to hold the arm beside the body so as to avoid any movement and supports it with the opposite hand. It occurs most frequently in young adults. Similar injury in a elderly person usually leads to a fracture.

Physical Examination
1. **Inspection.** The rounded contour of the shoulder is lost (Fig. 15–5). The arm is held in an adducted position by the side of the body.
2. **Palpation** reveals diffuse tenderness in the shoulder region during the immediate post-trauma period. Instead of a bony greater tuberosity, there is a gap under the acromion. The head of the humerus may be felt under the coracoid process if it is an anterior dislocation.
3. **Range of motion.** Active and passive movements are very painful and markedly restricted.
4. **Special tests**
   a. Radial and ulnar arteries are palpated to rule out any vascular complications.
   b. Sensations over the lateral aspect of the shoulder are tested to see if the axillary nerve is damaged. This nerve also supplies the deltoid muscle. It may be difficult to confirm deltoid paralysis because of severe pain.
   c. Sensations, muscle power, and reflexes of the involved arm are examined to rule out brachial plexus lesion.

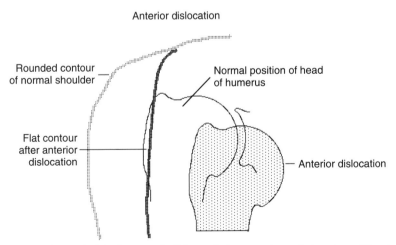

Fig. 15–5   When the head of the humerus is dislocated, the normal rounded contour of the shoulder looks flat.

Investigations

Plain anteroposterior x-rays may be misleading and not show the displaced head of the humerus, especially in the posterior dislocation. Associated fracture of the greater tuberosity or neck of the humerus can be confirmed by this view. The axillary view is necessary for diagnosis of shoulder dislocation.

Management

Shoulder dislocation should be **reduced** as soon as possible because:
1. It is a very painful condition and needs immediate relief.
2. Functional outcome is better if it is reduced early.

In the young adult, the most frequent complication after dislocation is **recurrent dislocation,** whereas in the older age groups, it is stiffness. Hence, postreduction management is different for young adults and for elderly patients.
1. In young adults, the shoulder is immobilized by bandaging it to the body for 3–4 weeks. This will give a chance for the soft tissues to heal and hopefully prevent **recurrent dislocation.**
2. For the elderly patient, the arm is kept in a sling and passive exercises are started early to prevent stiffness. The range and intensity are increased as tolerated by the patient.

Surgical

Open reduction is required when:
1. Closed reduction fails or is not possible.
2. Dislocation of the shoulder with fractured neck of the humerus or fractured greater tuberosity occurs.
3. Late unreduced dislocation occurs.

Complications

Recurrent dislocation is more common in young adults because subsequent dislocations occur with less severe trauma. Ultimately, the patient is able to "pop" his joint out at will and reduce it without difficulty. On examination, the patient may have a positive **apprehension test.** The arm is abducted and externally rotated. Just before the joint is about to dislocate, an expression of anxiety appears on the patient's face since he knows the joint is about to dislocate. Treatment of recurrent dislocation is by surgical repair.

SUBACROMIAL BURSITIS

Subacromial bursitis is a painful inflammation of the subacromial bursa. Other similar syndromes are impingement syndrome, calcific tendinitis, painful arc syndrome, supraspinatus tendinitis, and partial or minor tear of the rotator cuff. Clinically, all these conditions may be difficult to distinguish from one another, since all may present with symptoms of "painful arc." During abduction the patient complains of pain from 60°–120° of the range. Abduction from 0°–60° and from 120°–180° is painless. Management of all of these conditions is conservative and very similar.

Anatomy

The subacromial bursa and rotator cuff are squeezed between the head of the humerus and the coracoacromial arch when the arm is abducted beyond 45°–60° (Fig. 15–6). Normally,

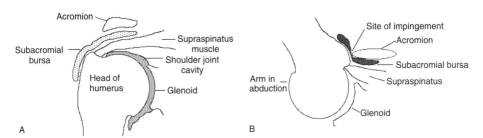

Fig. 15–6   Anatomy of subacromial bursa. *A,* Normal subacromial bursa. *B,* When the arm is abducted, the subacromial bursa is compressed between the acromion and greater tuberosity of the humerus.

full abduction is achieved by external rotation of the humerus, which helps to ease the subacromial bursa under the coracoacromial arch. Abduction of the arm becomes painful if there is swelling or inflammation in the subacromial region because of increased pressure on the inflamed structures.

Pathology
Inflammation in the subacromial region may be brought on by:
1. **Overuse** of the arm in the abducted position, e.g., swimming butterfly or freestyle, painting a ceiling, or tennis.
2. **Degeneration of the rotator cuff.** Blood supply to the rotator cuff comes from muscular branches in the supraspinatus muscle and arteries from the bone along the insertion of its tendon (see Fig. 15–9). The blood supply to the rotator cuff in the region of anastamosis is precarious (**critical zone**), which may lead to degenerative changes in the rotator cuff later in life.

History
The patient may give a history of overuse or minor trauma. Dull ache is felt in the shoulder region and may extend down to the middle of the arm or even the wrist, depending on the severity of the condition. **Pain** is worse at night and may interfere with sleep. Movements of the shoulder aggravate the pain, especially abduction. Sometimes, pain may be severe enough to compel the patient to go to an emergency room in the middle of the night. Pain and limitation of movements may make it difficult for the patient to comb the hair or hook her bra.

Physical Examination
1. **Inspection.** During early stages of the disease, the shoulder looks normal. Later, in the chronic stage, there may be wasting of the deltoid and supraspinatus muscles due to disuse.
2. **Palpation.** There may be **tenderness** in the subacromial region over the lateral aspect of the shoulder.
3. **Range of motion**
   a. **Active** movements are affected more than passive. Abduction beyond 50°–60° is painful. Later, other movements may be restricted, too. Active abduction of the arm against resistance reproduces pain in the shoulder (Fig. 15–7).

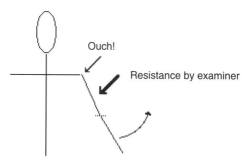

Fig. 15–7 Active abduction of arm against resistance is painful in subacromial bursitis and tendinitis of the rotator cuff.

   b. **Passive — Painful arc** is demonstrated by passive abduction. Movement from 0°–60° is painless, but that from 60°–120° causes shoulder pain. If passive abduction is continued beyond 120°, it again becomes painless.
4. **Special tests.** It is difficult to test for muscle strength whenever there is pain. An inability to abduct may be because of pain or due to rupture of the rotator cuff. To distinguish between these two conditions, the subacromial region is injected with local anesthetic to eliminate pain. If active abduction is possible after this, complete tear of rotator cuff is not likely.

Course
The course is marked by exacerbations and remissions.

Differential Diagnosis
It may not be possible to distinguish between impingement syndrome due to subacromial bursitis, supraspinatus tendinitis, or a partial or minor rotator cuff tear. Because conservative treatment of these conditions is similar, there is little need to distinguish them.
1. **Calcific tendinitis.** These patients may present with very severe pain and tenderness in the shoulder area. X-rays show calcium deposits in the subacromial region near the greater tuberosity.
2. **Fracture of greater tuberosity.** There is history of recent trauma to the shoulder, bruise, and localized tenderness on examination. All movements are painful. X-rays confirm the diagnosis.
3. **Bicipital tendinitis.** Tenderness is more anterior, over the long head of the biceps. Pain is felt on supination of the forearm against resistance.
4. **Degenerative joint disease** of acromioclavicular joint. Pain and tenderness are localized over the acromioclavicular joint.
5. **Cervical radiculopathy.** Radiculopathy of the fifth cervical nerve gives rise to pain in the shoulder region. It is aggravated by movements of the neck rather than of the shoulder. Spasm of paraspinous muscles may be present. Biceps reflex may be diminished or absent, with weakness of the biceps muscle.

Investigations
1. **Plain x-rays** are normal during early stages of the disease. Later, there may be sclerosis and osteophyte formation over the inferior surface of the acromion and reduced

space between the acromion and greater tuberosity. The greater tuberosity near the insertion of supraspinatus may show cystic changes. Plain x-rays also help to rule out calcific tendinitis and degenerative joint disease of the acromioclavicular joint.
2. **Electromyography** is indicated if cervical radiculopathy or brachial plexus lesion is suspected.

Management
1. **Medications**
   a. NSAIDs help reduce pain and inflammation.
   b. Local injection of steroids may be used to reduce inflammation and pain. It should be avoided in young athletes because of risk of damaging the rotator cuff.
2. **Ancillary**
   a. **Preventive measures.** Pain is a protective mechanism. Any repetitious activity that gives rise to pain should be avoided completely or reduced to a reasonable level. Subacromial bursitis is more likely after repetitive activities in which the shoulder is abducted to >90° for prolonged periods. Health education programs, especially for athletes involved in overhead activities, are very important. These may include:
      i. Instructions in shoulder **biomechanics**
      ii. **Warm-up** and **flexibility exercises** before the main sports activity
      iii. Reducing the level of activity if it produces pain. Add **rest** periods if activities are continued for prolonged periods.
   b. **Therapeutic measures** include physical therapy.
      i. Local **heat** or **ice** helps in reducing pain.
      ii. **Exercises** are started with passive exercises to increase ROM. As pain decreases and ROM increases, Codman's pendulum exercises and active assisted exercises are started. Later, exercises to strengthen the various muscle groups are prescribed. If pain gets worse after exercise, then that is an indication to back off.
3. **Surgical.** Indications for surgical treatment include:
   a. **Failure of conservative measures** is the major indication to consider operative treatment. Physical therapy program, NSAIDs, local injections of steroids, and avoidance of precipitating activities should be carried out for a prolonged period first.
   b. **Complete tear** of the rotator cuff which interferes with essential functions in a young athlete may require surgical repair. However, many elderly people function well with complete tear of the rotator cuff. Subacromial bursitis and rotator cuff pathology may coexist or may present with similar clinical features. If a complete rotator cuff tear is suspected, an orthopedic consultation is warranted.
   Surgical **procedures** that may be considered are:
   a. Resection of osteophytes on the inferior surface of the acromion
   b. Coracoacromial ligament resection
   c. Anterior acromioplasty (removal of part of the acromion)
   d. Repair of rotator cuff

ROTATOR CUFF TEAR

The rotator cuff plays an important role in abduction of the shoulder. Inflammation and tear of the cuff affect abduction and function of the upper extremity.

Anatomy

The rotator cuff is formed by tendons of the supraspinatus, infraspinatus, teres minor, and subscapularis muscles (Fig. 15–8). They **stabilize** the glenohumeral joint and prevent excessive upward movement of the head of the humerus. The supraspinatus muscle arises from the supraspinous fossa of the scapula. The muscle and its tendon pass under the acromion and insert into the greater tuberosity of the humerus. It is separated from the acromion, coracoacromial ligament, and deltoid muscle by the subacromial bursa. Supraspinatus and middle fibers of the deltoid are the main abductors of the arm. Supraspinatus initiates abduction and maintains the head of the humerus against the glenoid.

The infraspinatus muscle arises from the infraspinous fossa and inserts into the greater tuberosity. The teres minor muscle originates from the lateral border of the scapula and inserts into the greater tuberosity distal to the infraspinatus. These two muscles rotate the humerus laterally. Subscapularis muscle is situated anteriorly and arises from the costal surface of the scapula. The subscapular bursa lies deep to it, between it and the neck of the scapula. It is an internal rotator and adductor of the humerus.

Pathology

The supraspinatus tendon receives its blood supply from:
1. Muscular branches of the supraspinatus muscle
2. Osseus branches of the head of the humerus

These arteries anastamose just proximal to the insertion of the supraspinatus tendon into the greater tuberosity. Blood supply to this area may at times be insufficient, and hence, it is described as a **critical zone** (Fig. 15–9). This same area is also likely to be compressed against the acromion during abduction and prone to degeneration.

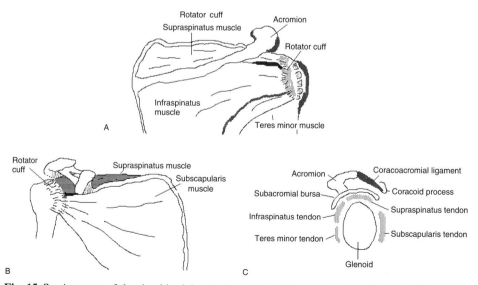

Fig. 15–8 Anatomy of the shoulder joint. *A*, Rear view; *B*, front view; *C*, side view. The rotator cuff is formed by tendons of supraspinatus, infraspinatus, and teres minor. The tendon of subscapularis muscle is in front of the shoulder joint.

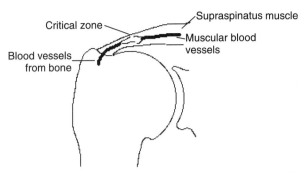

Fig. 15–9 The rotator cuff receives its blood supply from the muscular branches of the supraspinatus muscle and blood vessels from the head of the humerus entering through the insertion of the supraspinatus tendon over the greater tuberosity. The part of tendon where these two blood vessels meet is called the critical zone.

Overhead activities with the arm in abduction are one of the precipitating factors for rotator cuff problems. Freestyle or butterfly swimming and painting ceilings lead to repetitive trauma of the rotator cuff. Osteophytes projecting from the acromioclavicular joint may further narrow the space under the arch and increase impingement. This leads to inflammation, degeneration, and tear of the rotator cuff. Inflammation in the confined space under the acromion and coracoacromial arch gives rise to **painful arc syndrome.** The swollen, inflamed tissue has to pass under the coracoacromial arch and gets squeezed between the arch and the humerus. This explains painful limitation of abduction. Tendon degeneration later may lead to tear of the rotator cuff.

History

The patient may give a history of an activity that requires strong contraction of the supraspinatus and develops acute severe pain in the shoulder. In older patients, even a minor trauma may rupture the already degenerated tendon. However, pain may not be very severe in the elderly with a degenerated rotator cuff. Radiation of pain depends on the severity of the lesion. Initially, all movements may be painful. In most patients, however, there is a long-standing history of painful shoulder with exacerbations and remissions. This suggests chronic inflammation in the supraspinatus tendon and subacromial bursa. Patients may not remember the exact circumstances at the time of onset or the precipitating event for the rupture.

Physical Examination

1. **Inspection.** No abnormal findings are obtained on inspection during the early phase of tear. Deltoid and supraspinatus muscles may show wasting later because of disuse.
2. **Palpation** may reveal tenderness just distal (in the subacromial region) or proximal to the acromion (over the lateral end of the supraspinous fossa), especially in the early stages.
3. **Range of motion**
   a. **Active**—All active movements are painfully restricted during the initial stages. As pain subsides, greater range of active movements is possible. Weakness of abduction depends on the extent of the tear. In complete tears, an attempt at abduction produces shrugging of the shoulder.

b. **Passive**—During the acute stage, even passive movements may be painful. Later, contracture of adductors and internal rotators may lead to limitation of abduction and external rotation.
4. **Special tests**
   a. Injection of **local anesthetic** around the insertion of the supraspinatus tendon relieves pain. If limitation of abduction was due to pain, the patient should be able to actively abduct the arm after this injection. If there is a complete tear of the supraspinatus tendon, the patient will not be able to abduct, even though pain is relieved.
   b. In less extensive tears or later after the pain subsides, the **drop sign** may be elicited. The arm is passively abducted to 180°, and the patient is asked to let it come down slowly to the neutral position. Around 90° of abduction, the arm falls abruptly because of weakness. The smooth lowering of the arm is replaced by sudden drop. Alternatively, the patient may be asked to maintain the arm at 90° of abduction against gravity. A gentle tap on the hand will make the arm fall to the neutral position (Fig. 15–10).
   c. The patient is not able to **abduct the arm against resistance** because of pain or weakness of the abductors (Fig. 15–7).

Investigations

1. **Plain x-rays** are usually normal in the early stage of the disease. In chronic cases, there is less space between the humeral head and acromion. This space is normally occupied by the supraspinatus tendon. Degenerative changes, such as sclerosis and cysts, appear on the undersurface of the acromion and over the greater tuberosity near the insertion of the supraspinatus tendon.
2. **MRI** can show inflammation or tear of the rotator cuff and is replacing arthrography as a diagnostic test.
3. **Arthroscopy** can confirm the diagnosis of tear, and some surgical procedures can be carried out at the same time.
4. **Arthrography.** Contrast media injected in the shoulder joint usually does not enter the subacromial bursa, unless there is complete rupture of the supraspinatus tendon (Fig. 15–11). There is a small percentage of normal individuals in whom the shoulder joint communicates with the subacromial bursa.
5. **Double-contrast arthrography.** Injection of air and contrast helps delineate the size and location of the tear better in some cases.

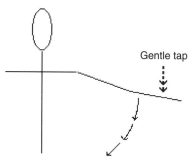

Gentle tap

Fig. 15–10 Drop sign. The abductors of the shoulder are weak in patients with rotator cuff tear. They are not able to maintain the arm in active abduction against gravity, and the arm falls when it is tapped gently.

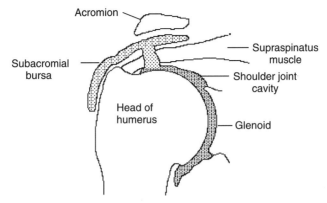

Fig. 15–11 Arthrography in complete tear of the rotator cuff. The cavity of the shoulder joint is separated from the subacromial bursa by the rotator cuff. When there is complete tear of the rotator cuff, dye injected into the shoulder joint flows freely into the subacromial bursa.

Management

Conservative treatment of this condition is very similar to that of subacromial bursitis. If the patient's lifestyle does not demand strong abduction at the shoulder and relief of pain is the main goal, nonsurgical treatment will give a satisfactory result.

Surgical repair of the tendon should be considered in young, active individuals with a complete tear. There is some controversy regarding timing after injury when the operation should be done. Anterior acromioplasty and excision of the acromioclavicular ligament may be considered as a desirable ancillary procedure at the time of repair of the supraspinatus.

BICIPITAL TENDINITIS

Anatomy

The long head of the biceps muscle arises from a small area at the superior end of the glenoid fossa (Fig. 15–12). The tendon passes over the head of the humerus and then lies

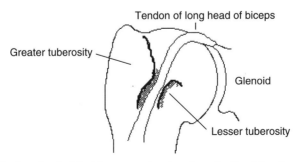

Fig. 15–12 The long head of the biceps muscle arises from the tip of the glenoid and then goes over the head of the humerus and within the bicipital groove.

between the lesser and greater tuberosities in the bicipital groove. This portion of the tendon is covered by a synovial sheath. The synovial cavity surrounding the biceps tendon communicates with the synovial cavity of the shoulder joint (Fig. 15–13). The synovial sheath facilitates movements of the tendon. The tendon of the long head of the biceps is held in the bicipital groove by the transverse humeral ligament. The short head of biceps arises from the tip of the coracoid process. Muscle bellies of the long and short heads unite in the arm. The tendon of biceps brachii crosses the elbow joint and inserts into the radial tuberosity.

The biceps muscle crosses two joints—the shoulder and elbow—and thus acts on both of them. Its major actions are to flex and supinate the forearm. The tendon of the long head also helps to stabilize the head of the humerus by preventing it from sliding upward.

Pathology
As with the rotator cuff, degenerative changes are seen in the long head of biceps by the fifth decade. Overuse and trauma may initiate **synovitis** around the long head of biceps. Adhesions form between the tendon and the synovial sheath, giving rise to pain on movements. Inflammation and degeneration may lead to fraying and ultimately to **rupture** of the tendon.

Symptoms
Symptoms may be brought on by repeated use of the shoulder. **Pain** is felt over the anterior aspect of the shoulder joint. In more severe cases, it may radiate down the front of the arm. It is aggravated by movements of the shoulder and is usually worse at night during sleep.

Physical Examination
1. **Inspection** yields normal findings.
2. Palpation elicits tenderness over the biceps tendon in the bicipital groove. The tendon is located between the greater and lesser tuberosities of the humerus (Fig. 15–12). The elbow is flexed to 90° with the shoulder in neutral rotation and with the palpating fingers over the anterior aspect of shoulder. The forearm is moved gently to rotate the humerus into position of external and internal rotation. The long head of biceps will slip under the palpating fingers and give rise to pain if there is bicipital tendinitis. Tenderness over lateral aspect of the shoulder may also be felt if there is coexisting rotator cuff pathology or subacromial bursitis.

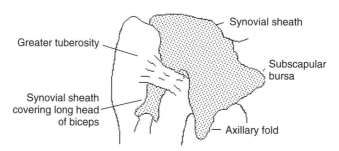

Fig. 15–13 The long head of biceps muscle is enclosed in synovial sheath of the shoulder joint when it traverses through the bicipital groove. Inflammation of the synovial sheath surrounding the biceps tendon is called bicipital tendinitis.

3. **Range of motion**
   a. **Active**—Forward flexion and abduction may be painful.
   b. **Passive**—Extension at the shoulder stretches the tendon and is painfully limited. External rotation presses the tendon and its synovial sheath against the lesser tuberosity, giving rise to pain.
4. **Special tests**
   a. When the elbow is flexed to 90° with the shoulder in neutral rotation and the arm by the side, the patient is asked to **supinate the forearm against resistance.** Since the long head of biceps supinates the forearm in this position, pain on this maneuver confirms bicipital tendinitis.
   b. **Forward flexion** of the shoulder against resistance reproduces pain over the anterior aspect of the shoulder.
   c. Injection of local **anesthetic** in the synovial sheath of the long head of biceps relieves the pain and restores all movements. The intertubercular groove is located between the greater and lesser tuberosities of the humerus. It is easier to palpate with the arm in slight external rotation. The needle is directed posteriorly. Local anesthetic should flow easily. Injection into substance of the tendon should be avoided.

Differential Diagnosis
1. **Rotator cuff pathology** may coexist or be mistaken for bicipital tendinitis. Pain and tenderness are more lateral over the supraspinatus tendon in the subacromial region in rotator cuff pathology. Abduction against resistance is painful and supination of the forearm is not affected.
2. In **degenerative arthritis** of the acromioclavicular joint, the pain is felt more proximally over the joint. Adduction of the shoulder is painful.

Investigations
Diagnosis is mainly clinical. Special views of the bicipital groove may show irregularities of the floor to suggest the diagnosis.

Management
1. **Medications**
   a. NSAIDs to control inflammation and pain
   b. Local injection of long-acting steroid
2. **Ancillary**
   a. **Rest.** Activities that precipitate tendinitis should be discontinued.
   b. **Physical therapy. Local heat** in the form of hot packs, shortwave diathermy, or ultrasound helps to relieve pain. Gentle **passive ROM exercises** are started to prevent contractures. Active exercises are started as tolerated by the patient.

RUPTURE OF THE LONG HEAD OF BICEPS

Pathology
Degeneration of the tendon occurs with advancing age. Roughness of bone under the tendon contributes to fraying and ultimate rupture.

Symptoms

Lifting a heavy weight may rupture the tendon. Sometimes, there is no definite history of trauma when the tendon has degenerated slowly over a long period of time. Sudden pain is felt over the anterior aspect of the upper arm. The patient may feel a snap or tearing sensation.

Physical Examination

1. **Inspection.** The biceps muscle loses its proximal attachment (Fig. 15–14), and the muscle belly gets displaced distally into the lower half of the arm, forming a bulging mass with a depression between it and the deltoid muscle. There may be swelling or bruise if there was bleeding due to rupture of blood vessels.
2. **Palpation.** There may be tenderness over the anterior aspect of the shoulder where the long head of the biceps tendon is normally located. The bulge in the distal arm feels soft and flabby because of lack of tone in the muscle belly.
3. **Range of motion.** Active elbow flexion during the initial stages is painful and weak. Later (after months), the short head of biceps, brachialis, and brachioradialis muscles are able to provide sufficient power for elbow flexion.

Management

1. **Medications.** Analgesics are prescribed to relieve pain.
2. **Ancillary.** Gentle passive ROM **exercises** are started to prevent contractures. Active exercises are started as tolerated by the patient. Later, exercises to increase strength of other elbow flexors are taught to compensate for the long head of biceps.
3. **Surgical repair** is considered for a young person involved in vigorous sports or occupation requiring strong elbow flexion.

ADHESIVE CAPSULITIS

Frozen shoulder and **adhesive capsulitis** are considered two different clinical entities by some. Frozen shoulder develops as a stiff shoulder after a painful shoulder condition like subacromial bursitis, biceps tendinitis, or partial tears of the rotator cuff. Adhesive capsulitis, on the other hand, is believed to start as inflammation of the synovium of the shoulder joint and leads to intra-articular adhesions, especially in the axillary fold.

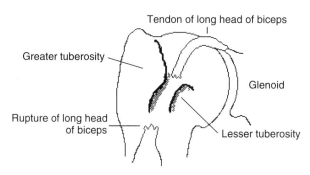

Tendon of long head of biceps

Greater tuberosity

Glenoid

Rupture of long head of biceps

Lesser tuberosity

Fig. 15–14 Rupture of the long head of biceps.

Anatomy
Movements of the glenohumeral joint are possible because of a lax joint capsule and shape of the bones forming the joint. There is a fold of capsule and synovial membrane at the distal end of the shoulder joint in axilla, called the axillary fold or dependent fold (Fig. 15–15). This loose fold allows the arm to be abducted. When this fold is obliterated by adhesions, abduction is limited.

Etiology
The exact etiology of this disease is unknown. Prolonged immobilization due to other painful conditions of the shoulder or myocardial infarction may play an important role in the development of frozen shoulder.

Pathology
Arthroscopy has shown erythema and synovial thickening in early stages of the disease. Later, fibrinous adhesions form, which may organize into fibrous tissue. Joint space is reduced, bringing the head of the humerus very close to the glenoid. The dependent fold of synovial membrane gets obliterated.

History
The onset is gradual, with **limitation of movements** and **pain** in the shoulder region as the two main symptoms. Initially, it may mimic subacromial bursitis (impingement syndrome) because of painful restriction of abduction in the midrange. There may be difficulty with reaching the hip pocket, combing hair, or hooking the bra. Pain and limitation of ROM gradually worsen without treatment and may ultimately lead to a very stiff shoulder. In very late stages, pain subsides but stiffness persists.

Physical Examination
1. **Inspection.** Normal swing of the arm during walking may be limited on the affected side. Later, when the shoulder has lost all movements, there may be **wasting** of the deltoid and other muscles due to disuse atrophy. The arm is kept adducted, close to the body, in neutral or internally rotated position.
2. **Palpation.** The shoulder area is tender as long as there is inflammation. Tenderness and pain subside when inflammation is controlled.

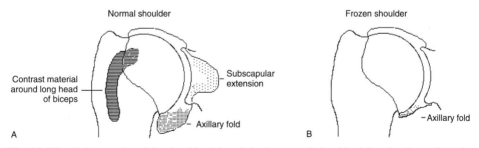

Fig. 15–15 Arthrography of the shoulder joint. *A,* In the normal shoulder joint, the dye collects in the axillary fold and subscapular extension and around the long head of biceps tendon. *B,* In adhesive capsulitis, the capacity of the joint cavity is markedly reduced. The axillary fold has very little dye because of adhesions.

3. **Range of motion**
   a. **Active**—Initially, active movements are affected more than passive. External rotation and abduction are restricted to a greater extent than other movements.
   b. **Passive**—During the stage of inflammation, movements are restricted and painful. Later, when inflammation subsides and fibrosis sets in, all movements are restricted and there may be little pain.

Course
The course is usually slow, taking months to develop. Once it has developed, it may take months of therapy to improve.

Differential Diagnosis
Subacromial bursitis and adhesive capsulitis may present as pain on active abduction. External rotation is affected more, and tenderness is diffuse all over the shoulder region in adhesive capsulitis.

Investigations
Diagnosis is mainly clinical, but the following investigations may be ordered:
1. **Plain x-rays** are not very helpful since there are no abnormal findings.
2. **Arthrography** of the shoulder shows reduced capacity of the joint. The normal shoulder joint can take 15–18 ml of contrast material (Fig. 15–15A), but in adhesive capsulitis, it may not be able to take >10 ml. The dependent fold of the synovial membrane is obliterated (Fig. 15–15B). Normally, this space is filled with contrast material, but in adhesive capsulitis, the dependent fold is not visualized.
3. **Arthroscopy** can show different stages of the disease, from inflammation and synovial thickening to fibrosis and obliteration of the dependent synovial fold.

Management
1. **Prevention.** Maintaining ROM of shoulders in patients who are likely to develop frozen shoulder, e.g., after myocardial infarction, may avoid much pain and therapy later.
2. **Medications. NSAID**s relieve pain and reduce inflammation. Local injection of steroids is given in the most painful and tender areas or in the joint cavity.
3. **Ancillary.** Local **heat** in the form of hot packs or ultrasound help relieve pain and allow passive stretching and active **ROM exercises** by a physical therapist. During the acute painful stage, very gentle exercises are prescribed so as not to aggravate pain. Later, as the patient is able to tolerate, activities and exercises are increased.
4. **Surgical.** If the patient fails to improve after a prolonged course of conservative treatment, **manipulation under anesthetic** should be considered. Manipulation should not be done if there is marked osteoporosis of the proximal end of the humerus or a history of fractured neck of the humerus.

CALCIFIC TENDINITIS

Deposits of calcium salts in the subacromial region are sometimes seen on x-rays. These deposits may or may not be the cause of pain in the shoulder.

Pathology
Deposition of calcium is part of a natural process of healing after degeneration of tissues. Since degenerative changes are common in the supraspinatus tendon near its insertion, calcium deposits may be seen in this region. Presence of calcium can initiate inflammatory changes in the overlying subacromial bursa.

History
The onset may be very sudden with excruciating pain or subacute with many episodes of a less severe nature. Usually, there is no history of injury. Pain increases in severity over a few days and then begins to subside.

Physical Examination
1. **Inspection.** During the acute stage, there may be some swelling and redness around the shoulder.
2. **Palpation** of the skin over the shoulder may be warm to touch. The subacromial region is markedly tender during acute exacerbation.
3. **Range of motion.** All active and passive movements are severely restricted because of pain. In the chronic stage, abduction is painful in the midrange.
4. **Special tests**
   a. Injection of local **anesthetic** in the subacromial region will give immediate relief of pain.
   b. The calcium hydroxyapatite material can be **aspirated** and examined under the microscope to confirm the diagnosis.

Differential Diagnosis
1. **Gout.** Patients with gout usually give history of previous similar attacks in other joints.
2. **Septic arthritis** is ruled out by examination of fluid aspirated from the joint. If infection is suspected, injection of cortisone preparation is contraindicated.
3. **Infection of subacromial bursa** should be handled in the same way as septic arthritis.

Investigations
Plain **x-rays** show calcification near the greater tuberosity.

Management
1. **Medications**
   a. Injection of **local anesthetic** in the subacromial region helps to relieve pain.
   b. **Needling** with a large-bore needle is done to aspirate or release calcium hydroxyapatite crystals.
2. **Ancillary.** Initially, the arm is put in a **sling** to provide rest for a few days. Local **ice** or heat is applied to reduce inflammation. **ROM exercises** are started as soon as the patient can tolerate in order to prevent stiffness of the shoulder.
3. **Surgical** treatment is rarely required, only when conservative measures fail to relieve symptoms.

Bibliography

1. Bonafede RP, Bennett RM: Shoulder pain. Guidelines to diagnosis and management. Postgrad Med 82(1):185–193, 1987.

2. Hawkins RJ, Abrams JS: Impingement syndrome in the absence of rotator cuff tear (stages 1 and 2). Orthop Clin North Am 18:373–382, 1987.
3. Itoi E, Tabata S: Conservative treatment of rotator cuff tears. Clin Orthop 275:165–173, 1992.
4. Lyons AR, Tomlinson JE: Clinical diagnosis of tears of the rotator cuff. J Bone Joint Surg 74-B:414–415, 1992.
5. Murnaghan JP: Adhesive capsulitis of the shoulder: Current concepts and treatment. Orthopedics 11:153–158, 1988.
6. Neviaser RJ: Diagnosis and management of rotator cuff tears. J Musculoskel Med 9(2):62–69, 1992.
7. Neviaser RJ, Neviaser TJ: The frozen shoulder: Diagnosis and management. Clin Orthop 223:59–64, 1987.
8. Rogers LF, Hendrix RW: The painful shoulder. Radiol Clin North Am 26:1359–1371, 1988.
9. Spiegel TM, Crues JV: The painful shoulder: Diagnosis and treatment. Prim Care 15:709–723, 1988.
10. Tearse DS: Shoulder problems in athletes. Postgrad Med 97(2):67–85, 1995.

16

Elbow

Jay Subbarao, M.D., M.S.

Anatomy

The elbow joint is formed by the distal end of the humerus and proximal ends of the radius and ulna (Fig. 16–1). The trochlea of the humerus articulates with the articular surface on the olecranon and coronoid processes of ulna. The elbow is a hinge joint that moves in only one plane and has flexion and extension movements. The head of the radius articulates with a prominence over the lateral side of the distal end of the humerus, called the capitellum. The radial head also articulates with the lateral side of the proximal ulna. These two joints—radiocapitellar and radioulnar—allow rotation of the forearm, i.e., pronation and supination.

All these joints are enclosed by the same fibrous capsule and synovial membrane. The capsule of the joint is thin and lax to allow movements. The joint stability is primarily provided by localized thickenings of the capsule which form the medial and lateral collateral ligaments. The radial head is kept in close contact with the ulna by the annular ligament.

Movements of the elbow are controlled by specific muscles (Table 16–1).The medial epicondyle of the humerus gives origin to flexors of the wrist and fingers and pronator teres muscles, whereas extensors of the wrist and fingers originate from the lateral epicondyle. The radial, median, and ulnar nerves cross the elbow and pass through fibromuscular arches. Compression syndromes can develop in these areas and result in neuropathies with different symptom complexes, e.g., cubital tunnel syndrome or pronator teres syndrome.

In children, epiphyseal separations occur because the junction of the shaft and epiphysis is not strong. It is important to know the age at which centers of ossification for these epiphyses appear and the age at which they fuse with the diaphysis (Table 16–2).

History

A detailed history regarding duration and location of pain, its onset, and aggravating and relieving factors should be obtained. **Pain** from elbow pathology is well localized to the elbow region. Pain in the elbow region may be referred from the cervical region, brachial plexus, or heart. It is important to know if the symptomatic side is the patient's dominant extremity or not. If the patient gives a history of **injury,** it will help to find out the position of the elbow at the time of injury, point of impact, and direction of forces. **Age** of the patient and the vocational and avocational **activities** that result in elbow dysfunction should be noted. A tennis player or baseball pitcher may develop pain syndromes specific to these activities. If the joint is **swollen,** inquire about pain and swelling of other joints.

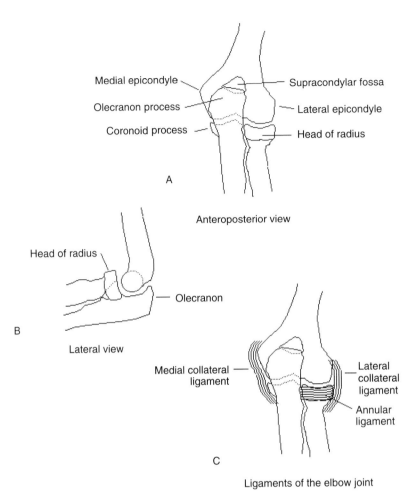

Fig. 16–1 Anatomy of the elbow joint. *A*, Anteroposterior view; *B*, Lateral view; *C*, Ligaments of the elbow joint.

Physical Examination

1. **Inspection.** Alignment of forearm with the arm is observed. Normally, there is a 5°–15° angle (valgus) between the axis of the arm and that of the forearm—the "carrying angle." It is greater in women than men. When the elbow is fully extended, the hand is more lateral (farther from the body) than the elbow. This angle is increased in valgus **deformity.** A diffuse **swelling** may be due to effusion in the elbow joint, bruise, or fracture.

2. **Palpation.** Skin **temperature,** tenderness, and characteristics of any swelling are noted during palpation. **Localized tenderness** is very useful in determining the anatomic structure involved. Bony points—the medial and lateral epicondyle and the olecranon—are palpated. When the elbow is flexed to 90°, these three points make a triangle, but when the joint is fully extended, they are in one line. The head of the radius can be palpated just distal to the lateral epicondyle. It can be felt to rotate as the forearm is

Table 16–1   Muscles Controlling Movements of the Elbow

Movement	Muscles	Predominent Nerve Root Innervation
Flexion	Brachialis Biceps brachi Brachioradialis	Cervical 5 and 6
Extension	Triceps	Cervical 7
Supination	Biceps Supinator	Cervical 5 and 6
Pronation	Pronator teres Pronator quadratus	Cervical 6 Cervical 8

pronated and supinated. The ulnar nerve is behind the medial epicondyle.

3. **Range of Motion.** The range of flexion and extension of the elbow is measured from a neutral position (0°) when the arm is in line with the forearm. The range is from 0°–150° when the forearm is brought as close to the arm as possible. The neutral position for measurement of pronation and supination is with the elbow close to the body and flexed to 90°. In this position, the movements of the shoulder are prevented from contributing to pronation and supination of the forearm. The fingers and thumb are in sagittal plane with the thumb on top. For pronation, the hand is rotated so that the palm faces down, and for supination, the palm faces upward. The range is from 0°–80° to either side from neutral. Good painless ROMs of the elbow are essential for proper placement of the wrist and fingers for functional activities, e.g., washing the face or feeding. Crepitus may be palpable on movements of the elbow.

4. **Special Tests.** The diameter of the arm should be measured at definite distance from a bony point (e.g., tip of the olecranon). This value can be compared to the opposite side and also used as a reference for follow-up visits. Injury in childhood with fracture of the elbow may give rise to valgus deformity of the elbow and late ulnar nerve palsy. The most common site for compression of the ulnar nerve is at the elbow. It passes through a fibromuscular arch in the flexor carpi ulnaris. Sensation and muscles innervated by the ulnar nerve in the hand and forearm should be examined. Compression neuropathy of the median and radial nerves is not as common as ulnar neuropathy at the elbow. The radial nerve passes through the supinator muscle and the median nerve through the pronator teres, where they can be compressed. Fractures around the elbow in children are notorious for injury to blood vessels, and **circulation** of the hand and forearm should be checked often. Sometimes, pain in the elbow

Table 16–2   Age at Elbow Epiphyses

Epiphysis	Age When It Appears	Age When It Fuses With The Diaphysis
Radial head	6 yrs	18 yrs
Lateral epicondyle	12	16
Capitellum and outer half of trochlea	2	16
Trochlea, inner half	10	16
Medial epicondyle	5	18
Olecranon	10	16

may be referred from **cervical nerve root** compression or **intrathoracic** lesion such as myocardial infarction.

Investigations
1. **Plain x-rays.** Anteroposterior and lateral views usually are sufficient for most conditions.
2. Special imaging techniques. Magnetic resonance imaging and bone scan are commonly done to evaluate soft tissue or intra-articular pathology.
3. Aspiration of the elbow joint is done for diagnostic and therapeutic purposes. The joint is approached either medial or lateral to the olecranon.
4. Electromyography and nerve conduction tests help to localize the lesion when the patient complains of tingling, numbness, or weakness in the distribution of a peripheral nerve or nerve root.

TRAUMA

Injury or spasm of the brachial artery is a dreaded complication of fracture of the distal end of the humerus and dislocation of the elbow joint. A detailed examination of nerves and blood vessels around the elbow is very important after any injury. This should be done at the time of initial examination, repeated before and after any treatment, and redone often during recovery.

Supracondylar Fracture of the Humerus
This injury is one of the commonest fractures seen in children. It should be considered a "true emergency" because this injury can result in vascular compromise and Volkmann's ischemic contracture. Early reduction of the fracture and close watch on circulation of the extremity may prevent these very serious complications. Malunion with cubitus varus or cubitus valgus deformity, myositis ossificans, and tardy ulnar nerve palsy are some of the late complications of this fracture.

Dislocation of the Elbow
A fall on an outstretched hand with the elbow partially flexed or a direct trauma may dislocate the elbow. The dislocation may be complicated by fracture of the olecranon or coronoid process of the ulna. Uncomplicated dislocation is reduced by manual traction under anesthesia. Anteroposterior and lateral x-ray views of the elbow are obtained before and after reduction of the dislocation. The elbow is immobilized for 3 weeks with close watch on the neurovascular status of the distal extremity. Active assisted and active ROM exercises are started as soon as immobilization is discontinued, followed later by strengthening exercises for elbow flexors and extensors and muscles of the hand. Forcible stretching of the elbow is avoided to minimize the risk of myositis ossificans.

Intra-articular Fractures
Intercondylar fractures of the humerus and fracture-dislocations of the elbow are managed aggressively and immobilized for the shortest possible time to avoid stiffness of the elbow. Open reduction and internal fixation is used to reduce the fracture fragments accurately, and ROM exercises are initiated as soon as possible. Post-traumatic degenerative arthritis is a common late complication after intra-articular fractures.

Fractured Neck of Radius

Fracture of the head and neck of the radius commonly occur after a fall on an outstretched hand. Most fractures are undisplaced and impacted. If there is an angulation deformity of >30° between the head and shaft of the radius or marked comminution of the head, then excision of the head of the radius may be carried out.

Epiphyseal Injuries

Epiphyseal injuries occur in children whose epiphyses have not yet united with the diaphysis. Accurate and early reduction and external or internal fixation are done to prevent premature closure of the epiphyseal plate and subsequent deformity.

Injury to Collateral Ligaments

Acute sprain and strain of the collateral ligaments of the elbow are not uncommon. They are diagnosed by localized swelling and tenderness. Plain x-rays are done to rule out any bony injury. On occasions, stress films of the joint are done under anesthesia to exclude complete tears. Most strains and sprains heal with rest, ice, and immobilization for a short time, which is followed by exercises to regain ROM and function.

Pulled Elbow

This injury, also known as **nursemaid's elbow,** is produced by forces that result in subluxation of the head of the radius. The annular ligament is interposed between the radial head and capitellum. There may be a history of a parent's pulling a reluctant, crying child by its hand and giving a sudden jerk. This injury is most common around the age of 2 years, when the radial head is flush with the shaft and slips out distal to the annular ligament. It is rarely seen after age 8 years.

There is localized tenderness over the lateral aspect of the elbow. The child is not able to fully extend the elbow. All passive movements of the elbow are painful, especially extension and supination. X-rays of the elbow are normal, but wrist x-rays may show downward displacement of the radius. The head of the radius should be reduced and the arm immobilized in a sling for a few days. The chance of recurrence can be minimized by avoiding traction on the forearm.

Rupture of the Biceps Tendon

Rupture of the biceps tendon at the elbow is rare. It occurs when the elbow is forcibly flexed against strong resistance. The patient experiences severe pain at the elbow and is not able to actively flex the elbow. There is tenderness over the antecubital fossa. The belly of the muscle is seen in the upper arm because of its proximal retraction. It is treated conservatively unless the patient needs strong flexion of the elbow for vocational or avocational activities. The elbow is immobilized in 90° of flexion and supination, followed by active exercises to regain movement and strength.

CHRONIC REPETITIVE TRAUMA

Inflammation of tissues as a result of **repetitive movements** or **overuse** may occur in the vicinity of lateral and medial epicondyles of the humerus. These patients present with pain in that region or the proximal elbow. Lateral epicondylitis is much more common than medial.

Lateral Epicondylitis
Lateral epicondylitis and **tennis elbow** have very similar clinical features.

Anatomy
The common extensor tendon is attached to the lateral epicondyle and gives origin to the extensor carpi radialis brevis, extensor digitorum communis, extensor digiti minimi, and extensor carpi ulnaris muscles. The extensor carpi radialis brevis and extensor carpi ulnaris muscles extend the wrist, and the other two muscles extend the fingers. There is a separate muscle for extension of the index finger (extensor indicis proprius).

Etiology
Inflammation of the tissues near the epicondyle is presumed to be the cause of the symptoms. The tendon of origin, periosteum, or lateral collateral ligament are some of the structures that may be involved. Repeated strain in certain occupations or activities, such as playing tennis, may bring on this inflammation. Some have postulated entrapment of the radial nerve or one of its branches as the cause of tennis elbow.

History
The onset of symptoms and exacerbations is usually related to overuse. The patient complains of pain slightly distal to the lateral epicondyle and in the proximal forearm. The pain is aggravated by strong contraction of the extensors of the wrist and supination of the forearm against resistance. These muscles are required in playing tennis or turning a screwdriver.

Physical Examination
1. **Inspection.** There are no abnormal findings on inspection.
2. **Palpation.** There is localized **tenderness** over the common extensor tendon just distal to the lateral epicondyle. In true epicondylitis, the tenderness is over the bone rather than the muscle.
3. **Range of motion** in all joints is normal.
   a. **Active**—Active extension against resistance of the index or middle finger or of the wrist reproduces pain and is very weak because of the pain. Active supination of the forearm against resistance may be painful.
   b. **Passive**—Stretching of the common extensor tendon or supinator muscle may also reproduce the pain. The patient's elbow is extended, forearm is fully pronated, and wrist is flexed to stretch these structures and reproduce the pain.

Investigations
All blood tests and x-rays are normal. Local injection of an **anesthetic** helps to confirm the diagnosis by relieving the symptoms and signs of tennis elbow.

Management
The goals of treatment are to decrease inflammation and pain and to promote healing. Since overuse is the most frequent cause of this condition, **rest** is the most important modality. A detailed analysis of the patient's occupation and recreational activities will assist in planning treatment and prevention of future exacerbations. The activity that precipitated the onset should be avoided or reduced. **NSAIDs** and **ultrasound** help in reducing the inflammation. If this fails to relieve pain, **injection** of local anesthetic with a cortisone preparation may help. An epicondylar **splint** that reduces stress on the common extensor origin is rec-

ommended for tennis players and those who cannot avoid repetitive movements. In rare cases, surgical release of the extensor origin may be required to relieve the symptoms.

Medial Epicondylitis
Medial epicondylitis is less common than lateral epicondylitis, but it has a similar pathophysiologic basis for symptoms and similar management. The common flexor tendon takes its origin from the medial epicondyle. The muscles arising from the medial epicondyle are the pronator teres, flexor carpi radialis, palmaris longus, and flexor carpi ulnaris. Golfers and pitchers commonly present with pain and tenderness over the medial epicondyle. The symptoms are reproduced by flexion of the wrist and pronation of the forearm against resistance. In young pitchers (Little Leaguer's elbow), avulsion fracture of the medial epicondyle should be ruled out by x-rays.

Osteochondritis Dissecans
This condition, also known as **Panner's disease,** is avascular necrosis of the capitellum. The exact etiology of this condition is not known. Ninety percent of the lesions occur in males. Occasionally (5%), it affects both sides. It is rarely seen before age 5 years. The child presents with a history of pain, swelling, and locking of the elbow. X-rays demonstrate a defect in the capitellum and a loose body in the joint. Surgical removal of the loose body is indicated if there is history of locking. Conservative treatment consists of ROM and strengthening exercises.

OLECRANON BURSITIS

Olecranon bursitis is also known as **student's elbow.** The olecranon bursa is situated superficial to the tendinous insertion of triceps brachii into the tip of the olecranon. Acute inflammation in the bursa may be due to infection or hemorrhage. Chronic bursitis may occur in association with rheumatoid arthritis or prolonged pressure, e.g., students resting their elbows on desks or miners crawling on their elbows. The subcutaneous rheumatoid nodules occur over the subcutaneous border of the ulna more distal to the site of olecranon bursa.

   The bursa should be aspirated and fluid sent for culture and sensitivity testing if infection is suspected. Hemorrhagic bursitis will need only aspiration, firm bandage, and ice application. Infected bursa is treated with antibiotics and repeated aspiration or incision and drainage. Chronic bursitis in a student or miner needs relief from pressure by elbow pads and avoiding the activity that precipitated the inflammation. In rare cases, it may require surgical excision if conservative measures fail.

PERIPHERAL NERVE LESIONS

Ulnar Neuropathy

Anatomy
The ulnar nerve is located in a groove behind the medial epicondyle where it is covered by a fibrous sheath. This fibro-osseous tunnel is called the **cubital tunnel.** The roof of the tunnel is formed by the arcuate ligament. The ulnar nerve can be easily compressed between the

bone and the fibrous sheath, especially when the elbow is fully flexed or when the patient is lying on a hard surface, such as an operating table. A slowly progressive ulnar neuropathy may develop secondary to cubitus valgus deformity and excessive stretching of the nerve. More distally, the ulnar nerve passes through the two heads of flexor carpi ulnaris muscle, where it can also be compressed.

Clinical Features

The sensory symptoms of tingling and numbness are more common than the motor symptoms, because sensory fibers are more superficial. The ulnar nerve innervates the skin of the little finger and medial half of the ring finger. It also innervates all dorsal and palmar interosseous muscles, hypothenar, and third and fourth lumbrical muscles. A branch from the the ulnar nerve supplies flexor carpi ulnaris and the ulnar half of flexor digitorum profundus muscle. However, the branch to the last two muscles may originate proximal to the elbow and may not be involved in ulnar nerve lesion at the elbow.

The interosseous muscles are wasted in ulnar neuropathy. This is best seen in the first interosseous space between the first and second metacarpals. Weakness of these muscles can be tested by asking the patient to abduct the index finger against resistance. The hand is in midprone position, and the patient is asked to lift the index finger toward the ceiling. Strength of the adductor muscles is tested by putting a thin paper between index and middle fingers and asking the patient to hold it while the examiner tries to pull it away. If the palmar interosseous muscles (adductors of fingers) are weak, then the examiner will be able to pull the paper away without resistance (Froment's sign).

The ulnar nerve can be palpated in the groove behind the medial epicondyle. Normal nerve is not tender and does not elicit tingling in little finger on light percussion. When light tapping over the nerve causes tingling in its distribution, it is reported as a positive **Tinel's sign.** Sensation over the little finger and medial half of the ring finger may be diminished or absent.

Investigations

Nerve conduction velocity across the elbow is slow in ulnar entrapment neuropathy, and needle electromyography may show evidence of denervation in muscles supplied by the nerve. These tests help in confirming the diagnosis and localizing the problem.

Management

It is important to identify the source, level, and extent of nerve compression for effective management. The patient is taught how to avoid pressure on the nerve by proper posture, use of elbow padding, and other orthotic devices. This may be all that is necessary. Most postoperative ulnar neuropathies recover on their own. Selected cases may require decompression of the nerve by cutting the fibrous arch or by anterior transposition of the nerve. Patients with cubitus valgus deformity with tardy ulnar nerve palsy may require correction of the bony deformity.

Radial Neuropathy

The radial nerve can be compressed against the middle of the shaft of humerus in the spiral groove. This happens often when an intoxicated person falls asleep with his head on his arm (**Saturday night palsy.**) Displaced bone fragments or callus from a fracture of the midshaft of humerus can also damage the nerve in the spiral groove and give rise to a similar clinical picture. In the proximal forearm, the motor branch of radial nerve—posterior interosseous nerve—goes through two heads of supinator muscle. It may be compressed here to produce posterior interosseous nerve palsy or a milder syndrome resembling tennis elbow.

The radial nerve innervates a small area of the skin over the first dorsal interosseous space between the first and second metacarpals. The sensation may be diminished or absent in this region. Weakness of the extensor muscles of the wrist and fingers leads to **wrist drop.** The patient is not able to lift the wrist up against gravity and also is not able to extend fingers at the metacarpophalangeal (MCP) joints when the proximal and distal interphalangeal joints are flexed. The long extensors extend the fingers at the MCP joints. Electromyography and nerve conduction tests help to localize the lesion and determine its severity.

Most patients with Saturday night palsy recover on their own. The wrist is supported by a splint which prevents overstretching of the weak muscles until they recover their strength. The posterior interosseous nerve palsy usually recovers without any definitive treatment. Very few patients who present with symptoms similar to tennis elbow and who do not respond to the usual management may require surgical release of the radial nerve.

The median nerve may be subject to compression between the two heads of pronator teres and may present as pain and tenderness over the pronator teres, associated with weakness of the flexor pollices and abductor pollicis. A similar entrapment may occur proximal to pronator teres by a fibrous band (ligament of Struthers). There may be associated compression of the brachial artery, but the distinguishing feature is the weakness of pronator teres. The anterior interosseus nerve may be injured in dislocation of the elbow and will result in weakness of flexor pollicis longus, flexor digitorum I and II, and pronator quadratus, resulting in a "pinch sign." Electrodiagnostic studies are required to confirm the diagnosis.

MYOSITIS OSSIFICANS

Myositis ossificans refers to new bone formation in soft tissues around the elbow joint. Myositis ossificans is usually post-traumatic and is commonly seen after supracondylar or intercondylar fracture or dislocation of the elbow joint. It is especially likely to occur after forceful manipulation of the joint. **Heterotopic ossification** is a metaplastic change in soft tissues without a definite history of trauma. It is seen in a number of neurologic disorders, e.g., quadriplegia, stroke, Guillain-Barré syndrome, and also after burns.

Etiology
The exact etiology of this condition is unknown.

History
During the acute stage, the patient complains of pain and swelling. These may persist for weeks and then gradually subside.

Physical Examination
1. **Inspection.** The anterior aspect of the elbow and proximal forearm are swollen.
2. **Palpation.** There is increased warmth and tenderness during the acute phase. Later, a hard mass may be palpable.
3. **Range of motion.** All movements are painfully restricted.

Differential Diagnoses
Infection should be ruled out during the acute phase. WBC count should be normal, and alkaline phosphatase is elevated. X-rays may show deposition of calcium in soft tissues around the joint in myositis ossification.

Investigations
1. **Alkaline phosphatase** is elevated.
2. **Plain x-rays** may be normal initially for few weeks. Later, calcium deposition is seen in the soft tissues around the joint. Ossification of the mass may be observed months after onset.

3. Three-phase **bone scan** will show increased uptake in the soft tissues in very early stages of the disease.

Course
From 3–10% of patients may end up with **ankylosis** of the joint.

Management
Initially, the joint should be treated with local ice and immobilization. NSAIDs and etidronate disodium have been used to decrease calcification with varying degrees of success. Forceful stretching of the elbow joint is contraindicated. After the acute stage, gentle ROM exercises are started. Later, exercises to strengthen muscles of the forearm and hand and activities to improve hand function are added. Surgery is contraindicated in early stages of the disease but may be considered after a year or more to remove organized bone tissue if the function of the joint is severely limited.

ARTHRITIDES

Rheumatoid Arthritis
The elbow joint may be involved in rheumatoid arthritis. Pain, stiffness, and swelling of the joint are present. The swelling is visible on the posterior aspect of the joint on both sides of the olecranon. Chronic synovitis results in destruction of the cartilage, ligamentous laxity, and deformity. All movements of the joint are painful.

The elbow joint is supported by a **sling** when it is acutely inflamed, painful, and swollen. Gentle passive ROM **exercises** are started, followed later by active-assisted and active exercises. In selected cases, **synovectomy** or excision of radial head are done to increase ROM and decrease pain. Total joint replacement **arthroplasty** may be considered for severe involvement of the elbow.

Degenerative Joint Disease
Degenerative joint disease of the elbow is not common, but it may occur after fracture involving the joint or in certain metabolic disorders (e.g., ochronosis, hemochromatosis, Wilson's disease, and Gaucher's disease).

Infectious Arthritis
Infectious arthritis of the elbow joint is not as common as that of the knee. The most common organisms are gonococci, staphylococci, and pseudomonas. Chronic infectious arthritis due to tuberculosis or fungi are rarely encountered. Synovial fluid aspiration and analysis confirm the diagnosis and dictate selection of antibiotics.

Bibliography

1. Bennett JB: Lateral and medial epicondylitis. Hand Clin 10:157–163, 1994.
2. Coonard RW: Tendonopathies at the elbow. Instr Course Lect 40:25–32, 1991.
3. Gellman H: Tennis elbow (lateral epicondylitis). Orthop Clin North Am 23:75–82, 1992.

17

Hand and Wrist

Arun J. Mehta, M.B., F.R.C.P.C.

The hand is an intricate organ without which humans could not manipulate their environment. It is one of the most important parts of the body in performing ADLs. It is also one of the most commonly injured structures. The hand is able to function efficiently only if other joints of the upper extremity assist it in reaching its destination and have normal sensation and motor control.

Differential Diagnosis

Tingling and Numbness
1. Median nerve (**carpal tunnel syndrome**). Patients complain of tingling and numbness at the tips of the thumb, index, and middle fingers or the whole hand. It is usually worse at night or while holding a pen or steering wheel.
2. **Peripheral neuropathy.** Usually, tingling and numbness are present in both hands and both feet. Tendon reflexes may be absent or depressed.
3. **Ulnar nerve.** Compression neuropathy of the ulnar nerve commonly occurs at the elbow. Sensation of the little finger is usually involved, with weakness or wasting of the interosseous muscles.
4. **Cervical radiculopathy.** Cervical 6, 7, and 8th nerve roots supply the skin of the hand. Nerve root involvement usually gives rise to pain from the neck down to the hand and can also cause tingling and numbness. The neurologic signs are restricted to one particular nerve root involved.
5. **Cerebrovascular accident** or **transient ischemic attack.** Vague and intermittent sensory symptoms in the hand or forearm may occur during early stages of a CVA, during TIA, or as a residual of a stroke.
6. **Thoracic outlet syndrome.** It usually affects the lower trunk of the brachial plexus, with tingling and numbness of the little finger and weakness of the hand.

Pain
Localized pain may be due to:
1. **Trauma.** History of injury with pain may be due to sprains, fractures, and dislocations.
2. **Infection** around the nailbed, tendon sheath or palmar space may present with warm, painful swelling and marked tenderness.
3. **Inflammation** of joints or tendon sheaths may be part of a generalized disease process, e.g., rheumatoid arthritis.

4. **Degenerative joint disease.** Heberden's nodes over the distal interphalangeal (DIP) joint and swelling around the carpometacarpal (CMC) joint of the thumb are common in degenerative joint disease in the hand.

Pain over **radial aspect of the wrist** may be due to:

1. Fracture of the scaphoid
2. Degenerative joint disease of CMC joint of the thumb
3. DeQuervain's disease—Tenosynovitis of the abductor pollicis longus and extensor pollicis brevis
4. Fracture at the base of the first metacarpal
5. Degenerative joint disease of the radiocarpal joint

Pain **over DIP joint** may be due to:

1. Degenerative joint disease—Heberden's nodes
2. Avulsion of extensor tendon
3. Paronychia
4. Psoriatic arthritis

Diffuse, severe pain affecting the **whole hand** may be due to:

1. **Reflex sympathetic dystrophy.** The patient complains of very severe, diffuse, burning pain in the initial stages.
2. **Compartment syndrome** due to compression of blood vessels and nerves in the forearm secondary to tight cast or swelling

Referred pain in the hand may be from:

1. **Cervical radiculopathy** due to involvement of cervical 6, 7, or 8th nerve roots. Pain usually radiates from the neck or shoulder down along the sensory distribution of the root.
2. **Cardiac** pain may be felt in the arm or forearm.
3. **Brachial plexus**—e.g., in brachial plexitis or Pancoast's tumor

Deformity

1. **Trauma**—fractures or dislocations
2. **Joint disease**—e.g., rheumatoid arthritis
3. **Peripheral nerve disease**—e.g., wrist drop due to radial nerve palsy

Swelling

Localized swelling may be due to:

1. **Trauma**—hematoma, dislocation, or fracture
2. **Degenerative joint disease**—especially of DIP joints (Heberden's nodes) or metacarpophalangeal (MCP) and CMC joints of the thumb
3. **Infection** of the nailbed (paronychia) or pulp space of fingertip.
4. **Inflammatory joint disease.** Rheumatoid arthritis frequently affects MCP and proximal interphalangeal (PIP) joints.

Generalized swelling may be due to:

1. **Trauma.** The whole hand may swell after severe injury.
2. **Infection** of the palmar space or common synovial sheath of the flexor tendons
3. **Reflex sympathetic dystrophy** is associated with severe burning pain in the hand.
4. **Impaired venous or lymphatic return**—e.g., after mastectomy or involvement of axillary lymph nodes in malignancy

Anatomy

The skin of the hand on the palmar aspect is thicker and less mobile than that on the dorsal aspect. This thickness is necessary for holding objects. Any swelling due to infection or inflammation is seen more easily on the dorsal aspect because of the skin's looseness over the dorsum of the hand.

Three nerves— the median, ulnar, and radial—innervate the skin. The radial and ulnar arteries supply the hand. They are both on the palmar aspect. Venous drainage is by the veins along the arteries and those on the dorsum of the hand.

The eight carpal bones in the wrist are arranged in two rows of four bones each. The proximal row articulates with the radius and an articular disc. This articular disc separates the distal end of the ulna from the proximal row of carpus. Five metacarpals articulate with the distal row of carpus. The fingers—index, middle, ring, and little—are formed by three phalangeal bones in each. The thumb has only two phalangeal bones and is the shortest of all the phalanges with the widest webspace. Its size, together with the mobility of the first metacarpal, allow the thumb to oppose other fingers to grasp objects. It would be difficult to hold an object, such as a glass of water, if the webspace were decreased.

History

Onset, duration, progress, aggravating and **relieving factors,** and relation to time of the day or activities are queried for each symptom the patient has described. In case of recent trauma, it is important to know the exact time of injury, the place where it occurred, and how it occurred (**mechanism of injury**). In rheumatoid arthritis, joints are stiff in the morning and gradually become more flexible. Progression of symptoms may help in diagnosis and management. Severe pain lasting for months suggests reflex sympathetic dystrophy, whereas severe pain lasting for a few weeks may indicate brachial plexitis. Intermittent pain, swelling, and stiffness are usually seen in rheumatoid arthritis.

Development of **deformities** over a period of time may affect **function** of the hand. Fine functions, such as writing or buttoning, may be difficult to perform because of pain, deformity, or neurologic conditions. A history of which functions are affected, to what extent, and for how long is important for developing a treatment plan. Whether the patient's **dominant** or **nondominant hand** is affected also makes a difference in management. Inquire about the activities the patient performs at **work** and during **leisure.** A nonfunctional hand may prevent a person from working and earning a livelihood. Details of **previous injuries** and **operations** help in diagnosis and management. **Review of systems** is important if involvement of the hand is part of a systemic disease.

Physical Examination

Both upper extremities should be exposed for proper examination of the hand. The patient may need to undress to the waist if symptoms in the hand are thought to be secondary to **cervical spine, breast, brachial plexus,** or **shoulder** pathology. If a systemic problem is suspected, the lower extremities and other major systems should be examined.
1. **Compare both sides.** Subtle changes may be missed if the normal side is not observed.
2. **Inspection.** The hand is observed from the **palmar** and **dorsal** aspects and from the **sides.** It may be subdivided for convenience into **wrist, metacarpal,** and **phalangeal** regions.
   a. **Posture.** How the hand is held when the patient enters the office may give an important clue as to the severity of pain. The hand supported by the opposite hand and held in front of the chest may indicate severe pain.
   b. **Skin. Color** and **scars** over the palmar and dorsal aspects and **hair** over the dorsum of the hand are noted. Changes in skin color due to exposure to cold may suggest Raynaud's phenomenon.

   c. **Swelling** occurs more easily over the dorsum of the hand because of its loose skin. Even with infection on the palmar aspect, swelling is seen over the dorsum. The skin creases on the dorsal aspect are obliterated by the swelling. **Diffuse swelling** involves the dorsal aspect of the whole hand, including the fingers. It is seen in infections of the palmar spaces, paralyzed hand, lymphatic or venous obstruction, or reflex sympathetic dystrophy. **Localized swelling** may occur on the dorsolateral sides of an interphalangeal joint or MCP joint due to effusion in these joints. It is not observed on the palmar side because of a fibrocartilaginous plate or on the dorsum because of the extensor tendon. Swelling due to ganglion and tenosynovitis are also confined to the involved structure.

   d. **Deformity.** Long flexors of the fingers are able to contract maximally only when the hand held in slight (10°–15°) extension (dorsiflexion) in relation to the forearm. The thumb and first metacarpal lie in slight abduction and flexion in relation to the plane of the palm. Note the relationship of phalanges with the metacarpals and with each other. Is there any angulation in the shaft of the metacarpal indicating a fracture? The fingers are held in slight flexion. Are there any fingers or parts of fingers missing? The metacarpals are curved in their longitudinal axis with convexity toward the dorsum of the hand. They are also arranged in such a way that they form a hollow in the center of the palm. This hollow is accentuated by thenar and hypothenar eminences on either side. These eminences are formed by the muscles of the thumb and little finger.

   e. **Atrophy.** If there is atrophy of the muscles for any reason, the hollow of the palm is flattened. Thenar and hypothenar muscle atrophy is seen best by viewing it from an angle, whereas wasting of first dorsal interosseous muscle is observed from the radial side of hand.

   f. **Nails** are observed from the side and dorsal aspect. The angle between the nail and skin is 160° when viewed from the side. It is increased when there is clubbing of the nails.

3. **Palpation.** The skin on the palmar side is thicker and attached very firmly to the deeper structures, whereas skin on the dorsal aspect is thinner and loosely attached.

   a. **Temperature** of the skin is noted.

   b. **Tenderness.** Is it localized or diffuse? Tenderness over a small area helps to localize the pathology. Localized pain felt by the patient when the examining finger is very lightly passed over a foreign body under the skin helps pinpoint its location. Pain on light touch suggests **hyperesthesia.** Localized tenderness in cases of trauma may indicate a fracture. Diffuse hyperesthesia is seen in reflex sympathetic dystrophy.

   c. **Swelling.** Examination of a swelling should include its site, size, surface (smooth or irregular), margins, consistency (soft, firm, or hard), fluctuation, and mobility or attachment (to joint synovium, tendon sheath, or bone).

   d. **Deformity** observed during inspection is confirmed by palpation.

   e. **Scar** is palpated to see whether it is tender, soft, or firm and whether it is attached to any deeper structures. Does it interfere with any function or movement of any joint or tendon.

   f. **Arteries.** Pulsations of the ulnar and radial arteries are palpated.

   g. **Tendons.** Some tendons can be palpated easily on the dorsum of the wrist and hand.

4. The hand can be divided into **three regions** to make it easier to examine:

   a. **Wrist region.** On the radial side of the dorsum of the hand, two groups of tendons form a triangular space called the **anatomic snuffbox** (*see* Fig. 17-4). The patient is asked to extend the thumb in the plane of the palm. The tendons seen toward the palmar side are the extensor pollicis brevis and abductor pollicis longus. The tendon on the dorsal side is the extensor pollicis longus. These tendons form the boundary of the anatomical snuffbox. Tenderness in this area after a fall suggests fracture of the **scaphoid** bone. In **deQuervain's disease** or **tenosynovitis** of the tendon sheath of the extensor pollicis brevis and abductor pollicis longus, a tender swelling is felt in this area.

The **styloid process** of the **radius** is palpated and its relation to the level of **ulnar styloid** is compared. The lateral border of the distal radius is followed toward the wrist. The bony projection felt at the very end of the radius is the styloid process. Slight lateral flexion toward the ulnar side makes it easier to palpate the radial styloid. The ulnar styloid process is distal and palmar to the prominent head of the ulna. Its palpation is facilitated by slight radial deviation of the hand. The radial styloid is slightly distal to the ulnar. This relationship is altered in fractures of the wrist (**Colles' fracture**).

On the palmar aspect of the wrist, two tendons may be palpable near the central portion. The one on the ulnar side is the palmaris longus and on the radial side is flexor carpi radialis longus. The median nerve lies deeper and toward the ulnar side of palmaris longus tendon.

  b. **Metacarpal region.** The **extensor tendons** of the fingers can be seen and palpated over the dorsum of the hand. The **metacarpal bones** are also palpable in this region. Localized tenderness or deformity suggests fracture of the metacarpal. These structures are not palpable over the palmar aspect because of overlying muscles and tendons.

The first metacarpal should be followed proximally toward its base and **carpometacarpal** (CMC) **articulation.** A common cause of tenderness in this region is degenerative arthritis of the CMC joint, which is very common in people over 60 years of age. When this metacarpal is followed distally, one can palpate the **metacarpophalangeal (MCP) joint** of the thumb. This joint is also commonly involved in degenerative joint disease. Heads of the metacarpals form the knuckles. Part of the articular surface of the head can be palpated when the proximal phalanx is flexed. The synovial membrane of the MCP joints should be palpated for tenderness and swelling. This is best done over the sides of the extensor tendons where they cross the joint.

  c. **Phalanges.** Tenderness over interphalangeal joints suggests inflammation. The DIP joints are commonly involved in degenerative joint disease, whereas MCP joints are affected in rheumatoid arthritis.

5. **Range of Motion.** ROM may be affected because of:
  a. Pain
  b. Swelling
  c. Soft tissue contracture
  d. Bony deformity
  e. Tendon rupture
  f. Muscle weakness

In all these conditions, active movements are restricted. However, in tendon rupture and muscle weakness, passive ROM is normal. In normal individuals, passive ROM may be slightly (10°–20°) more than the active range. ROM of each joint should be compared with that of the opposite side. ROM is measured from the **neutral position** of each joint (0°). In neutral position, the fingers are all straight, in line with the metacarpals, and together. The thumb lies close to the index finger in the palmar plane. The metacarpals are in line with the radius and ulna. In the anatomically neutral position, the palm is facing the front. However, for measuring pronation and supination, this is the position of full supination. The neutral position for pronation and supination is when the thumb is facing the front and the palm is toward the thigh. Abduction and adduction of the fingers are measured from the axis of the third metacarpal and middle finger.

Brief ROM exam can be done by asking the patient to perform circumduction (combined flexion, extension, and radial and ulnar deviations) at the wrist and making and opening the fist. If there is limitation of ROM, the distance from the fingertips to the distal crease of the palm is measured. Normally, the fingertips can touch the distal crease.

Active movements are performed by the patient. These movements needs to be explained to the patient in simple language without technical words such as flexion and extension. Alternatively, the examiner can demonstrate the movement. The proximal segment is fixed by the examiner. The final range is measured from the neutral as 0°.

Passive ROM is also measured from the neutral position and after immobilizing the proximal segment with one hand of the examiner. The distal segment is held by the other hand and moved in various directions. If the active ROM is normal, passive range need not be examined.

6. **Special Tests**
   a. **Function.** Some common functions of the hand can be tested by asking the patient about writing, buttoning, and feeding. Help of an occupational therapist may be sought if a more detailed functional examination is required.
   b. **Neurologic examination.** A regional or complete neurologic examination is necessary if the patient complains of tingling, numbness, weakness, incoordination, or atrophy of muscles of the hand. The hand is affected in median, ulnar, or radial nerve problems as well as brachial plexus or cervical 6, 7, or 8th nerve root involvements. CNS conditions such as amyotrophic lateral sclerosis, multiple sclerosis, or stroke can also affect the hand.

Investigations
1. **Plain x-rays** help in the diagnosis and management of fractures, dislocations, arthritis, reflex sympathetic dystrophy, and other conditions.

Table 17–1 Approximate Normal Range for Wrist and Hand Joints

Wrist	Flexion 80°	Extension 70°
	Ulnar deviation 40°	Radial deviation 20°
Finger joints		
MCP	Flexion 90°	Extension 30°
	Abduction 20°	Adduction 20°
PIP	Flexion 100°	Extension 5°
DIP	Flexion 80°	Extension 15°
Thumb		
As one unit	Flexion 50°	Extension 50°
	(along the plane of the palm)	
	Abduction 80°	Adduction 0°
	(in plane at right angles to palm)	
Opposition to tips of all fingers		
MCP*	Flexion 40°	Extension 0°
IP	Flexion 90°	Extension 15°

*There is no abduction or adduction at the thumb MCP joint.

2. **Electromyography** and **nerve conduction studies** are indicated for carpal tunnel syndrome, ulnar neuropathy, and cervical radiculopathy.
   Other appropriate investigations are ordered depending upon differential diagnosis.

Management
The hand is notorious for developing stiffness of joints within days if immobilized, especially if a swollen hand is immobilized. A normally functioning hand is so important in the ADLs, at work, and at play that a stiff, nonfunctioning hand is a major disability. Even if only a part of the hand is not doing its job right, it interferes with activities. That is why it is so important to prevent any disability related to the hand.

CARPAL TUNNEL SYNDROME

Carpal tunnel syndrome (CTS) is the most common compression neuropathy encountered. The median nerve is compressed in the carpal tunnel, giving rise to tingling and numbness of the hand, clumsiness, and sometimes pain.

Anatomy
The median nerve, together with nine flexor tendons, pass through the fibro-osseous tunnel at the wrist. The bony part of the tunnel is formed by carpal bones. On the palmar side, the transverse carpal ligament, a thick fibrous ligament, completes the tunnel (Fig. 17-1). The flexor tendons are surrounded by a synovial sheath. The median nerve and the tendons enter the palm at the distal end of the tunnel. In the hand, the median nerve divides into motor and sensory branches. Sensory branches supply the skin of the thumb, index, middle, and radial half of the ring fingers (Fig. 17-2). The motor branches supply the abductor pollicis brevis, opponens pollicis, and part of the flexor pollicis brevis muscles. These muscles form the thenar eminence.

Etiology
Median neuropathy results from increased pressure in the fibro-osseous carpal tunnel. In more than half of patients, the exact etiologic factor causing increased pressure cannot be determined (**idiopathic**). It may result from increased volume of the contents or decreased size of the canal. **Tenosynovitis** due to **overuse** or **rheumatoid arthritis** as

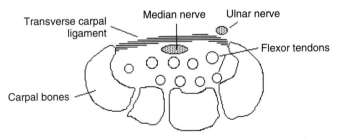

Fig. 17–1 Transverse section of wrist at the level of the carpal tunnel showing median nerve and nine flexor tendons within the tunnel. The ulnar nerve is outside the fibro-osseous tunnel.

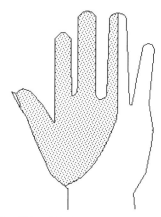

Fig. 17–2 Skin of the hand innervated by the median nerve.

well as swellings (e.g., ganglion) within the canal can compress the median nerve. CTS may be a late complication of **Colles' fracture.** Peripheral nerves are more susceptible to pressure in patients with diabetes, alcohol abuse, and chronic renal failure, and CTS occurs more frequently in these conditions. Occupations that require repeated flexion and extension of the fingers and wrist or use of vibratory tools predispose to development of CTS.

Pathology
The extent of damage to the median nerve depends on the severity and duration of pressure in the canal. In mild cases, there may be **neurapraxia** (physiologic block to nerve conduction without any structural changes). **Demyelination** and **axonal degeneration** are found in more severe cases. Nocturnal symptoms are explained by venous engorgement causing increased pressure within the tunnel. Edema may be the reason for median neuropathy that occurs during pregnancy and clears up after delivery.

History
CTS is more common among **women** between **40–70 years** of age. Onset of symptoms may be related to a new job or hobby that involves repeated movements of wrist and fingers, e.g., crocheting. The patient usually visits her physician months after the onset. Sometimes, acute compression of the median nerve occurs after bleeding or infection in the region. **Tingling** and **numbness** of the hand are the most common symptoms. These may be poorly localized and not necessarily restricted to the sensory distribution of the median nerve.

During the early stages, the patient wakes up from sleep because of a tingling sensation in the hand or feels her hand going numb while driving a car or holding a newspaper. **Nocturnal** symptoms are relieved by shaking the hand. It is important to know how often the patient wakes from sleep because of these symptoms. **Pain** may be felt in the wrist, forearm, or, at times, the shoulder. Proximal extension of pain may make the diagnosis of CTS more difficult. Difficulty in carrying out **fine motor activities,** like writing, is reported by some. Patients may also complain of **dropping things** they are holding.

Ask about the following conditions which may be associated with CTS:

1. Overuse, occupational or recreational
2. Diabetes or alcohol abuse
3. Injury to wrist, fracture
4. Pregnancy
5. Inflammatory arthritis

Physical Examination

1. **Inspection. Atrophy** of thenar muscles may be seen in severe and long-standing cases. Mild atrophy can be observed by looking at the hand from the radial side and tangentially along the surface of the palm.
2. **Special tests**
   a. **Sensation** in the distribution of the median nerve may be affected (*see* Fig. 17-2). Touch, two-point discrimination, and pinprick are tested over the tips of all fingers. In CTS these sensations are diminished or absent over the thumb, index, middle, and radial side of the ring finger.
   b. **Muscle strength** of the **abductor pollicis brevis** is compared on both sides. The patient is asked to push her thumb against resistance of the examiner's finger. The thumb is close to the index finger, and the patient attempts to abduct it in a plane at right angles to the palm. Strength of **opponens pollicis** is tested by asking the patient to touch the tip of thumb to the tip of little finger while the examiner tries to separate them. Both of these muscles may be weak in CTS.
   c. **Wrist flexion (Phalen's) test** is performed by asking the patient to maintain both wrists in maximum flexion for 30–60 seconds. This maneuver brings on the symptoms of tingling on the affected side.
   d. Gentle tapping with a finger over the palmar aspect of the wrist may give rise to tingling in the median nerve distribution (positive **Tinel's sign**).

Course

Symptoms in most patients progress slowly over months and reach a plateau. A small group of patients develops acute CTS. Initially, the symptoms are nocturnal or brought on by overuse of the wrist and fingers. Later, the frequency increases, waking the patient more often from sleep. Clinical examination may yield completely normal findings in early stages. Later, wrist flexion (Phalen's) test becomes positive and sensory loss over the fingertips appear. Atrophy of the thenar muscles is seen much later in the course of the disease.

Complications

Permanent degeneration of the median nerve may occur if the compression is not relieved in time.

Differential Diagnosis

1. **Peripheral neuropathy** usually presents with tingling and numbness in the fingers and toes. Symptoms of peripheral neuropathy are not related to activity and usually affect toes, too. The nerves are more susceptible to compression neuropathy in patients with diffuse peripheral neuropathy so that CTS syndrome and peripheral neuropathy may be present in the same patient. Nerve conduction studies (NCS) and electromyography (EMG) can help in distinguishing between these two conditions.

2. **Cervical radiculopathy.** The sixth cervical nerve root innervates the skin over the thumb and radial aspect of the hand and forearm. Impingement of this nerve root in cervical spondylosis gives rise to pain radiating down to the forearm and thumb and numbness in the thumb. In this condition, there is some pain and restriction of movements of the neck; biceps and brachioradialis reflexes may be affected; and sensory changes may extend into forearm. EMG and NCS are useful in diagnosis.
3. **Transient ischemic attack** (TIA), or a minor **cerebrovascular accident,** involving the hand can cause tingling and numbness, loss of dexterity, and weakness. Symptoms of TIA are not nocturnal or related to use of the hand. They last for a few minutes to a few hours and may involve more than the hand. CTS symptoms are intermittent.

Investigations
1. **Electromyography** (EMG) and **nerve conduction studies** (NCS) help in confirming the diagnosis and determining the severity of damage to the median nerve. It is not absolutely necessary to do these tests before surgery. However, evidence of wallerian degeneration of nerve fibers, as shown by fibrillations and positive sharp waves on EMG, is a good reason for surgical decompression. These tests may also help in evaluating postoperative recurrence of symptoms.
2. **X-rays** are necessary to rule out fracture or dislocation if there is a history of injury to the wrist.

Management
Initial treatment for most patients is conservative. Acute CTS secondary to infectious tenosynovitis, recent fracture, or dislocation are exceptions and may need emergency treatment. In mild cases with nocturnal or intermittent paresthesias, patients are asked to **avoid activities** involving repeated wrist and finger movements and use a **wrist splint** at night. If there is no relief after 2–3 weeks, local **steroid injection** should be considered. This can be repeated once or twice after an interval of 1–2 weeks if there is partial relief of symptoms. Steroid injection is contraindicated in the presence of local infection. **Surgical decompression** is done after conservative treatment has failed.
1. **Medications**
   a. **NSAIDs** are prescribed for pain and nonspecific inflammation. They may relieve some swelling in the carpal tunnel.
   b. **Local injection of steroid** is given after a trial of splint and NSAID has failed to relieve symptoms. It is also indicated in patients who are poor surgical risks and have pain due to CTS. Steroid injection may not help when there is muscle atrophy or severe sensory loss. The skin over the palmar aspect of the hand and distal forearm is prepared. The needle is introduced about 1 cm proximal to the distal wrist crease and on the ulnar side of the palmaris longus tendon. The wrist is slightly dorsiflexed. The needle is introduced at an angle of 30°–40° with the forearm and is pointed toward the carpal tunnel. The subcutaneous tissue and carpal tunnel are infiltrated with 1 ml of 1% lidocaine without epinephrine. About 0.5–1 ml (20–40 mg) of prednisolone is injected in the carpal tunnel.
2. **Precautions** are necessary when considering steroid injection:
   a. Do not inject the median nerve or any tendon. If the patient complains of tingling or pain in the median nerve distribution, stop immediately. A total nerve degeneration can follow injection into the nerve. Do not exert much force while injecting. The injection material should flow easily.

b. Do not inject > 1–1.5 ml in the carpal tunnel; otherwise, the symptoms may be exacerbated because of increased pressure. For the same reason, avoid injecting in a very tense wrist.

c. **Do not inject if infection is suspected.**

3. **Ancillary.** Wrist splint, extending from the proximal forearm to proximal palmar skin crease, is worn, especially at night. There are readymade (off-the-shelf) splints available which work well for most patients. For a few who cannot use these, an occupational therapist or orthotist can make a custom splint.

4. **Surgery.** Surgical decompression is carried out by cutting the transverse carpal ligament. Indications for operation include:

   a. Failure of conservative measures

   b. Acute CTS

   c. Severe and constant numbness and mild to moderate atrophy of thenar muscles

   d. Evidence of axonal degeneration on EMG and marked delay on NCS

   e. Patient is unable to work because of symptoms

   f. Frequent and severe nocturnal symptoms

FRACTURES

Fractures of the distal end of radius, scaphoid, and metacarpals are frequently encountered.

Distal End of Radius

Fracture of the distal end of the radius occurs in older individuals, usually women with osteoporosis.

Mechanism of Injury

A fall on an outstretched hand is a common mechanism of injury. The patient tries to protect himself or herself by reaching out with the hand, which hits the ground first.

Classification of Fractures

The fracture fragment may or may not be displaced. The distal fragment is usually displaced dorsally and proximally (Fig. 17-3). The articular surface of the radius, which normally faces slightly toward the palmar aspect of the forearm, now is angulated and turned toward the dorsal aspect of the forearm. This deformity is seen in a **Colles' fracture.** If the deformity is opposite of this and the distal fragment is displaced toward the palmar aspect, it is called **Smith's fracture.** It is important to determine if the fracture line involves the joint surface or not (intra-articular).

History

The patient is usually an elderly woman who gives a history of falling on an icy or slippery surface or tripping over a rug at home. There is immediate pain in the wrist, and the patient is not able to use that hand.

Physical Examination

1. **Inspection** shows swelling around the wrist and later bruising. The deformity is described as a "**dinner fork**" deformity because of dorsal displacement of the distal fragment (Fig. 17–3).

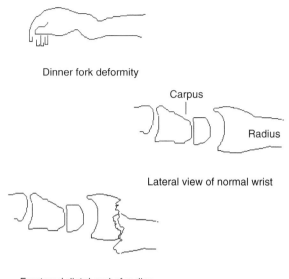

Dinner fork deformity

Lateral view of normal wrist

Fractured distal end of radius

Fig. 17–3 Deformed, normal, and fractured wrist.

2. **Palpation.** There is marked tenderness at the fracture site.
3. **Range of motion.** All movements of the wrist and fingers are painful and restricted.

Investigations

X-rays may show a transverse fracture line about 1–2 inches from the articular surface. In comminuted fractures, there are more than one fragments of the distal end of the radius with or without involvement of the articular surface. The type and extent of displacement are noted.

Complications

Acute median nerve compression may occur as a result of bleeding within the carpal tunnel or after the cast is applied. This, however, is not common. Later, median neuropathy (**carpal tunnel syndrome**) can occur if the fracture unites with a persisting deformity (**malunion**). **Degenerative arthritis** of the wrist joint is common especially after intra-articular fracture.

Management

If there is no displacement of fracture fragments, a below-elbow cast is applied. Displaced fragments need to be reduced and put in a cast. These fragments are likely to be redisplaced when the swelling goes down after a week or two. Repeat x-rays are done to see if the alignment is maintained. The final cast is usually removed after 6 weeks and joints are mobilized. Some complicated fractures may require open reduction and internal fixation.

FRACTURE OF THE SCAPHOID

This fracture can be missed because the patient may not have much pain initially and a hairline fracture may not be visible on x-rays.

Anatomy
Sometimes, blood vessels enter the scaphoid bone from its distal end only. In these individuals, the blood supply to the proximal fragment of scaphoid may be cut off because of the fracture, and they may develop avascular necrosis of the proximal fragment.

Mechanism of Injury
Fall on an outstretched hand is the usual mechanism of injury.

Clinical Features
Fracture of the scaphoid occurs commonly in adults of younger age than those with fractures of the distal radius. There may not be enough pain to suspect a fracture, and the patient may not be x-rayed because of very little pain, no swelling, and no deformity. Localized tenderness in the **anatomical snuffbox** may be the only sign (*see* Fig. 17-4). The joint line between the radius and scaphoid is located by palpating along the lateral border of the radius. Tenderness is present just beyond the styloid process of the radius, in the space between the tendons of extensor pollicis brevis and longus.

Investigations
Fracture of the scaphoid is best seen on oblique views of the wrist. Initial **x-rays** may not show the fracture line, and if it is clinically suspected, x-rays should be repeated after 10 days to 2 weeks after injury. Sometimes, **bone scan** is ordered to see if there is increased uptake in the region of the scaphoid for early diagnosis.

Course/Complications
Union of the scaphoid fracture may be very slow. If there is avascular necrosis of the proximal fragment, nonunion can occur. This complication may lead to degenerative arthritis in the radiocarpal joint.

Management
The wrist is immobilized until the fracture shows signs of union. It sometimes takes months. Internal fixation with a screw may be necessary for delayed union.

FRACTURES OF THE METACARPALS

The metacarpals may break as a result of a direct blow on the hand or during a fistfight. The fracture occurs at the neck of the metacarpal, near the distal end, or in mid-shaft. In fracture near the neck, the distal fragment angulates toward the palmar side. This type of fracture is commonly seen in the fifth metacarpal. Most of these fractures do not require reduction and heal well after a few weeks of protection. Closed reduction may be required for severe deformity. The first metacarpal may break near its base. The fracture line passes through the joint, and the distal fragment slides proximally (Bennett's fracture). This fracture is very unstable and requires internal fixation.

RHEUMATOID ARTHRITIS

Rhematoid arthritis of the hand is a bilateral, symmetrical, inflammatory arthritis affecting the wrist, metacarpophalangeal (MCP) joints, and proximal interphalangeal (PIP) joints.

History

Morning stiffness and **pain** in joints affects **function** of the hand. Opening a water tap, buttoning, or writing may be impossible during exacerbations. It is important to find out which function is difficult to perform. Chronologic evolution of **deformities** should be noted.

Physical Examination

1. **Inspection.** Swelling of joints is more readily visible over the dorsal aspect of the hand because the skin is thin and loose.
   a. **Wrist**—**Swelling** due to synovitis of the wrist joint is seen over the dorsum and sides and is restricted to the carpal region. Tenosynovitis of the flexor and extensor tendons can also cause swelling visible in this region. However, swelling due to tenosynovitis extends proximally over the distal forearm and into the hand, unlike that due to wrist involvement. The head of the ulna becomes more prominent because of dorsal subluxation.
   b. **MCP joints**—The depressions between metacarpal heads (**knuckles**) are obliterated when MCP joints are swollen. Common deformities in rheumatoid arthritis include **palmar subluxation** of metacarpal heads (when proximal phalanx is displaced toward the palm) and **ulnar deviation** of the fingers.
   c. **Fingers**—Swelling of the **PIP joint** is described as spindle-shaped or fusiform. **Deformities** that can occur are of two types:
      i. **Buttonhole** (Boutonnière) deformity is a flexion deformity at the PIP joint with hyperextension at the distal interphalangeal (DIP) joint.
      ii. **Swan neck** deformity involves hyperextension at the PIP joint and flexion at the DIP joint.
2. **Palpation.** Skin temperature is increased during exacerbation of disease. Inflamed tissues are **tender.** Swelling of the joint may be due to intra-articular **effusion** during the acute stage or **synovial thickening** during the chronic stage.
3. **Range of motion.** Active and passive movements in a joint may be restricted because of pain, swelling, or soft tissue contracture. In tendon rupture, passive ROM may be normal and active movement is not possible.

Course/Complications

Pain, morning stiffness, and swelling are seen in the early stage of disease. Deformities develop later on. The course is usually marked by exacerbations and remissions.

Tenosynovitis of the flexor tendons at the wrist may compress the median nerve and give rise to **carpal tunnel syndrome.** Inflammation around the tendons can lead to **rupture of the tendon,** most frequently the extensor tendon of the fifth finger.

Investigations

X-rays of the hand show:
1. **Swelling** of soft tissue surrounding the joint. In the early stages, this is due to effusion in the joint. Later, thickened synovium due to chronic inflammation gives rise to soft tissue swelling on x-rays.
2. **Demineralization** of bone close to the inflamed joints due to hyperemia
3. **Uniform narrowing of the joint space** due to destruction of the articular cartilage (in contrast to irregular narrowing in degenerative joint disease)

4. Marginal **erosions** of the bone close to the attachment of synovial membrane
5. **Deformities** during late stage of disease
   Uniform narrowing and marginal erosions are important signs for diagnosis of rheumatoid arthritis.

Management
Medications are described in Chapter 4.
   Ancillary. Paraffin baths help relieve pain and stiffness of the hand for a short time. Rest is provided by **splints** to reduce inflammation. **Exercises** are prescribed to maintain and improve ROM and strength. **Adaptive equipment** helps improve function of the hand.
   Surgical. The goal of surgical correction of deformities should be to improve function and appearance and to relieve pain. Replacement arthroplasties for MCP joints and repair of ruptured tendons are some of the operations that may be considered for the rheumatoid hand.

TENOSYNOVITIS

Tenosynovitis (tenovaginitis or tendovaginitis) is inflammation of the synovial sheath surrounding the tendon. It gives rise to pain that is aggravated by active movements of the tendon or by passive stretching. There may be a tender swelling in relation to the tendon involved.

Etiology
   Inflammation of the synovial sheath of tendons may be acute or chronic. Both types can occur as a result of:
1. **Overuse.** Repetitive movement is a common cause of this condition.
2. **Inflammatory.** Arthritis, e.g., rheumatoid arthritis, may involve the synovial sheath.
3. **Infection.** *Staphylococcus aureus* and *Neisseria gonorrhoeae* are common organisms found in patients with acute infectious tenosynovitis. Chronic infection may be due to tuberculosis.

Management
Treatment of tenosynovitis depends on the cause. **Infection** is treated with appropriate antibiotics and splint. Sometimes, incision and drainage of pus may be necessary. For diagnosis and management of chronic infections, biopsy, culture, and antibiotic sensitivity testing are done. Rheumatoid tenosynovitis is treated with rest, splint and local injection of steroids.

DeQuervain's Tenosynovitis
Inflammation of the tendon sheath of the abductor pollicis longus and extensor pollicis brevis gives rise to pain and tender swelling over the radial aspect of the wrist.

Anatomy
The abductor pollicis longus and extensor pollicis brevis muscles arise from the radius on the dorsal aspect of the forearm. Their tendons are located in a single synovial sheath over

the lateral aspect of the wrist near the radial styloid process (Fig. 17-4). They abduct and extend the thumb, as indicated by their names. Congenital anomaly of these tendons is usually present with inflammation.

Etiology
Any activity that requires repeated movements of the wrist and thumb, e.g., knitting or wringing clothes, can cause this condition.

Pathology
The tendon sheath is inflamed and thickened initially. Later, in long-standing cases, it may become fibrosed. The tendons are not affected.

History
DeQuervain's tenosynovitis is common in middle-aged women. They complain of **pain** over the lateral (radial) aspect of the wrist, which may radiate down to the thumb and sometimes up the forearm. Any movement involving active contraction of these muscles against resistance aggravates the pain. The patient is not able to use the thumb to hold anything because of pain. This is interpreted by the patient as **"weakness."**

Physical Examination
1. **Inspection.** A longitudinal **swelling** along the course of the tendons is sometimes visible. It is located over the lateral side of the wrist, near the styloid process of the radius.
2. **Palpation.** Localized **tenderness** over the tendon sheath. The swelling is free from the skin but attached to deeper structures. **Crepitus** may be palpable on movements of the tendons in long-standing cases.
3. **Range of motion**
   a. **Active abduction** and extension against resistance are very painful.
   b. **Passive** and active **adduction** of the thumb and wrist causes pain.
4. **Special tests.** The thumb is brought in front of the palm, and the fingers are folded over it. The hand is then adducted or flexed toward the ulnar side. This is called **Finkelstein's test** and reproduces the pain.

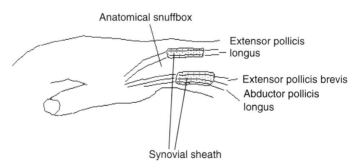

Anatomical snuffbox

Extensor pollicis longus

Extensor pollicis brevis
Abductor pollicis longus

Synovial sheath

.Fig. 17–4   Anatomical snuffbox and its boundaries.The boundaries are formed by the tendons of abductor pollicis longus and extensor pollicis brevis on the palmar aspect and tendon of extensor pollicis longus on the dorsal aspect. The radial artery runs in the floor of this space. Tenderness in the floor of the anatomical snuffbox after a fall on an outstretched hand suggests fracture of the scaphoid bone.

Differential Diagnosis

1. **Degenerative arthritis** of the **carpometacarpal** (CMC) **joint** of the thumb. The pain is felt on all movements of the thumb. The swelling is more distal and over the joint. The swelling in deQuervain's is elongated and near the radial styloid. There are no x-ray changes in deQuervain's.
2. **Ganglion** presents as a globular and painless swelling.
3. **Fracture of the scaphoid bone.** Long after the history of injury is forgotten, nonunion of this fracture may present with pain over the radial aspect of the wrist joint, which is aggravated by movements. There is localized tenderness over the anatomical snuffbox but no swelling.

Investigations

Diagnosis is clinical. X-rays may help in differentiating from degenerative joint disease of the CMC joint of the thumb or fracture of the scaphoid.

Management

Initial treatment consists of **rest** and **NSAIDs.** Physical therapy and local steroids are used for more severe cases.

1. **Medications**
   a. **NSAIDs** help reduce pain and swelling.
   b. Local injection of long-acting prednisolone in the synovial sheath and surrounding tissues is given to reduce inflammation. Injection in the tendon should be avoided.
2. **Ancillary**
   a. **Splint** or **cast** immobilizing the wrist and thumb is used for 2–3 weeks to give rest. The wrist is kept in slight dorsiflexion and radial deviation.
   b. Physical therapy initially to provide **local heat** is followed by gentle ROM exercises for the wrist and thumb when pain subsides.
3. **Surgical** treatment is considered when conservative measures fail. It consists of incision or excision of the synovial sheath.

Trigger Finger

Narrowing of the fibrous flexor sheath and presence of a nodule in the long flexor tendon of a finger make it difficult for the finger to flex and extend. Locking of the finger, pain, and palpable nodule are common presenting features.

Anatomy

The long flexors of the fingers pass through a fibrous flexor sheath (Fig.17-5). This arch of fibrous tissue keeps the flexor tendons close to the bone. The synovial sheath surrounding the tendons facilitates their movement.

Etiology

The exact etiology is unknown, but **repeated trauma** or **rheumatoid disease** is often blamed. In some patients, there may be an association with diabetes mellitus.

Pathology

The fibrous flexor sheath is thickened, making it difficult for the flexor tendons to slide through the narrowed arch. The fibers in bunch up, forming a nodule in the tendon (Fig. 17-5).

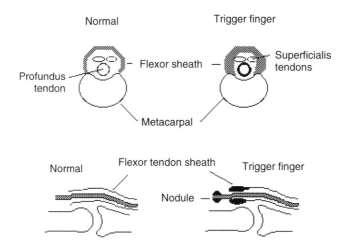

Fig. 17–5 In trigger finger, the fibrous flexor sheath surrounding the flexor tendon is thickened. Fibers of the flexor tendon bunch up into a nodule which is sometimes palpable. This nodule has difficulty sliding through the fibrous flexor sheath during movements of the finger.

History
Trigger finger is common in the middle finger of middle-aged women. During early stages, the patient has difficulty flexing the finger. After flexing the finger part of the way, it seems to require more effort and then **snaps** suddenly into full flexion. Later, similar difficulty is encountered on extension. These movements are **painful.** Sometimes, the finger gets **locked** in flexion and requires the help of the other hand to snap it into extension.

Physical Examination
1. **Inspection.** The sudden jerky movement of the finger can be observed on active flexion or extension of the finger.
2. **Palpation.** There may be a palpable, tender **nodule** over the palmar aspect at the level of MCP joint or head of the metacarpal. This nodule moves on flexion and extension of the finger.
3. **Range of motion**
   a. **Active** movement, especially flexion, is restricted, and the finger may need the assistance of the opposite hand to achieve full range.
   b. **Passive** movements may face some resistance when the nodule has to pass under a thickened fibrous flexor sheath.

Differential Diagnosis
Rupture of a tendon is suspected when the patient is unable to flex or extend the finger. Trigger finger is a chronic process that gradually gets worse. Active movements are usually possible at least during part of the range.

Management
1. **Medications. Local injection** of long-acting prednisolone is given in and around the synovial sheath. Injection in the tendon and blood vessels should be avoided. The tender nodule is located by palpation. The needle is inserted at an angle toward the nodule, and surrounding tissues are infiltrated.

2. **Surgical** treatment is considered when conservative measures fail. It consists of incision of the fibrous flexor sheath near its attachment to the metacarpal.

DEGENERATIVE JOINT DISEASE

Degenerative joint disease is very common in the distal interphalangeal (DIP) joints of fingers and carpometacarpal (CMC) and metacarpophalangeal (MCP) joints of the thumb. Degenerative joint disease of DIP joints is also known as **Heberden's nodes,** whereas that of proximal interphalangeal (PIP) joints is known as **Bouchard's nodes.** Pain and stiffness of the joints interfere with their function. There are no systemic symptoms, and x-rays show typical changes of degenerative joint disease.

Etiology
A strong genetic influence is suspected because the disease runs in families and is more common in sisters and daughters of affected women.

Pathology
The pathologic features are similar to those seen in degenerative joint disease of any other joint (*see* Chapter 8). There is destruction of cartilage with irregular narrowing of the joint space. Osteophytes develop later.

History
Onset of the disease is usually **after 45 years** of age. **Women** are affected 10 times more often than men. Most often, the onset is insidious without much pain. **Pain** is felt over the involved joints and is aggravated by excessive use. The patient has difficulty pinching and holding things because of pain. There is **morning stiffness** for a few minutes on waking which wears off after activity.

Physical Examination
1. **Inspection.** There is **swelling** over the joint, which is more noticeable over the dorsal aspect. **Heberden's nodes** are seen over the dorsolateral aspect of the DIP joints, one on either side of midline. The swelling around CMC and MCP joints of the thumb is more diffuse. **Deformity** occurs late in the disease and consists of lateral deviation or flexion deformity of the DIP joint. The CMC joint may **subluxate** radially.
2. **Palpation.** Localized **tenderness** over the involved joints is present during flareups. The DIP joints of the fingers and MCP joint of the thumb are easy to locate. The CMC joint of the first metacarpal is at the base of the first metacarpal, near the apex of the anatomical snuffbox. It articulates with the trapezium. Palpate the shaft of the first metacarpal, and then follow it to its base with a palpating finger over the dorsal aspect. The CMC joint is located by moving the first metacarpal over the trapezium, which remains stationary.
3. **Range of motion.** Both active and passive ROM are restricted because of pain and deformity.
4. **Special tests.** To detect disease of the **CMC joint** of the thumb, the first metacarpal is held firmly and pushed proximally toward the trapezium. Passive movement of the thumb during this pressure elicits pain when this joint is involved.

Course
Most patients have mild exacerbations and remissions with a slowly progressive course over the years.

Differential Diagnosis
1. **Traumatic** conditions, e.g., avulsion fracture of the extensor tendon to distal phalanx, can be differentiated by history of injury and involvement of only one finger.
2. **Inflammatory arthritis,** like rheumatoid arthritis, affects mainly MCP joints, wrist, elbow, and feet, whereas degenerative joint disease affects DIP joints and CMC joint of the thumb.
3. **Erosive osteoarthritis** has a much more acute and severe onset of pain and swelling of DIP joints. It progresses much faster clinically and radiographically.

Investigations
Plain **x-rays** of the hand show **subchondral sclerosis,** asymmetrical **narrowing of joint space,** and **osteophyte** formation in the involved joints. The joint contour becomes wavy. More advanced disease may show lateral **subluxation** of DIP joints of the finger or CMC joint of the thumb.

Management
Initial treatment consists of **NSAIDs,** local **heat,** and avoidance of activities that might aggravate the pain. A **splint** may help protect the CMC joint from excessive strain and help reduce symptoms. Local injection of **steroids** is added to these measures for acute flare-ups. **Surgical** treatment is considered when conservative measures fail.
1. **Medications**
   a. **NSAIDs** are prescribed for control of pain and inflammation. Acetaminophen may be prescribed for patients who cannot tolerate NSAIDs.
   b. **Local injection of steroid** preparation is used for CMC joint involvement when NSAIDs and physical therapy fail to relieve symptoms. The joint line is localized, and the patient is asked to extend and **abduct** the thumb against resistance to reveal the extensor pollicis longus tendon. The needle is inserted on the palmar side of this tendon in the line of the joint, and 0.5 ml of long-acting steroid for intra-articular use is injected. Injection of the DIP joint is given from the dorsal aspect. The joint line is located by flexion and extension of the distal phalanx. The joint is kept in a slightly flexed position, and the needle is inserted at the posterolateral aspect to avoid the extensor tendon. Injection of 0.25–0.5 ml of steroid preparation should be sufficient.
2. **Ancillary**
   a. Physical therapy in the form of **paraffin bath** for the hand helps relieve pain. Exercises and activities requiring strong contraction of muscles against resistance may increase pain.
   b. Occupational therapist can teach the patient **joint protection techniques** and provide equipment to reduce stress on the affected joints.
3. **Surgical.** Arthrodesis or arthroplasty of the CMC joint of the thumb may be necessary if conservative measures fail.

GANGLION

Ganglion is a very common cystic swelling that occurs near the wrist or other joint. It is benign and may not change in size for years.

Etiology
It is believed to occur as a result of mucinous degeneration of the connective tissue.

Pathology
The cyst consists of fibrous wall covering a cavity filled with thick fluid. It may be unilocular or multilocular. Usually, there is a fibrous cord connecting the cyst with the capsule of a joint or synovial sheath of one of the tendons.

History
A **swelling** around the wrist may be an incidental finding, since most ganglions do not give rise to any symptoms. The onset is usually during the second to fifth decade. It is more common in women. A ganglion may attract the patient's attention by causing pain after an unusual activity or by a feeling of weakness or heaviness.

Physical Examination
1. **Inspection.** Ganglia are most common over the dorsal aspect of the wrist. Some occur over the palmar aspect of the wrist and popliteal fossa. A swelling with a smooth dome-shaped surface may be visible, especially when the skin over it is stretched.
2. **Palpation.** The surface of the swelling is usually smooth but can be bumpy. It is not tender unless inflamed. The swelling can be moved around slightly under the skin. It is attached to either the capsule of a joint or synovial sheath of a tendon. The consistency is firm because fluid in the cyst is under tension.
3. **Range of motion** of the nearby joint is not affected unless the swelling is very large or the ganglion is inflamed and painful.

Course
Some ganglia subside on their own without treatment, whereas others may remain the same size for years without causing any problems. Those that continue to grow and cause symptoms require treatment.

Complications
1. Infection in the cyst presents with pain, tenderness, and restriction of movements.
2. Pressure on a nerve, e.g., median, can give rise to carpal tunnel syndrome.

Differential Diagnosis
1. **Lipoma** or **fibroma** may be difficult to distinguish clinically.
2. **Tenosynovitis.** Swelling due to tenosynovitis is along the tendon sheath and is longitudinal. Pain on passive stretching of the tendon and pain on movement against resistance are usually present in tenosynovitis.

Investigations
Plain **x-rays** of the wrist are normal but may be done before surgical excision.

Management
Treatment is not necessary for most patients. If the swelling grows too fast or too large, causes pain, weakness, or discomfort, or exerts pressure on a nerve or artery, then treatment should be considered.
1. **Medications.** Aspiration and injection of **steroids** can be tried. Infection of the cyst should be ruled out before injection of steroids.
2. **Surgical.** Excision of the cyst may be an extensive procedure because of extensions of the cyst and the long stalk attached to the joint capsule. The whole cyst with the stalk and part of the joint capsule needs to be removed to prevent recurrence.

DUPUYTREN'S CONTRACTURE

The palmar aponeurosis develops contracture, leading to flexion deformity of the fingers.

Anatomy
The thick deep fascia in the central part of the hand is called the **palmar aponeurosis.** It is triangular in shape with its apex toward the wrist. The palmaris longus tendon is attached to it at its apex. The deep fascia over the thenar and hypothenar muscles is much thinner than the palmar aponeurosis. Fibrous bands extend from the aponeurosis to the subcutaneous fat. This decreases the mobility of the overlying skin and helps hold objects in the hand.

Etiology
The exact etiology is not known. Dupuytren's contracture commonly affects **males** of northern European descent. Some other associated factors are **diabetes, trauma, alcohol** abuse, and family history.

Pathology
The **early stage** is characterized by proliferation of fibroblasts and production of collagen. This process starts in the fibrofatty tissue between the skin and palmar aponeurosis. It gradually involves the palmar aponeurosis and skin and forms **nodules** in the palm near the bases of the ring and little fingers. The blood vessels to the nodules and the overlying skin are obliterated. This process gradually extends and forms a band of abnormal connective tissue, which lies along the long axis of the flexor tendon of the finger and superficial to it.

In the **advanced stage,** the fibrous tissue adheres to the overlying skin and may also involve the tendon sheath of the long flexors of the finger. Flexion contracture develops at the metacarpophalangeal (MCP) and proximal interphalangeal (PIP) joints. Ultimately the joint capsule contracts, and permanent changes in the articular surfaces of the bones occur. The deformity of the finger interferes with use of the hand and may result in disuse atrophy of muscles of the hand and forearm.

History

Early stage. Dupuytren's may be an incidental finding since there is not much pain or deformity. The **onset** is very **insidious** in **third to fifth decade.** There may be history of diabetes, alcohol abuse, or trauma to the palmar aspect.

Late stage. The patient develops a gradually increasing **flexion contracture** of the ring and/or little finger which interferes with function of the hand.

Physical Examination

1. **Inspection.** In the **early stage,** there may be some **puckering** of the skin over the nodule. Later, this extends along the band of fibrous tissue under the skin. The involved finger is kept in slight flexion at the MCP joint. The **flexion contracture** gets worse, usually over a period of years, and involves the MCP and PIP joints. The distal interphalangeal joint remains in neutral position. In very **advanced stages,** the fingertip touches the palm.
2. **Palpation.** A nontender nodule is palpable at the base of the ring or little finger. The skin over the nodule becomes thickened and adherent. Later, a firm, fibrous band can be felt along the line of long flexors of the finger.
3. **Range of motion**
   a. **Active.** During early stages, extension at the MCP joint is limited. Extension at the MCP and PIP joints is markedly limited in late stage of disease.
   b. **Passive.** Initially, the contracture can be stretched by force. As time passes, the tissues become very tight and contracture cannot be corrected.

Course/Complications

The disease is very slowly progressive. It may take years to develop maximum deformity, when the fingertip touches the palm and interferes with function of the hand.

Differential Diagnosis

1. **Spastic contracture** of fingers can occur in hemiplegics. All long flexors of the fingers and wrist are usually involved. The flexion deformity of fingers can be partially corrected by flexing the wrist in hemiplegics, whereas the finger with Dupuytren's cannot be extended after wrist flexion.
2. **Ulnar nerve paralysis** gives rise to flexion deformity of the little and ring fingers. It is worse in the little finger than ring finger. There is hyperextension at the MCP joint in ulnar neuropathy and flexion at the interphalangeal joints. The skin over the palmar aspect has no nodules or bands, and fingers can be passively extended.

Management

1. **Ancillary** treatments may be tried in the early stage of disease to slow the progression of contracture and in the postoperative period to prevent recurrence:
   a. Underwater **ultrasound** may help by warming up the tissues before stretching.
   b. Passive **stretching** and **ROM exercises.** Dynamic splinting can provide gentle continuous stretching.
2. **Surgical.** Once contracture is established and progressing, conservative treatment does not help. Two types of operations are available:
   a. **Subcutaneous fasciotomy,** a relatively minor operation, is done for early cases.

The rate of postoperative complications is low. However, recurrence rate of contracture is high.

   b. **Fasciectomy.** Excision of abnormal fibrous tissue is a more extensive operation with higher incidence of postoperative complications and better long-term results.

Intensive **ROM exercises** should be started early after the operation and continued for a long time. **Delayed wound healing** and **recurrence** of the contracture are two common complications.

REFLEX SYMPATHETIC DYSTROPHY

Also known as **causalgia, Sudeck's atrophy,** and **shoulder-hand syndrome,** reflex sympathetic dystrophy (RSD) is characterized by severe burning pain in the hand or foot, hyperesthesia, swelling, and vasomotor changes. These symptoms and signs may last for months. The hand may end up severely contracted, shriveled, and useless.

Etiology
Many hypotheses have been proposed to explain all the phenomena seen in this condition. The basic mechanism seems to be an imbalance in the autonomic regulation. A triggering event increases the autonomic outflow, which leads to pain and vascular dilatation. How exactly this comes about is explained by various hypotheses. Injury probably initiates a reflex; the pain sensation sets up a reverberating cycle along the internuncial neurons in the spinal cord, which perpetuates pain and increased vascularity. In patients with stroke, a central mechanism is postulated for a similar reflex arc.
   Precipitating events include:
1. Cerebrovascular accident
2. Myocardial infarction
3. Hand or foot injury, e.g., fracture or soft tissue strain
4. Operation, e.g., carpal tunnel release
5. Nerve injuries

Pathology
Increased vascularity leads to edema and swelling of the soft tissues of the hand. Since active movements aggravate pain, the patient does not move the hand. This inactivity leads to more swelling, and chronic edema encourages deposition of fibrous tissue and contractures, ultimately leading to a stiff, nonfunctional hand. Increased blood flow to the bones gives rise to osteopenia. Initially, it may be spotty around the blood vessels only or near joints, but later it becomes diffuse, affecting all the bones of the involved part of the extremity.

History
The onset of **pain** may be sudden and follow soon after one of the precipitating events, or it may be gradual, starting many weeks or months later. Pain is very **severe** and **burning** in character. It is felt in the hand or foot and, at times, may extend proximally. The pain is not confined to any dermatomal or nerve distribution. It is aggravated by movements, touch, or, in severe cases, even loud noise. The patient cannot find any relief. Some wrap the hand in a wet towel and keep it in one fixed position to avoid exacerbating the pain. In

the **shoulder-hand syndrome,** the patient also complains of pain in the shoulder on the same side. The shoulder pain is usually not as severe as in the hand.

Physical Examination
1. **Inspection.** The whole hand, including fingers, is swollen. The **swelling** is more marked on the dorsum of hand. The skin is **hyperemic** initially and may become dusky red later. In the last stage, the skin may be atrophic and pale. The hand is held close to the body with fingers slightly flexed.
2. **Palpation.** The characteristic feature on palpation is severe pain on light touch (**hyperesthesia** or **allodynia**). The part touched remains painful even after the stimulus is withdrawn (**hyperpathia**). There is pitting edema over the dorsum of the hand, but the swelling of the fingers is solid (nonpitting).
3. **Range of motion.** The patient is reluctant to move the hand or fingers, either actively or passively, because of pain. During the acute stage, the patient is unable to hold anything in the hand. Later, he or she may not be able to move the fingers because of contractures. There may be some restriction in ROM of the shoulder on the same side.

Course
The course of RSD is supposed to have three stages, although there are no clear distinctions between these stages. One stage gradually merges into the next.

Stage 1: There is intense burning pain in the hand and fingers with swelling and vasomotor changes. The skin is warm and sweaty. On examination, the patient has hyperesthesia, and the hand is held in one position without moving. This stage lasts from several weeks to few months.

Stage 2: Distinctions between this stage and other stages are hazy. Pain may subside to some extent. Wasting of skin and muscles begins. The skin is cool and dusky. X-rays show spotty osteoporosis.

Stage 3: There is marked atrophy of skin and muscles. Joint contractures develop. The skin is cold, pale, and atrophic.

Complications
1. Completely useless, contracted hand
2. Addiction to narcotics may develop.

Differential Diagnosis
All the symptoms and signs are not present in all patients. There are partial syndromes which may make the diagnosis difficult.
1. **Trauma.** Sometimes pain, swelling, and tenderness after an injury may persist longer than usual, especially in patients who are reluctant to move their fingers and hand. These patients should be treated with vigorous physical and occupational therapy to prevent RSD.
2. **Early inflammatory arthritis.** RSD may be bilateral, but it does not usually affect elbow or knee joints. Inflammatory arthritis is a systemic disease with morning stiffness, fatigue, and other joint involvement. Raynaud's phenomenon, if present, may be confused with vasomotor disturbances of RSD.
3. **Carpal tunnel syndrome (CTS).** Diminished sensation, muscle weakness, and wasting characterize CTS, whereas in RSD, pain, swelling, and hyperesthesia are prominent. Symptoms and signs of CTS are confined to the median nerve distribution, i.e.,

lateral three and one-half fingers and the thenar muscles. In RSD, all the fingers and whole hand are affected.

4. **Infection** of a palmar space may present with pain and swelling of the hand. The pain is throbbing and accompanied by fever. Tenderness is confined to the involved area. Total and differential WBC count may help confirm the diagnosis.

Investigations

1. **Plain x-rays** may show **soft tissue swelling** initially for 3–6 weeks after onset. Later, **spotty demineralization** is seen, which is more marked near the joints (moth-eaten appearance). These changes may be difficult to distinguish from disuse atrophy. The joint space is well-maintained, and there are no juxta-articular erosions.
2. **Bone scan** with technetium-99m shows increased uptake near the joints. Similar findings are obtained in rheumatoid arthritis. Changes in bone scan occur before x-ray changes.
3. **Stellate ganglion block** can be used as a therapeutic and diagnostic procedure. Relief of pain within 15 minutes suggests RSD.

Management

Best results are obtained when vigorous treatment is started early. Unusually, severe pain with hyperpathia should suggest RSD. The initial strategy is to control pain and start physical and occupational therapy. These patients require prolonged therapy lasting for months. If there is no relief within 2–3 weeks, oral steroids and/or sympathetic ganglion blocks should be considered.

1. **Medications**
   a. **Analgesics.** Nonnarcotic analgesics may not be effective in controlling pain. Analgesics should be given on a regular schedule and not on an as-needed basis (prn). The patient will be able to cooperate in physical therapy if there is some relief of pain. An NSAID with acetaminophen and codeine may be a good combination with which to start. Stronger analgesic may be required if this does not control the pain.
   b. **Steroids.** Patients are started on 40–60 mg/day of prednisone. The dose is rapidly tapered within 2–3 weeks.
   c. **Stellate ganglion block** is given for upper extremity involvement and **epidural injection** for the lower extremity. If there is temporary relief, this may be repeated 3–4 times.
2. **Ancillary.** Multiple physical and occupational therapy modalities are used. The goals are to reduce pain and swelling and increase sensory input. According to the "gate control" theory of pain, increased sensory input along large-diameter fibers inhibits pain sensation. The number of hours a patient spends in therapy depends on the severity of the disease and the patient's tolerance. The duration of therapy can be increased gradually up to even 6–8 hours/day.
   a. **Paraffin baths** are used for prolonged periods and repeated a few times during the day. This may be substituted or alternated by blowing hot air. This works as a temporary analgesic and helps increase sensory input.
   b. Active ROM **exercises** for wrist and fingers are done after paraffin baths. If the patient has pain and stiffness of the shoulder, then local heat and exercises are prescribed for the shoulder.
   c. **Elevation** of the hand and **intermittent pneumatic compression** help to reduce swelling.

d. **Transcutaneous electrical nerve stimulation (TENS)** is used to increase sensory input in large-diameter nerve fibers and to inhibit pain.

e. **Splint** is used to immobilize the hand in a functional position and protect it, especially at night.

3. **Surgical** intervention is very rarely required. Sympathectomy may be considered after failure of all conservative measures and if sympathetic blocks help only temporarily.

Bibliography

1. Amadio PC: Scaphoid fractures. Orthop Clin North Am 23:7–17, 1992.
2. American Society for Surgery of Hand: The Hand, 2nd ed. Edinburgh, Churchhill Livingstone, 1983.
3. Docken WP: Clinical features and medical management of osteoarthritis at the hand and wrist. Hand Clin 3:337–349, 1987.
4. Flatt AE: Care of the Arthritic Hand, 4th ed. St. Louis, C.V. Mosby Co., 1983.
5. Gonzales SM, Gonzales RI: Dupuytren's contracture. West J Med 152:430–433, 1990.
6. Hodgkins ML, Grady D: Carpal tunnel syndrome. West J Med 148:217–220, 1988.
7. Holbrook JL: Arthritis of the hand and wrist: Management options for some common arthritic conditions. Postgrad Med 87 (5):255–262, 1990.
8. Johnson EW, Pannozzo AN: Management of shoulder-hand syndrome. JAMA 195:152–154, 1966.
9. Kraemer BA, Young VL, Arfken C: Stenosing flexor tenosynovitis. South Med J 83:806–811, 1990.
10. Loder RT, Mayhew HE: Common fractures from a fall on outstretched hand. Am Fam Physician 37:327–338, 1988.
11. Neviaser RJ: Tenosynovitis. Hand Clin 5:525–531, 1989.
12. Pellegrini VD Jr: Osteoarthritis at the base of thumb. Orthop Clin North Am 23:83–102, 1992.
13. Phalen GS: The carpal tunnel syndrome: Seventeen years' experience in diagnosis and treatment of 654 hands. J Bone Joint Surg, 48-A:211–228, 1966.
14. Pomerance JF: Painful basal joint arthritis of the thumb: II. Treatment. Am J Orthop 24:466–472; 1995.
15. Schwartzman RJ, McLellan TL: Reflex sympathetic dystrophy. Arch Neurol 44: 555–561, 1987.
16. Smith DL, Campbell SM: Reflex sympathetic dystrophy syndrome. West J Med 147:342–345, 1987.
17. Subbarao JV, Blair SJ: Reflex sympathetic dystrophy syndrome. Phys Med Rehabil State Art Rev 9:31–50, 1995.
18. Whitley JM, McDonnell DE: Carpal tunnel syndrome: A guide to prompt intervention. Postgrad Med 97(1):89–96, 1995.
19. Young L, Bartell T, Logan SE: Ganglions of the hand and wrist. South Med J 81:751–760, 1988.

.

18

Hip

Arun J. Mehta, M.B., F.R.C.P.C.

The hip joint is the largest ball-and-socket joint in the body. Compared to the shoulder, it is more stable but has less ROM. Bony structure and ligaments contribute toward stability of the joint. Painfree movements of the hip are necessary for many ADLs, including walking, sitting, transferring from sitting to standing, squatting, and others. Some of the conditions affecting the hip joint, sacroiliac joint, and adjoining structures are considered in this chapter.

Differential Diagnosis

History
Patients with hip problems may present with a history of pain and/or difficulty with some activity such as walking, going up and down stairs, or tying shoelaces. Individual hip conditions may occur at specific times in a person's life (Table 18–1).
1. **Pain** due to hip pathology is usually located in the **groin.** Sometimes patients with hip disorders may present with diffuse pain in the thigh or **knee** region. The hip and knee joints are supplied by the obturator nerve, which leads to this difficulty in localizing the pain. Pain in the gluteal region may be reported as hip pain by some patients. However, this is usually due to lumbosacral pathology.
2. **Difficulty in walking.** Is it painful to walk? Is it painful when the patient starts walking? How far can he or she walk without discomfort? What does the patient do when pain occurs? Does it get better or worse as the patient continues to walk?
3. **Activities of daily living.** Some activities, such as tying shoelaces or squatting, require nearly normal ROM in the hip joint. These activities may be difficult or impossible when there is limited ROM in the hip joint. During **sexual** intercourse, the female partner requires some abduction at the hips. If this is painful or limited, this activity may need to be curtailed or modified. **Sleeping** on the affected side may be difficult for patients with degenerative joint disease of the hip or trochanteric bursitis.

Physical Examination
For proper examination of the hip region, the patient should wear the minimal clothes, preferably a bikini.

Inspection
The patient is observed while standing, walking, sitting, and lying. The examination procedure should be streamlined so that the patient does not have to change positions several times. Observation is carried out from the front, side, and back (Fig. 18–1).

Table 18–1 Hip Conditions Seen in Various Age Groups

Age (yrs)	Diagnosis
0–1	Congenital dislocation of the hip
4–10	Infection
	Coxa plana (Perthes' disease)
12–15	Slipped femoral epiphysis
>25	Secondary degenerative joint disease
>45	Primary degenerative joint disease
>50	Fracture of neck of the femur
	Metastasis

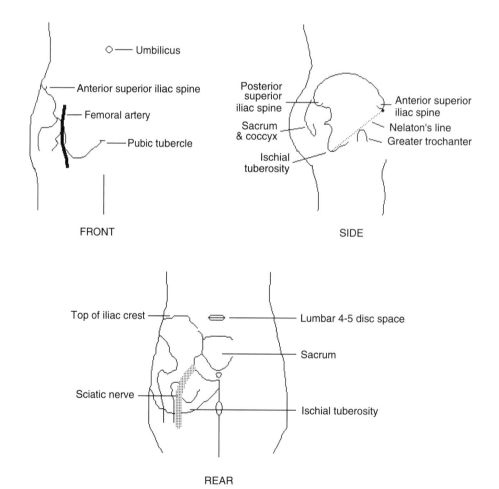

Fig. 18–1 Hip structures to observe and palpate during examination.

1. **Gait.** Observe the patient as he or she walks into the office. Observe again after the patient has removed his or her clothes. During normal walking, each step is of equal length, and the same amount of time is spent weight-bearing on each foot.

   a. **Antalgic Gait**—When there is pain on weight-bearing, we try to reduce the time of single-stance phase (time spent weight-bearing on one foot) on the affected side to reduce pain. This leads to shorter single-stance phase (Fig. 18–2A). A second adjustment made to reduce forces acting on the hip joint is bringing the center of gravity of the body closer to the center of the hip joint. This is achieved by leaning over to the painful side (Fig. 18–2B). These changes in gait are seen in any painful condition of the lower extremity.

   b. **Trendelenburg gait**—Normally when we stand on the right foot, the right gluteus medius muscle contracts to balance the body, which elevates the left side of the pelvis. If the gluteus medius is weak, the pelvis on the opposite side drops down (positive Trendelenburg test). When a patient with a weak gluteus medius muscle walks, everytime the patient puts weight on the weak side, the pelvis on the opposite side drops—i.e., Trendelenburg gait.

2. **Skin.** Look for any discoloration, breakdown, swelling, or abnormal skinfolds. In infants, abnormal skinfolds may indicate congenital dislocation of the hip. The skinfolds on the thighs and the gluteal folds on both sides are compared for their level and depth.

3. **Bony landmarks.** The anterior superior iliac spine and iliac crest can be seen easily in thin patients. Compare the level of the highest points of the iliac crests and anterior superior iliac spines of both sides. If these bony points are not level, there may be a deformity of one hip or more distal part of the lower extremity. Dimples of Venus lie over the posterior superior iliac spines and are observed from the posterior aspect. Curvature of the lumbar spine (**lumbar lordosis**) is exaggerated in hip flexion contracture (Fig. 18–3). This compensatory mechanism brings the lower extremity in neutral position.

4. **Soft tissue contours.** Look for muscle spasm or atrophy of gluteal muscles.

5. **Sitting** in a chair. Does the patient sit evenly with weight distributed equally on both buttocks? How does the patient manage to untie the shoes? Ordinarily, when we bend forward with feet on the floor to untie shoelaces, we flex >120° at the hip joints. If there is significant hip pathology, it will be very difficult to perform this task.

Palpation

The patient can be standing or lying for palpation. Levels of different bony points can be determined better when the patient is standing. Look for any increase in skin **temperature** and **tenderness** over different areas being palpated.

1. **Front.** Confirm the position of the anterior superior iliac spines (Fig. 18–1A). They are the most anterior and distal bony landmarks palpable on the iliac crests. Keep each thumb on the anterior superior iliac spine, and see if they are at the same horizontal level. About 2 cm distal to the anterior superior iliac spine, the lateral femoral cutaneous nerve pierces the deep fascia. There may be tenderness in this area in compression neuropathy of this nerve (meralgia paresthetica).

   Move the fingers along the inguinal ligament and feel for the pulsations of the **femoral artery.** The head of the femur is deep to the femoral artery. If it is dislocated, pulsations may be difficult to feel because there is no firm structure against which one can compress the vessel. The femoral vein and nerve lie on either side of the artery but are not palpable. Inguinal and femoral **hernia** and enlarged inguinal **lymph nodes** can present with a swelling and pain in this region.

   Continue medially to the pubic symphysis. The **adductor longus** muscle arises from

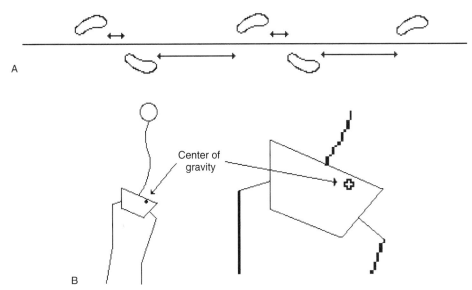

Fig. 18–2   Antalgic gait. *A*, A patient with painful hip pathology tries to shorten the weight-bearing phase (single-stance phase) on the painful side. This results in unequal length of footsteps. *B*, A patient experiencing pain on weight-bearing because of hip pathology tries to shift the center of gravity toward the affected hip joint.

the superior ramus of the pubis near the pubic symphysis. It may be strained during athletic activities with pain and tenderness in this area.

2. **Back and side.** This part of the hip examination is carried out with the patient on his or her side. The **greater trochanter** is partially covered by the gluteus medius muscle. Its position can be confirmed by moving the thigh. Localized tenderness in this area indicates trochanteric bursitis or other hip pathology. The level of the tip of greater trochanter is compared with the opposite side and its relation to the anterior superior iliac spine and ischial tuberosity of the same side. The highest point of the iliac crest is at the level of the space between the spinous processes of the L4 and L5 vertebrae.

Palpate along the iliac crest to the **posterior iliac spine.** These bony landmarks are over the middle of sacroiliac joints and S2 vertebra. The sacroiliac joints are not palpable because they are deeper or in front of the posterior superior iliac spines. The **ischial tuberosity** is palpable near the gluteal fold. This bony prominence may be difficult to palpate since it is covered by the gluteus maximus muscle. Flexion of the hip exposes them for easier palpation. Body weight is transmitted through ischial tuberosities when we sit. Bursitis or callus may present with pain and tenderness in this region.

The **sciatic nerve** leaves the gluteal region and enters the back of the thigh behind the gluteus maximus and midway between the greater trochanter and ischial tuberosity. Tenderness over the sciatic nerve may suggest compression of one of the roots forming the nerve.

Range of Motion

The hip is considered to be in neutral position when the lower extremity is in line with the rest of the body and the toes are pointing toward the ceiling. The line joining the anterior superior iliac spines is perpendicular to the axis of the trunk. ROM is measured from the

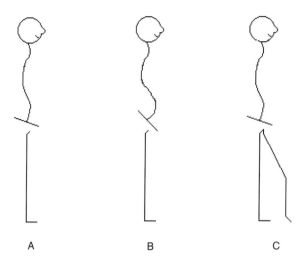

Fig. 18–3 Flexion contracture of the hip joint: *A*, Normal lordosis. *B*, Flexion contracture of the hip is obscured by increasing the lordosis of the lumbar spine. *C*, Flexion contracture becomes obvious when lumbar lordosis is corrected.

neutral as 0°. It is important to see that the pelvis or spine does not move when ROM tests for the hips are performed. One hand is kept on the pelvis on the opposite side of the hip being tested to check when the pelvis starts moving.

1. **Passive**

Flexion—The patient lies flat on his back, and the thigh is bent forward. The range of flexion in the hip joint with knee flexed to 90° is 120°. If the knee is kept straight, then flexion at the hip is limited to 90° because of the hamstring muscles. Flexion deformity at the hip joint is determined by **Thomas' test** (Fig. 18–4). The deformity is obscured by exaggerated lumbar lordosis. The opposite (normal) hip is flexed to its maximum limit to straighten the lumbar lordosis. One hand of the examiner is kept under the lumbar spine to determine if this is achieved. If there is a flexion deformity, the involved hip will take up a position of flexion. The degree of flexion deformity is the angle between the thigh on the affected side and the horizontal. Normally, a person is able to keep the thigh on the examination couch while the opposite thigh is flexed to the maximum.

Abduction—Normal range of abduction at the hip joint is up to 45°. The patient lies on his back with legs in neutral position. One hand of the examiner is placed on the opposite anterior superior iliac spine to detect any movement. With the other hand under the calf or the heel of the patient, the extremity under examination is moved away from the neutral position. The angle formed by the lower extremity with the neutral position is the degree of abduction.

Adduction—From the same starting position as for the abduction test, the lower extremity is taken over the opposite extremity. The angle is measured with the neutral as 0°. Normal adduction is up to 30°.

Rotations—External and internal rotations can be tested in three positions:

a. Patient lies on the back with both lower extremities in neutral position. The examiner holds the foot or leg and turns it outward (external rotation) or inward toward the midline (internal rotation). The most prominent part of the patella is observed. The degree of movement is measured as a change from the neutral.

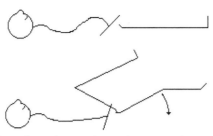

Fig. 18–4 Thomas' test is performed to confirm and measure the extent of flexion contracture at the hip joint. With the patient lying on his or her back, the normal hip is flexed to flatten the lumbar lordosis. The thigh on the affected side takes up the position of flexion. The angle formed by the thigh on the affected side and the examining table is the angle of flexion contracture at the hip joint.

   b. With the patient on his back, the hip and knee are flexed to 90°. One hand of the examiner is kept on the knee, and the other holds the heel. From this neutral position, the hip is rotated externally by pushing the heel beyond the midline toward the opposite leg. Internal rotation is in the opposite direction. The angles are measured from the neutral with the leg in line with the body.

   c. Patient sits on the examination couch with the legs dangling. The rotations are performed in the same way as in test *b*.

      Normal range for external rotation is 0°–45°, and for internal rotation it is 0°–35°.

      Extension—The patient lies on the abdomen in a prone position. The knee is flexed to 90°. The examiner holds the ankle and lifts the lower extremity backward. The angle made by the thigh with the couch is the range of extension. Normal range is 0° to 15°–30°. Extension can also be measured with the patient lying on the opposite side, and the other hip is extended

2. **Active.** Active movements are performed by the patient to check the ROM and strength of muscle contraction. Any difference between active and passive ROM is helpful in diagnosis of muscle weakness and some soft tissue problems. Muscle strength can be tested by asking the patient to perform the movement **against resistance.** These tests are described below.

Special Tests

1. **Neurologic** examination is necessary when the following conditions are suspected:
   a. Pain is referred from the spine.
   b. A neurologic condition affects the gait.
   c. Entrapment neuropathy is giving rise to pain in the hip or thigh region.
2. **Sensation.** Superficial touch and pain sensations are tested. The area of abnormal sensation is compared with the normal sensory distribution according to roots and peripheral nerves. The thoracic 10th nerve root supplies the skin at the level of the umbilicus. Inguinal and scrotal regions are innervated by the 12th thoracic nerve root. The lower third of thigh, just above the knee, is supplied by the 3rd lumbar root (same as the hip joint). Pain due to involvement of lumbar 5th and sacral 1st roots radiates down from the gluteal region along the back of the thigh and is felt in the leg and foot.
3. **Muscle strength** is tested to determine if any muscle or group of muscles is weak. Knowledge of nerve roots and peripheral nerves innervating different muscles helps in localizing the pathology.

a. **Flexors**

Muscle	Roots	Nerve
Iliopsoas	L2, 3, 4	Femoral and ventral rami

The patient sits with legs over the side of the couch. The patient is asked to raise his or her thigh. Resistance is applied by the examiner's hands on the patient's lower thigh.

b. **Abductor**

Muscle	Roots	Nerve
Gluteus medius	L4, L5, S1	Superior gluteal

If the right side is being examined, the patient lies on the left side. The patient is asked to raise his or her right lower extremity vertically up against the examiner's hand, providing resistance to this movement. Trendelenburg test is another method of testing gluteus medius function.

c. **Adductors**

Muscles	Roots	Nerve
Adductor longus	L 2,3,4	Obturator
Adductor brevis	L 3,4	Obturator
Adductor magnus	L 3,4	Obturator

With the patient on his or her back and with the legs slightly abducted, the patient is asked to bring the legs together. Resistance is applied to both thighs by the examiner's hands to prevent the patient from bringing the lower extremities together.

d. **Extensors**

Muscle	Roots	Nerve
Gluteus maximus	L5, S1, S2	Inferior gluteal

The patient lies face down with the knee flexed to 90°. He or she is asked to raise the thigh off the couch. The examiner applies resistance to the back of the thigh with the hands.

4. **Leg-length discrepancy.** Difference in leg lengths may occur due to pathology in the head or neck of the femur, the shaft of the femur, or shaft of the tibia. **Real shortening** is measured from the anterior superior iliac spine to medial malleolus and compared with the opposite side. **Apparent shortening** is due to **adduction** deformity and is measured from the umbilicus to the medial malleolus. The patient lies on his or her back with the spine straight and both lower extremities in similar position. If one extremity has an **abduction** contracture, the other extremity is placed in the same degree of abduction. One end of the tape measure is placed at the tip of the anterior superior iliac spine. The tape is stretched along the front of the thigh, medial aspect of the knee, and up to the tip of the medial malleolus. This distance, between the anterior superior iliac spine and medial malleolus, is compared with the opposite side.

The following tests are carried out to localize the site of shortening in the lower extremity:

a. Draw a line between the anterior superior iliac spine and ischial tuberosity. If the top of the greater trochanter is higher than this line, then the pathology is in the neck or head of the femur.

b. Measure the length from the top of the greater trochanter to the lateral tibial condyle. Compare this length to the opposite side to find out if there is a difference in length of the shaft of femur.

c. The length from the tibial condyle to the lateral malleolus determines if shortening is in the shaft of the tibia.

CONGENITAL DISLOCATION OF THE HIP

Early diagnosis of congenital dislocation is of utmost importance. If diagnosed and treated appropriately before the child starts walking, the hip will develop normally, radiologically and functionally, in >95% of patients. However, if treatment is postponed, chances of a good outcome diminish. If treatment is started after age 5 or 6 years, almost all will develop painful, degenerative arthritis in their early adult life. Congenital dislocation of the hip is not very obvious on clinical examination or on x-rays during infancy, which makes early diagnosis very difficult. Deliberate attempts should be made by the physician to look for congenital dislocation of the hip (CDH) in every infant in order to achieve a good outcome.

Etiology

Normal development of the head of the femur and acetabulum occurs only when both of these structures remain in contact with each other. If they become separated, then neither of them develops normally.

Predisposing factors:

1. **Mechanical.** The **first born** has a higher incidence of congenital dislocation of the hip than subsequent children. Tight maternal tissues may prevent movement of the hip joint of the fetus. **Oligohydramnios** and **breech presentation** are also associated with an increased incidence of congenital dislocation of the hip, probably for a similar reason.
2. **Physiologic.** Congenital dislocation of the hip is more common in **girls** than in boys (8:1). Female children may be affected more by maternal hormones than male fetuses, leading to laxity of ligaments.
3. **Genetic.** Familial tendency is seen in about 20% of patients with congenital dislocation of the hip.
4. **Environmental.** After birth, some infants (of Native North American tribes) are wrapped up tightly in blankets with their thighs and legs straight in neutral position. This position prevents flexion and abduction at the hips and may contribute to congenital dislocation of the hip.

Pathology

A **dislocation** (luxation) is considered to occur when the articular surface of the head of the femur has no contact with that of the acetabulum. When there is partial contact, it is said to be a **subluxation.** The hip joint develops normally when the head of femur and acetabulum are in contact with each other. This contact is maintained well in flexion and **abduction** of the hip joint, whereas extension and **adduction** promote subluxation and dislocation in susceptible infants.

Pathologic changes are progressive and become increasingly difficult to correct over time. The infant may be born with a lax capsule of the hip joint, which may later lead to subluxation or dislocation. There is proximal and lateral migration of the femur, with shortening of adductor and iliopsoas muscles. The capsule of the joint becomes thickened. Later, a false joint develops between the head of the femur and the ilium. Degenerative arthritis occurs at a very early age in these patients, who continue to walk on dislocated hips.

History

The deformity is not obvious at birth, and the mother may not notice any abnormality. After the child has been walking for some time, a limp may be noticed by the parents. Pain in the hip develops during adolescence or early adulthood because of degenerative arthritis.

Physical Examination

Routine physical examination to rule out congenital dislocation of the hip is very important for early diagnosis. This exam should be carried out on all newborns and at subsequent followup visits. The physical signs vary with age of the patient and extent of pathologic changes. There may be no abnormal signs in the newborn infants, which makes the examination at followup visits all the more important. Presence of other musculoskeletal deformities (e.g., torticollis or metatarsus adductus) should make the physician look for congenital dislocation of the hip more carefully.

In Infants

1. **Inspection.** A newborn infant may not show any abnormal sign on inspection. The gluteal folds and skin creases over the medial aspect of thigh may be different on two sides (**asymmetrical skinfolds**).
2. **Range of motion.** On **passive** movement, there is gradually increasing limitation of **abduction** as the infant grows.
3. **Special tests**
   a. **Barlow test** is carried out when the hip is still not dislocated. This test helps to show that the hip joint is not stable. The knees and thighs of the infant are grasped by the examiner between the thumb and fingers. The knee and hip joints are flexed to 90° each, and the hip is in maximum **abduction.** The thigh is gently pressed downward while the hip is **adducted.** If the hip is unstable, it will dislocate with a click (Fig. 18–5).
   b. **Ortolani's click test.** If the hip joint is already dislocated, this maneuver helps to reduce the head of the femur in the acetabulum. Both tests, Ortolani and Barlow,

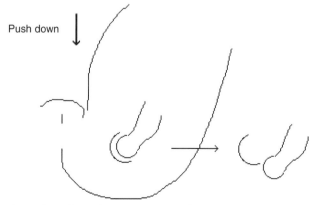

Push down

Fig. 18–5 Barlow's test is performed with the hip in 90° of flexion and maximum abduction. The femur is pushed down while trying to adduct the hip. This maneuver will dislocate the hip joint if it is unstable.

are performed with the hips and knees flexed to 90°. During Ortolani's test, the hip is **abducted** and greater trochanter is gently pushed upward and medially. The hip joint can be reduced with a click when this test is positive (Fig. 18–6). Later, the hip cannot be reduced by this maneuver, and Ortolani test becomes negative even though the child has congenital dislocation of the hip.

c. **Telescoping.** There is abnormal movement of the head of femur on the ilium. The hip and knee are flexed to 90° each. The examiner fixes the pelvis by one hand and, with the other, holds the knee and thigh. He alternately pushes the knee down and pulls it up to look for abnormal movement.

In Children

A child with congenital dislocation of the hip starts to walk later than usual. Examination of a young child may show:

1. **Trendelenburg test.** The child walks with a limp. Normally, when we stand on one foot, the pelvis is balanced by hip abductors. In congenital dislocation of the hip, the abductors are not able to do this when the child stands on the affected side and the pelvis drops down on the opposite side (positive Trendelenburg test). Bilateral congenital dislocation of the hip leads to a waddling gait.

2. **Galeazzi's sign.** With the child on her back, the hips are flexed to 60°–70° with feet flat on the examination couch. The knee on the affected side is lower than that on the normal side because of proximal migration of the femur. (Fig. 18–7)

3. **Ortolani's test** becomes negative when the hip joint cannot be reduced because of more advanced pathologic changes.

Investigations

1. **Plain anteroposterior x-ray** of a newborn infant is very difficult to interpret because most of the pelvis is cartilaginous (Fig. 18–8). In a newborn, normal x-rays **do not** rule out congenital dislocation of the hip. Later, x-rays may show:

a. The femoral head is more proximal and lateral as compared with normal.

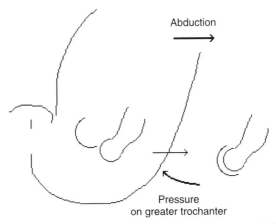

Abduction

Pressure
on greater trochanter

Fig. 18–6 Ortolani's test is performed by gently abducting the flexed thigh and lifting the head of the femur by pressure over the greater trochanter. The dislocated hip is reduced with a click when the test is positive.

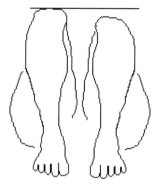

Fig. 18–7 Galeazzi's sign. The hips and knees are flexed, and the feet are kept flat on the examination couch. The child is observed from the end of the couch. The knee on the dislocated side is lower than the normal side.

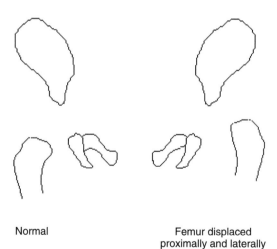

Normal

Femur displaced
proximally and laterally

Fig. 18–8 X-rays of the pelvis in a newborn are difficult to interpret because the pelvis is mostly cartilaginous. The changes suggestive of congenital dislocation are not apparent. Proximal and lateral migration, characteristic of dislocation, are not very obvious.

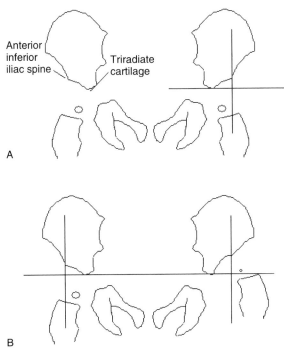

Fig. 18–9 X-rays in congenital dislocation of the hip. *A,* Normal pelvis at 6–12 months of age. On the *left* side, a vertical line is drawn through the anterior inferior iliac spine (Perkin's line), and a horizontal line is drawn through the triradiate cartilage of the acetabulum. In a normal hip, the center of ossification for the head of the femur lies in the lower and medial quadrant. *B,* In congenital dislocation of the hip, the center of ossification of the head of the femur lies in the upper and outer quadrant.

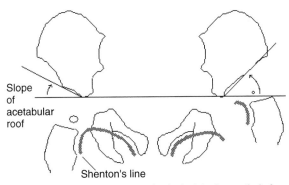

Fig. 18–10 Slope of the acetabular roof (acetabular index) is the angle it forms with the horizontal. It is increased in congenital dislocation of the hip. Shenton's line is the curved line formed by the medial side of the neck of the femur and the upper and inner margin of the obturator foramen. In normal infants, this line is a smooth curve. It becomes discontinuous in congenital dislocation of the hip.

A horizontal line is drawn through the triradiate cartilage of the acetabulum and a vertical line through the anterior inferior iliac spine. The normal head of the femur lies in the inferior and medial quadrant, whereas a dislocated head will lie in the upper and outer quadrant (Fig. 18–9).

b. The angle formed by the roof of the acetabulum with the horizontal is called the **acetabular index.** If this angle is >30°, it is abnormal. In congenital dislocation of the hip, the slope of the roof of acetabulum is increased (Fig. 18–10).

c. Normally, a smooth curved line can be drawn along the upper border of the obturator foramen and the medial surface of neck of the femur (**Shenton's line**). In congenital dislocation, because of upward migration of the femur, Shenton's line is broken or discontinuous (Fig. 18–10).

2. **Ultrasonography** is useful in diagnosis and management of congenital dislocation of the hip since there are no harmful effects of ionizing radiation.

3. **Arthrography** is requested when closed reduction is not successful. It may show why conservative treatment has failed.

Management

Congenital dislocation of the hip should be treated by an experienced orthopedic surgeon. Chances of a normal hip (radiologically and functionally) developing in congenital dislocation of the hip are very good if this condition is treated properly during the first year of life. Some of the options available are as follows:

1. Closed reduction and maintenance of reduction
2. Traction
3. Open reduction

Complications

Avascular necrosis of the head of the femur may occur as a complication of treatment. Degenerative arthritis occurs at an earlier age, especially when definitive treatment is delayed.

FRACTURES OF THE PROXIMAL FEMUR

Fracture of the neck of the femur is the most common fracture requiring hospital admission. The cost of treating these patients in the United States is estimated to be >$8 billion annually. About one in five patients die after sustaining this fracture.

Anatomy

The proximal end of the femur consists of the head, neck, and greater and lesser trochanters (Fig. 18–11A). The attachment of the capsule of the hip joint (Fig. 18–11B) forms an important demarcating border in classifying the types of fractures. The prognosis for healing of a fracture proximal to the line of attachment of the capsule is worse than for a fracture more distal to it. Fractures proximal to the attachment of the capsule are called **intracapsular.** Arteries to the neck and head of the femur (Fig. 18–12) pierce the capsule and travel along the neck in subsynovial tissue. They can be damaged by an intracapsular fracture, leading to avascular necrosis of the head of femur.

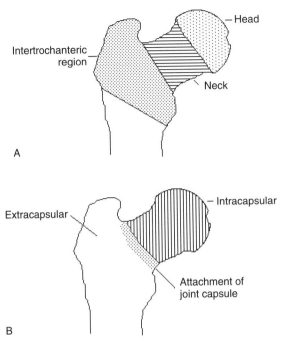

Fig. 18–11 *A,* Parts of the proximal end of the femur. *B,* The capsule of the hip joint is attached to the femur near the base of its neck. Fractures of the proximal end of the femur which are proximal to the line of attachment of the capsule are called intracapsular, and those distal to it are extracapsular. Intracapsular fractures have worse prognosis for healing than extracapsular fractures.

History/Mechanism of Injury

Usually, a minor fall or sudden twisting movement in an osteoporotic elderly person can break the neck of the femur. An elderly female patient with such a history develops **pain** in the groin and is not able to put any weight on the involved side.

Types of Fractures

1. **Intracapsular**—The fracture line is within the capsule of the hip joint (Fig. 18–11B). The blood supply to the head of the femur is more likely to be damaged if the fracture is close to the articular surface, since the arteries come from the base of the neck toward the head. Fractures involving the articular surface of the head are not very common.
2. **Extracapsular**—The fracture line goes through the trochanters. The blood supply to both the fragments is good, and hence, chances of healing are much better.

Physical Examination

1. **Inspection.** The affected lower extremity lies in **external rotation** and is **shorter** than the normal side. Rarely, there may not be any deformity at all.
2. **Palpation.** There is **tenderness** in the groin and over the greater trochanter on palpation.
3. **Range of motion**
   a. **Active** movements are not possible.
   b. **Passive** movements are very painful.

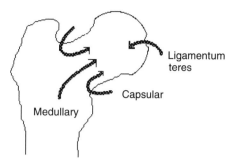

Fig. 18–12 Most of the blood to the head of the femur comes from the capsular and medullary arteries. These blood vessels may be damaged in fractures through the neck of the femur close to its head. The blood supply through the artery of ligamentation teres may not be enough to prevent avascular necrosis of the head of the femur.

Course

These fractures should be treated as orthopedic emergencies. Incidence of complications, such as avascular necrosis of the head of the femur, increases if definitive treatment is delayed. In the days before internal fixation for these fractures, patients would die due to complications of prolonged bedrest.

Complications

1. **Avascular necrosis** of the head of the femur. Chances of this complication increases if:
   a. Reduction of the fracture and immobilization is delayed
   b. Fracture line is closer to the articular cartilage
   c. Accurate anatomical reduction of the fracture fragments is not obtained
2. **Delayed union** or **nonunion** of the fragments
3. **Complications of bedrest**—e.g., pneumonia, pressure ulcers
4. **Degenerative arthritis** of the hip joint is late complication.
5. **Deep vein thrombosis**

Investigations

Plain x-rays, anteroposterior and lateral, usually are sufficient to diagnose the fracture.

Management

Fractures of the neck of the femur are treated surgically. Without internal fixation, the fracture requires prolonged bedrest, which may lead to serious complications.

These fractures are very prone to complications and should be handled by an orthopedic surgeon. Depending on the circumstances, he or she may carry out one of the following procedures:

1. Reduction of fracture under anesthetic and internal fixation with a nail or a nail and plate.
2. Arthroplasty is performed if the fracture line is very close to the head of the femur and the patient is elderly.

FRACTURES OF THE PELVIS

Anatomy
The bony pelvis forms a ring around the urinary bladder, urethra, rectum, and female reproductive organs. This ring is made up of the sacrum posteriorly, with the two hip bones on the sides and in front. It connects to the spine through the sacrum and to the lower extremities by hip joints. It protects important anatomical structures.

Mechanism of Injury
Pelvic bones are very strong and require violent forces to break. Elderly **osteoporotic** individuals and patients with **metastasis** are exceptions in that minor falls can fracture the pubic rami easily in these groups. Other common causes are **automobile accidents** and **falls** from a considerable height. Because of the severity of the injury, pelvic fractures are usually accompanied by fractures of other bones and visceral injury, e.g., rupture of the urethra.

Types of Fractures
1. **Stable.** The pelvic ring is intact, and the fracture is stable. There is no damage to the weight-bearing portion of the pelvis. There are two types in this group:
   a. **Avulsion fractures**—A small portion of bone is broken off near the origin of a muscle, e.g., anterior superior iliac spine.
   b. **Isolated fracture** of the pelvic ring—The pelvic ring is broken at only one place (Fig. 18–13A).
2. **Unstable.** The pelvic ring is broken at two places with displacement of fragments (Fig. 18–13B). This is a serious injury with great potential for complications and death.

History
The type and severity of injury give some indication as to what might have happened. The patient may complain of pain in the groin, lower abdomen, or low back depending on the part of the pelvis that is broken. The patient may not be able to give any history in cases of major trauma because of shock or unconsciousness.

Physical Examination
Priority is given to diagnoses of shock, internal hemorrhage, and visceral injury. Fracture of the pelvis should be suspected in all major trauma cases.
1. **Inspection.** There may be swelling and skin discoloration due hematoma or extravasation of urine. Shortening of the lower extremity is seen in patients with proximal displacement.
2. **Palpation.** There may be tenderness over pubic symphysis, groin, iliac crest, or lumbosacral region, depending on the part of the pelvis involved.
3. **Range of motion.** Movements of the lumbar region and hip are painful.

Differential Diagnosis
Other fractures, such as fracture of the neck or shaft of the femur, may mimic pelvic fracture.

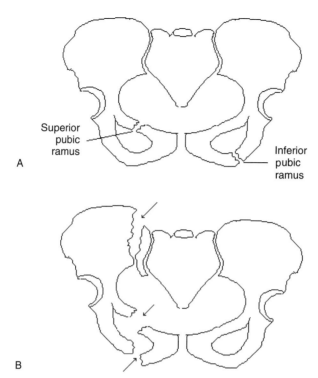

Fig. 18–13 Pelvic fractures. *A,* In stable, undisplaced fractures, the pelvic ring is intact. *B,* In unstable fractures, the pelvic ring is broken. These fractures may be associated with injury to internal organs or major blood vessels.

Complications
1. **Shock** is very common.
2. **Rupture of urethra or bladder** should be ruled out by catheterization. It may be difficult or impossible to catheterize a patient with a ruptured urethra. Blood-stained urine indicates injury to the urinary tract.
3. **Intrapelvic hemorrhage** from rupture of a major vessel

Investigations
Suspect fracture of the pelvis in all major trauma cases, and ask for **x-rays** of the pelvis. In all cases of pelvic fracture due to major trauma, rule out fractures of the proximal femur and lumbosacral spine. **Catheterization** should be attempted to rule out rupture of the urethra. **Cystogram** may be indicated if rupture of the urinary bladder is suspected.

Management
Discussion of unstable, displaced, or multiple fractures of the pelvis with vascular or visceral injuries is beyond the scope of this book. For single, undisplaced, uncomplicated fracture of a pubic ramus or ilium, treatment is:
1. **Medications.** Analgesics are used to control pain.

2. **Ancillary**
   a. **Bedrest** is advised until pain subsides. Frequent turning in bed is recommended to prevent pressure ulcers.
   b. Gradually increasing activities as tolerated are prescribed, such as sitting up in bed or sitting in a chair for increasing periods of time.
3. **Surgical** management is necessary for more complicated cases. It may take the form of:
   a. Treatment of shock
   b. Closed reduction and plaster spica of displaced unstable fractures
   c. Open reduction and internal fixation
   d. Exploration for vascular or visceral damage

DISLOCATIONS OF THE HIP

Anatomy
The hip is a very stable joint because of the shape of the acetabulum surrounding the head of the femur and the presence of strong ligaments. It takes a violent force to dislocate the hip. The sciatic nerve lies posteriorly in close proximity to the joint and is likely to be damaged in hip dislocations.

Mechanism of Injury
The hip may dislocate in an automobile accident, when the knee hits the dashboard in front-end collision. The hip and knee are flexed, and the hip joint is pushed backward. If the hip is abducted as well as flexed, then the posterior rim of the acetabulum may be fractured at the same time.

Types of Dislocations
1. **Posterior.** The head of the femur is displaced posteriorly. This is the most common type of dislocation and may be associated with fracture of the rim of the acetabulum and injury to the sciatic nerve.
2. **Anterior.** The head of the femur comes to lie anteriorly. This variety is not common.
3. **Central.** The head of the femur is driven through the acetabulum by a lateral force. It is actually a type of fracture of the pelvis (acetabulum) and is not very common.

History
The type of accident and position of the femur at the time of the accident give some indication as to the type of dislocation that may occur. Severe pain is felt in the hip region. If the sciatic nerve is damaged, the patient may complain of numbness or severe pain in the distribution of the nerve.

Physical Examination
1. **Inspection.** There may be swelling and deformity in the hip region. The posterior dislocation results in **shortening** of the lower extremity with adduction and internal rotation **deformity** at the hip.
2. **Palpation.** The groin, trochanteric, and gluteal regions are tender. The femoral pulse is difficult to palpate because the resistance provided by the head of the femur is missing

in posterior dislocations. The head of the femur may be palpable in the gluteal region or the groin, depending on the type of dislocation.

3. **Range of motion**
   a. **Active** movements are not possible.
   b. **Passive** ROMs are markedly restricted because of pain.
4. **Special tests. Neurologic exam** for sciatic nerve damage should be done before any anesthetic is given. It is possible that only the common peroneal part of the sciatic nerve is clinically involved. **Distal pulses** in the dorsalis pedis and posterior tibial are checked to rule out vascular injury.

Complications

1. **Sciatic nerve** injury may occur, especially in posterior dislocation. The nerve is vulnerable during closed or open reduction of the hip.
2. **Avascular necrosis** of the head of femur. The blood supply to the head may be damaged due to tear of the joint capsule or ligamentum teres.
3. **Degenerative joint disease** secondary to fracture of the articular surface of the acetabulum or avascular necrosis of the head is a common sequel.

Differential Diagnosis

Dislocation of the hip may be missed in the presence of a fracture of the femur or vice versa. In any major trauma, it is important to examine the whole body and order x-rays of the pelvis.

Investigations

1. **Plain x-rays.** The anteroposterior view may not show associated fracture of the rim of the acetabulum. Special views or CT scan may be needed.
2. **CT scan** helps to visualize bony fragments and their displacement.
3. **Electromyography** helps to determine the extent of sciatic nerve damage.

Management

1. Closed reduction under anesthetic
2. Open reduction
3. Open reduction and internal fixation of bone fragments

SOFT TISSUE CONDITIONS

Trochanteric Bursitis

Inflammation of the trochanteric bursa may give rise to pain in the hip, thigh, and knee region. It is a fairly common condition and can be easily mistaken for degenerative arthritis of the hip or lumbosacral spine. Since the treatment for these conditions is very different, it is very important to arrive at a correct diagnosis.

Anatomy

The trochanteric bursa is a large bursa separating the greater trochanter and gluteus maximus muscle (Fig. 18–14). The gluteus maximus muscle arises from the posterior part of

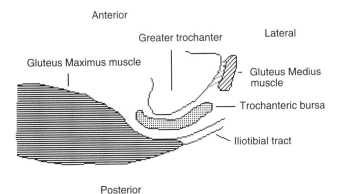

Fig. 18–14   Cross-section at the level of the trochanteric bursa. The bursa is covered by the gluteus maximus and is posterolateral to the greater trochanter.

the iliac crest and sacrum. Its fibers course anterolaterally and are inserted into the iliotibial tract and gluteal tuberosity over the upper, posterior part of the femur. Trochanteric bursa facilitates movement of the distal part of the gluteus maximus and iliotibial tract over the greater trochanter. Gluteus maximus muscle is an extensor and lateral rotator of the hip. It contracts during walking, running, rising from a chair, and climbing stairs.

Etiology
Trochanteric bursitis may occur together with degenerative disc disease of the lumbosacral spine, degenerative arthritis of the hip, or rheumatoid arthritis or after operation in the hip region. It may also occur as an **overuse** syndrome in people who bicycle or run long distance.

Pathology
There is aseptic inflammation of the bursa.

History
The **onset** may be insidious or sudden, with pain in the hip region. Inquiries regarding unusual or athletic activities should be made. Middle-aged and elderly groups are commonly affected. **Pain** is felt over the lateral aspect of the upper part of the thigh. It may radiate from the buttock to the knee and mimic radiculopathy. The pain is aggravated by lying on the same side and may wake the patient from sleep. Activities such as walking, running, and sitting cross-legged (with the leg over the opposite knee) also make the pain worse.

Physical Examination
1. **Inspection.** The patient may **limp** because of pain on walking.
2. **Palpation.** There is localized **tenderness** over the bursa. The bursa under the gluteus maximus muscle is located over the posterolateral aspect of the greater trochanter (Fig. 18–14), whereas the bursa under the gluteus medius muscle is over the tip of the greater trochanter.
3. **Range of motion**
   a. **Active abduction** against resistance aggravates the pain.
   b. **Passive adduction** and internal rotation may be limited because of pain.

4. **Special tests**
   a. **Patrick-Fabere test.** The patient is asked to put the heel on the affected side over the opposite knee. This maneuver flexes, abducts, and externally rotates the hip. The examiner then gently pushes the knee on the affected side outward and downward. The patient complains of pain if there is hip or sacroiliac pathology or trochanteric bursitis.
   b. Infiltration of the tender area with **local anesthetic** gives immediate relief of symptoms and confirms the diagnosis.

Differential Diagnosis
1. **Lumbar radiculopathy.** Low back pain is made worse by movements of the spine. There is tenderness and muscle spasm in the lumbosacral region. Straight leg raising test may be positive.
2. **Degenerative arthritis of the hip.** There is no localized tenderness, and all movements of the hip aggravate the pain.
3. **Meralgia paresthetica.** The patient complains of tingling, numbness, and pain over the lateral aspect of the thigh. Symptoms may be reproduced by palpation near the anterior superior iliac spine. There is diminished sensation over the lateral and anterior part of the thigh.

Investigations
X-rays of the hip are normal. Irregularity of the surface of the greater trochanter or soft tissue calcification may be seen in a small percentage of cases.

Management
1. **Medications. NSAIDs** may help by reducing inflammation and pain. Local injection of a **steroid** preparation at the site of maximum tenderness has been found to be very effective.
2. **Ancillary. Rest** is provided by reducing activities that aggravate the pain. **Local heat** and **exercises** to stretch the iliotibial band should be recommended.
3. **Surgical** treatment is rarely necessary. If bursitis is due to a protruding nail following hip operation, the hardware must be removed. If conservative measures fail to relieve symptoms, the thickened part of the iliotibial tract and the bursa can be excised.

Iliopsoas Bursitis
Iliopsoas bursitis is also known as **psoas** or **iliopectineal bursitis.**

Anatomy
The iliopsoas bursa is situated between the iliopsoas tendon and the capsule of the hip joint (Fig. 18–15). The psoas major muscle arises from the anterolateral surfaces of the lumbar vertebrae and their transverse processes. The iliacus muscle arises from the inner surface of the ilium. Both pass under the inguinal ligament and insert as a common tendon into the lesser trochanter. It is a flexor of the hip joint. The iliopsoas bursa may communicate with the hip joint cavity in some cases.

History
Pain is felt in the groin and anterior thigh. It is aggravated by movements of the hip, such as walking.

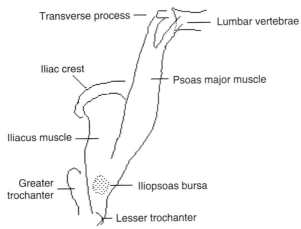

Fig. 18–15 The psoas major muscle arises from the lumbar vertebrae and their transverse processes. iliacus muscle arises from the iliac bone. The combined iliopsoas muscle is inserted into the lesser trochanter of the femur. The iliopsoas bursa is between the hip joint capsule and the iliopsoas tendon.

Physical Examination
1. **Palpation.** Tenderness is felt in the groin, below the inguinal ligament.
2. **Range of motion**
   a. **Active** flexion of the hip against resistance reproduces the pain.
   b. **Passive** extension and extreme flexion and adduction also give rise to pain.

Differential Diagnosis
1. **Inguinal lymphadenitis.** Tender lymph nodes are palpable in the groin. A primary site of infection or malignancy in the lower extremity or external genitalia should be sought.
2. **Degenerative arthritis** of the hip. Onset of symptoms is gradual, with a long history of intermittent pain which is worse on weight-bearing. X-rays show characteristic changes in the hip joint.
3. **Femoral hernia.** The swelling in the groin increases in size on coughing and may be reducible.

Investigations
1. X-rays help to rule out hip pathology.
2. Fluid from the bursa is sent for examination for crystals, culture, and sensitivity testing. It is very important to rule out hernia before attempting to aspirate any swelling in the groin.

Management
1. **Medications.** NSAIDs are prescribed to reduce inflammation and pain. Aspiration and injection of long-acting **steroid** preparation (if there is no infection) is given if NSAIDs fail to control symptoms.
2. **Ancillary.** All activities that aggravate the pain are restricted. Physical therapy to maintain and increase ROM of the hip joint may be helpful.

Ischial Bursitis

Ischial bursitis is also known as **ischiogluteal bursitis** and **weaver's bottom.**

Anatomy

The bursa is located over the ischial tuberosity. It is covered by the gluteus maximus muscle in the standing position. However, in the sitting position, the gluteus maximus muscle slides upward, and the bursa lies directly under the skin and subcutaneous tissue.

Etiology

Ischial bursitis was called a weaver's bottom because weavers had to sit for long hours on hard benches, which ultimately led to ischial bursitis. Nowadays, it may occur in people operating heavy equipment on rough roads.

Pathology

Vibration of the heavy equipment or pressure between the bone and a hard surface is believed to start the inflammation.

History

Pain on sitting, especially on a hard surface, is the usual presenting symptom. It is felt in the gluteal region and may radiate down the posterior aspect of the thigh. It is relieved by standing.

Physical Examination

1. **Inspection.** Usually, there are no visible signs of inflammation or swelling.
2. **Palpation.** The ischial tuberosity can be palpated near the medial end of the gluteal fold. There is localized, severe tenderness.
3. **Range of motion.** Forward bending and straight leg raising are painful because they increase pressure on the inflamed bursa.
4. **Special tests.** Injection of local anesthetic relieves the pain immediately.

Differential Diagnosis

1. **Lumbosacral strain.** Tenderness and muscle spasm are located in the lumbar region.
2. **Lumbar radiculopathy.** The sciatic nerve is close to the ischial bursa. Straight leg raising test may be positive in both conditions. Exquisite tenderness over the ischial bursa and absence of neurologic signs help distinguish between ischial bursitis and lumbar radiculopathy.
3. **Tear of hamstring tendon.** Semitendinosus, semimembranosus, and long head of biceps femoris muscles arise from the ischial tuberosity. Injury to any of these structures gives rise to pain and tenderness in the same region. History of athletic injury and pain on active extension of the thigh against resistance helps diagnose hamstring tendon injury.

Management

1. **Medications**
   1. Injection of **local anesthetic** is diagnostic and also therapeutic.
   2. Injection of long-acting **steroid** preparation locally is used if the local anesthetic fails to control symptoms.
2. **Ancillary**
   1. The patient is advised to avoid sitting for long periods on hard surfaces or operating heavy equipment on rough roads.
   2. Physical therapy. Ultrasound over the painful area helps relieve pain and inflammation.

Snapping Hip

An audible or palpable click or snap around the hip joint is called snapping hip. It may not require any treatment.

Pathology

The following structures may be implicated:
1. Thickened posterior border of iliotibial band
2. Trochanteric bursitis
3. Roughened greater trochanter

History

A snapping sensation is described on flexion, adduction, or internal rotation of the hip. There is usually no discomfort or pain. Presence of pain and limitation of activities are indications for treatment.

Physical Examination

1. **Inspection.** There is no abnormality on inspection.
2. **Palpation.** The examiner places the palm of the hand to feel the snapping structure. The trochanteric region should be palpated for tenderness.
3. **Range of motion.** Active and passive movements, such as sitting or squatting, should be performed to reproduce the snapping.

Differential Diagnosis

1. **Loose bodies** can cause pain and locking of the hip joint. X-rays may confirm the diagnosis.
2. A **subluxed hip,** on reduction into the socket, may give rise to sensation similar to snapping. The sensation of the head of the femur being reduced into the acetabulum as felt by the palpating hand is different from that of a snapping due to thickened fascial band.

Investigations

X-rays help to rule out subluxation and loose bodies in the joint.

Management

No treatment is necessary in most patients. Reassurance as to the benign nature of this condition is sufficient. If pain interferes with vocational or avocational activities, then the following treatments should be considered. **NSAIDs** are prescribed to reduce pain and inflammation. Physical therapy in the form of local **heat** and **exercises** to stretch the iliotibial tract may help. Local injection of **steroids** should be given if both NSAIDs and physical therapy measures do not give relief. **Surgical** release or excision of the thickened iliotibial tract is considered as a last resort.

DEGENERATIVE JOINT DISEASE OF THE HIP

Degenerative joint disease (DJD) of the hip, also known as **osteoarthritis** or **osteoarthrosis,** is a very common problem in people over age 60 years. The incidence of the disease increases with age. Degeneration of the hip occurs at a much earlier age when it is secondary to some other pathology, e.g., congenital dysplasia of the hip.

Anatomy/Biomechanics
The forces transmitted through the hip joint may reach up to 3 times body weight during normal walking. The load on the hip joint increases as the speed of walking increases or with running. These forces may aggravate symptoms when the articular cartilage is not normal.

Etiology
Secondary DJD may occur as a result of congenital malformation of the hip (dysplasia), deformity such as coxa vara or coxa plana, prior infection in the joint, fracture, or inflammatory disease such as rheumatoid arthritis. The cause of primary or idiopathic DJD is not known.

Pathology
The articular cartilage loses some of its water content over years. Dull and yellowish patches develop on the surface, there is some breakdown of collagen fibers, and small pieces of cartilage become loose and float around in the synovial fluid. Synovial inflammation results. The articular cartilage becomes thinner. This is seen on x-rays as diminished joint space. In some areas, bone under the cartilage is exposed. The subchondral bone becomes sclerosed as a result of increased stress. On x-rays, this shows up as **subchondral sclerosis. Cysts** and **osteophytes** are other common changes seen in pathologic specimens and on x-rays.

History
The onset of disease is much earlier (in the third or fourth decade) in secondary osteoarthritis of the hip. In primary disease, it may start with a mild **ache** in the groin after a long walk or early in the morning. The early-morning pain subsides after 10–15 minutes of activity. The pain gradually worsens over a period of years and may curtail walking. In the advanced stage of disease, pain wakes the patient at night, and he or she must resort to walking around for relief. In some patients, the pain is felt in the thigh or knee and creates difficulty in diagnosis. Pain and restriction of movements may interfere with tying shoelaces or sitting down in the tub for bathing.

Physical Examination
1. **Inspection.** The patient walks with **antalgic gait** (*see* Fig. 18–2). The patient shifts the body weight over to the affected hip and reduces the weight-bearing time on that joint. Flexion, adduction **deformity** may be observed in some of these patients.
2. **Palpation.** There may be some tenderness in the groin or pain on pressure over the greater trochanter.
3. **Range of motion.** Internal rotation and extension are usually limited with pain in the extremes of the range. Later, restriction of abduction in female patients may interfere with sexual intercourse.

Course
The course is slowly progressive over years. There may be periods with more pain and limitation of function followed by remissions.

Differential Diagnosis
1. Patients with **lumbosacral degenerative disc disease** may complain of pain in the gluteal region, which they may interpret as hip pain.

2. **Knee** pathology. Some patients with hip disease may complain of pain referred to the knee, and unless the hip is examined and x-rayed, the correct diagnosis can be missed.

Investigations

Plain x-ray shows **narrowing of joint space** and **subchondral sclerosis.** These changes are most marked in the superior and lateral aspect of the hip joint. **Bone cyst** and **osteophytes** are seen at the upper and lower margin of the acetabulum.

Management

Conservative management consists of NSAIDs, curtailment of weight-bearing activities, local heat, stretching exercises to increase ROM, and use of a cane in the opposite hand to reduce forces on the affected hip. If the patient is obese, losing weight helps to reduce pain and stress on the hip joint. Night pain and failure of conservative treatment are good indications for arthroplasty.

1. **Medications. NSAIDs** help relieve pain and allow the patient to increase activities. Patients who are not able to tolerate NSAIDs may be prescribed acetaminophen. For patients with more severe symptoms and limitation of function, intra-articular **steroid injection** should be considered.
2. **Ancillary.** During normal walking, the hip joint has to withstand forces equivalent to 2–3 times body weight. The hip can be relieved of a lot of these forces by reducing the body weight to as close to the patient's ideal body weight as feasible. Using a cane in the opposite hand also helps to reduce weight-bearing forces. Physical therapy in the form of local **heat** (ultrasound or shortwave diathermy), stretching **exercises** to increase ROM, and **gait training** with a cane also help relieve symptoms.
3. **Surgical.** Severity of changes on x-rays do not always correlate well with clinical symptoms and signs and should not be the main reason for operating on patients with degenerative arthritis of the hip. **Night pain** that wakes the patient from sleep and severe **limitation of function** are good indications for considering surgical treatment. Osteotomy of the upper end of the femur is not done very frequently. Replacement **arthroplasty** for the head of the femur and/or acetabulum is the treatment of choice.

TRANSIENT SYNOVITIS OF THE HIP

Transient synovitis, which is also known as acute transitory epiphysitis, idiopathic monarticular synovitis, or transitory coxitis, is a nonspecific inflammation of the synovial membrane of the hip joint.

Etiology

Its exact etiology is not known, but it may occur 2–4 weeks after an attack of upper respiratory infection or allergy.

Pathology

There is **effusion** in the hip joint and swelling of the synovial membrane. High intra-articular pressure may impair blood supply to the epiphysis of the femoral head. Transient synovitis is implicated as an etiologic factor in Perthes' disease. No organisms can be cultured from the joint fluid.

History
Transient synovitis is seen fairly frequently in children, especially boys, between the ages of 3 and 10 years. **Painful limp** is the most common presenting complaint. There is no history of fever, loss of appetite, or weight loss. Questions about upper respiratory tract infection a few weeks before the onset of hip pain should be asked. The patient may complain of pain in the groin, thigh, or knee region.

Physical Examination
1. **Inspection.** The patient walks with an **antalgic gait.** The thigh is kept in the flexed position, which leads to functional shortening of the lower extremity and **limp.** In more severe cases, **abduction** and external rotation deformity occur together with flexion. The capacity of the hip joint to hold fluid is maximal when the joint is flexed, and that is the reason for the patient's adapting a flexed position when there is effusion in the joint.
2. **Palpation.** Some **tenderness** may be present in the groin. Usually, there is no palpable swelling.
3. **Range of motion**
   a. **Active**—The patient is reluctant to move the affected lower extremity.
   b. **Passive**—Extension, **adduction,** and internal rotation are limited because of flexion, abduction, and external rotation deformity.

Course/Complications
The disease is self-limited. Signs and symptoms usually subside in 2–3 weeks. However, increased intra-articular pressure may interfere with blood flow to the epiphysis of the head of the femur and lead to **Perthes' disease.** This can happen as late as 2 years after the episode of transient synovitis. Followup x-rays at 6-month intervals are recommended.

Differential Diagnosis
1. **Septic arthritis.** It is very important to rule out infection, because treatment for septic arthritis is specific and if it is not treated properly and promptly the hip joint will suffer permanent damage. Systemic symptoms like fever, malaise, and loss of appetite should suggest infection. The ESR is high with a high WBC count. The hip joint should be aspirated and joint fluid sent for culture and sensitivity.
2. **Rheumatic fever.** The joint pain and swelling migrate from joint to joint in rheumatic fever.
3. **Rheumatoid arthritis** of the oligoarticular variety may be difficult to rule out in the early stages.
4. **Tuberculosis.** The course is very prolonged with abnormal joint fluid. X-rays show demineralization of bone, large effusion in the joint, and later lytic lesions.
5. **Perthes' disease.** Plain x-rays are normal initially and may take 2–3 months to show changes. Followup of these patients is important.

Investigations
1. **Blood tests.** WBC total and differential are done to rule out infection. They are normal in transient synovitis.
2. **Plain x-rays.** Hip joint effusion is difficult to diagnose on plain x-rays. Soft tissue swelling may be seen over the lateral aspect. Followup x-rays do not show any soft tissue or bone abnormality.

3. **Aspiration** helps to relieve intra-articular pressure, pain, and muscle spasm. Examination of joint fluid is the most important test to rule out septic arthritis or tuberculosis.

Management
1. **Medications.** Analgesics are given to relieve pain.
2. **Ancillary.** Bedrest and skin traction for a week or two are sufficient to relieve signs and symptoms of transient synovitis.

SLIPPED CAPITAL FEMORAL EPIPHYSIS

This condition is also known as slipped upper femoral epiphysis, adolescent coxa vara, epiphyseal coxa vara, and epiphyseolisthesis. It is the most common disorder of the hip in **adolescents,** and if not detected early and treated properly, it may lead to early degenerative arthritis of the hip.

Anatomy
The epiphysis of the femoral head appears from the 5th to 8th month and fuses by the 18th to 20th year. The articular surface of the femoral head is formed from this epiphysis.

Etiology
The exact etiology is not known. It is 2 to 3 times more common in **boys** than girls. It is believed to be related to the rapid growth period and imbalance between the growth hormone and sex hormones during adolescence. Half of the patients are obese with underdeveloped genitalia. A small percentage of patients may be slim and tall. Slipped capital femoral epiphysis is at times associated with following conditions:
1. Endocrine disorders
   Pituitary
   Thyroid
   Hypothyroid
2. Other conditions
   Down's syndrome
   Growth hormone therapy
   Rickets

Pathology
The normal epiphyseal plate is horizontal in children but becomes oblique during adolescence. This change may place increased mechanical stress on the growth plate at a time of excessive activity. The growth plate itself may be abnormal because of hormonal imbalance. The growth plate of the upper femoral epiphysis is widened and irregular. The epiphysis is displaced inferiorly and posteriorly in relation to the neck of the femur (Fig. 18–16)—i.e., the neck of the femur moves anteriorly and proximally. This leads to **adduction (coxa vara)** and external rotation deformity. Blood supply to the femoral head may be compromised, and **avascular necrosis** may develop. Later, if this displacement persists without any treatment, **degenerative arthritis** develops in the hip joint at an early age.

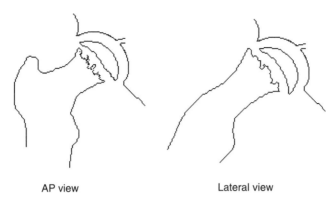

AP view   Lateral view

Fig. 18–16   Slipped capital femoral epiphysis. The AP view may not show any displacement of the epiphysis. There is irregular widening of the growth plate and some osteoporosis of the adjacent metaphysis. Slippage of the epiphysis is seen better on the lateral view.

History

The **age** at onset of symptoms is usually between **8–16 years.** The symptoms are usually mild and the onset insidious. The patient may complain of vague **discomfort** in the groin, thigh, or knee region, which is intermittent and brought on by walking or running. Rest relieves this discomfort. The symptoms may be brought on by minor trauma. Parents may notice a **limp,** especially when the patient is tired. Review of systems should include questions regarding endocrine and metabolic disorders. The patient may have had a rapid increase in body weight or height at the time of onset.

Physical Examination

1. **Inspection.** Most patients are **obese.** A few may be of normal or thin and tall build. During the painful stage, the gait is **antalgic,** with the foot on the affected side being more externally rotated than that on the normal side. Later, the gait becomes **Trendelenburg** type because of coxa vara deformity. No abnormal signs are seen in the hip region on inspection.
2. **Palpation.** There may be tenderness in the hip region during early stages of the disease.
3. **Range of motion.** Passive ROM shows **limitation** of **internal rotation** and **abduction.**
4. **Special tests**
   1. The affected leg may be slightly **shorter** than the other. If the shortening is due to coxa vara deformity, the greater trochanter will be higher than on the normal side.
   2. **Trendelenburg test** is positive because of coxa vara deformity which reduces the effective length of the hip abductors.
   3. Genitalia should be checked for **undescended testicles.**
   4. Visual field defects may suggest a pituitary tumor.

Course

The upper femoral epiphysis may continue to slip. The course of the disease is usually slowly progressive. Secondary degenerative arthritis of the hip sets in early due to altered mechanics.

Differential Diagnosis

1. **Transient synovitis.** X-rays are normal. Symptoms and signs subside after 2–3 weeks of bedrest and analgesics.
2. **Juvenile rheumatoid arthritis.** Other joints are involved, and blood tests may be abnormal.
3. **Septic arthritis** of the hip joint. Fever, increased WBC count, elevated ESR, and abnormal joint fluid examination are helpful in diagnosis of infection. The joint should be aspirated whenever infection is suspected.
4. **Legg-Calvé-Perthes disease** occurs in younger children, and x-ray appearances differ.

Investigations

1. **X-rays.** The anteroposterior view of the hip shows widening of the epiphyseal plate with irregularity of the surface (Fig. 18–16). The displacement of the epiphysis is not seen well in this view. A line drawn along the upper surface of the neck of the femur normally passes through the head of the femur. If the upper femoral epiphysis is displaced downward, this line does not transect the femoral head. True **lateral view** shows the epiphyseal displacement in a downward direction better than the AP view.
2. **CT scan.** The extent of the posterior slippage of the epiphysis is seen better on CT scan than on plain x-rays.

Management

Patients suspected of having slipped capital femoral epiphysis should be referred to an orthopedic specialist as soon as possible, because treatment is mainly **surgical.** Various treatments available are:

1. **Traction.** Initially bedrest and traction are used to reduce pain and muscle spasm.
2. **Internal fixation** to prevent further displacement and early fusion of the epiphysis
3. **Osteotomy** to correct deformity or as a treatment for degenerative arthritis

Complications

1. **Avascular necrosis** of the head of the femur occurs if the blood supply is damaged.
2. **Chondrolysis** is inflammation and destruction of the articular cartilage of the hip joint. This may present with pain and restriction of movements and lead to ankylosis of the joint.

LEGG-CALVÉ-PERTHES DISEASE

This disorder is also known as **osteochondrosis, Perthes' disease, coxa plana,** osteochondritis deformans juvenilis, and pseudocoxalgia. The blood supply to the femoral head gets cut off, causing necrosis of the ossification center. The head of the femur is deformed, and early degenerative arthritis of the hip may develop. Avascular necrosis of the femoral head in the adult is considered separately (see page 286).

Etiology

The blood supply to the epiphysis of the femoral head is cut off, but the cause is not known.
Predisposing factors include:

1. **Age.** It usually occurs between ages **4–12 years.**
2. **Sex. Male** children are affected 4 times more often than females.
3. **Race.** Children of **European** and **Asian** ancestry are involved more often.
4. **Complication.** It may occur in association with:
   a. **Trauma**—e.g., dislocation of the hip
   b. **Transient synovitis** of the hip—Increased intrasynovial pressure probably cuts off the blood supply to the femoral head.
   c. **Sickle cell disease**

Pathology

Nutrition to the center for ossification of the femoral head is supplied by blood vessels traveling along the neck of the femur. The articular cartilage covering this center gets its nutrition from the synovial fluid. When the blood supply is cut off, the cells in the ossification center die. However, the cells of the articular cartilage survive. The ossification center stops growing, but the articular cartilage continues to grow. Radiographically, this is seen as a smaller center for ossification with increased joint space (because of thicker articular cartilage than on the normal side) (Figs. 18–17 and 18–18).

Blood supply to the adjacent metaphysis is increased in reaction to the necrosis, leading to radiolucency of the femoral neck in comparison with the dead bone of the ossific center. New blood vessels grow in and around the dead bone, followed by new bone formation. The dead part of the ossific center is seen as a smaller, denser bone within a larger, radiolucent center of ossification (Fig. 18–19). This is called the **head-within-a-head** appearance. Up to this stage, the child may remain asymptomatic.

The clinical or symptomatic stage of the disease starts after a **fracture in the subchondral zone** of the head of the femur (Fig. 18–20A). The blood supply to the bone underneath the fracture is cut off a second time and undergoes changes similar to those seen after the first episode. The amount of bone involved depends on the extent of fracture. New blood vessels grow from the periphery and absorb the dead tissue. Finally, new bone is laid down to replace the old in a process called **creeping substitution.** During this stage, irregular areas of dense and radiolucent bone are seen on x-rays. This is described as **fragmentation** of the ossific center. The result of all these processes may be a deformed, enlarged femoral head (coxa plana) with thick femoral neck. Incongruity of the femoral head and acetabulum leads ultimately to early degenerative arthritis of the hip joint.

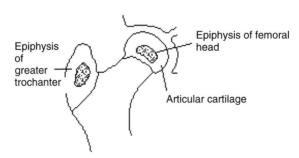

Fig. 18–17 X-ray appearance of normal hip joint of a 5–7-year-old child.

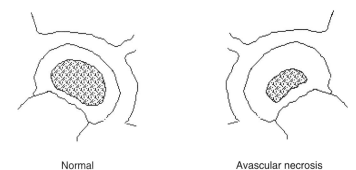

Normal   Avascular necrosis

Fig. 18–18 Growth of epiphysis stops when its blood supply is cut off, but the articular cartilage continues to grow. During the early stages of avascular necrosis of the epiphysis of the femoral head, the epiphysis looks smaller than the one on the unaffected side. There is apparent increase in joint space because of increased thickness of articular cartilage. Since the articular cartilage is not visible on x-rays, it is interpreted as joint space.

History

Onset is insidious with pain and/or limping. The **pain** may be felt in the groin, thigh, or knee. It is brought on by activity such as walking or running and is relieved by rest. Parents may complain that the child **limps,** especially when tired. There may be a history of mild trauma in a few patients.

Physical Examination

1. **Inspection.** The child walks with **antalgic gait.** The stance phase on the affected side is shorter—i.e., the patient puts weight on the affected side for a shorter time than on the normal side. **Atrophy** of thigh muscles may be noticeable.
2. **Palpation.** There may be some tenderness in the groin.
3. **Range of motion. Abduction** and internal rotation are particularly restricted. Extension is limited if there is muscle spasm in flexor muscles.
4. **Special tests**
   a. Measure the **circumference** of the proximal thigh to confirm muscle atrophy. Measurement is done at the same level on both thighs and compared.
   b. **Trendelenburg test** is positive during the early stages of disease because of inhibition of the **abductors** of the hip. Later, this test is positive because of the short thick neck of the femur and large greater trochanter, which effectively reduces the length of the **abductors** and thus strength of contraction.

Differential Diagnosis

1. **Transient synovitis** of the hip. Some patients may develop avascular necrosis after synovitis of the hip joint. Symptoms and signs are similar in both conditions. If symptoms persist or recur after treatment, followup x-rays are necessary to rule out avascular necrosis.
2. **Septic arthritis.** Fever, leukocytosis, and ESR may suggest bacterial infection. Aspiration of the joint and analysis of the joint fluid should be done without delay.
3. **Juvenile rheumatoid arthritis.** Inflammatory arthritis can be confused with Perthes'

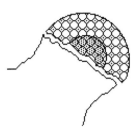

Fig. 18–19 Growth of the epiphysis resumes after revascularization. The avascular part looks more dense and presents a "head-within-a-head" appearance on x-rays.

disease during its initial stages. Involvement of other joints, joint fluid examination, and blood tests can differentiate the two conditions.
4. **Slipped capital femoral epiphysis** occurs at a later age, and x-ray findings are different.

Investigations
1. **Plain X-rays.** Anteroposterior and frog-leg lateral views are usually sufficient to make the diagnosis. There is a delay (of months) in the appearance of x-ray changes, and other investigations may be necessary during the early stages of the disease. The x-ray changes vary with the stage of the disease:
    a. **Synovitis**—Soft tissue swelling is seen without any changes in the bony structure.
    b. **Necrosis of the capital epiphysis**—The epiphysis is smaller than that on the opposite side and denser than the adjacent metaphysis. The joint space is wider because the articular cartilage continues to grow (Fig. 18–18).
    c. **Subchondral fracture** is seen better on frog-leg lateral view. There is a thin radiolucent area under the subchondral bone and parallel to it (Fig. 18–20A). The bone under this fracture undergoes a second episode of necrosis.
    d. **Fragmentation**—Revascularization and resorption of the necrotic bone are seen on x-rays as irregular small areas of radiodensities and radiolucencies (Fig. 18–20B).
    e. Stage of **healing**—Severity of changes seen in this stage depends on factors mentioned under Prognosis (below). The head of the femur may be larger, flattened, and mushroom-shaped. Part of the head extends beyond the acetabulum. The neck of the femur is broader and thicker (Fig. 18–20C).
2. **MRI** detects changes of necrosis earlier than plain x-rays and shows the extent of the area involved.
3. **Arthrography** helps in delineating the shape of articular cartilage and congruity of the developing head of femur and acetabulum.
4. **Technetium bone scan.** The avascular area does not pick up technetium.

Prognosis
The outcome depends on:
1. **Age of onset** of symptoms. Onset after the age of 5 or 6 years has a worse prognosis.
2. Extent of the **subchondral fracture.** With more extensive fracture, the area of the femoral head that will be affected is larger, and the prognosis is worse.
3. Final **shape of the femoral heads.** The more deformed the femoral head or less spherical its shape, greater are the chances of degenerative arthritis later in life.

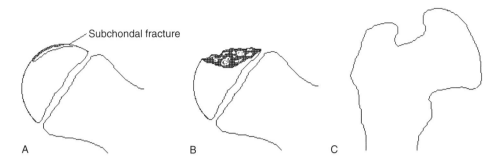

Fig. 18–20 Symptomatic phase of the disease. *A,* Pathologic fracture leads to a second episode of necrosis of the underlying bone. On lateral x-rays of the hip, the fracture is seen as a "crescent sign." A radiolucent line is seen under a rim of cortical bone. *B,* Fragmentation, revascularization and resorption of the necrotic bone are seen on x-rays as irregular small areas of radiodensities and radiolucencies. *C,* The final outcome depends on the extent of subchondral fracture and involvement of the epiphysis. The head of femur is flattened (mushroom-shaped) and incongruous with the acetabulum. Part of the head may project beyond the acetabulum (extrusion and subluxation). The neck of the femur is widened.

Complications
Degenerative arthritis of the hip develops early when the head of the femur is deformed.

Management
The patient should be referred to a specialist.
1. **Goals** of treatment are:
   a. **Reduce** soft tissue **inflammation** (during synovitis).
   b. **Increase ROM** of the hip joint and strength of muscles necessary for walking.
   c. Develop **femoral head** which is **spherical and congruous.**
2. **Medications. Analgesics** and **NSAIDs** are given for pain and muscle spasm.
3. **Ancillary**
   a. **Bedrest** and **traction** are prescribed during the stage of synovitis.
   b. A **brace** is prescribed for maintaining the femoral head in contact with the acetabulum so that it develops into a congruous, spherical shape. This is achieved by abduction and internal rotation of the hip joint. Many varieties of braces are used for this condition.
   c. **Physical therapy** is necessary for **increasing ROM** of the hip and **gait training** with brace and after the operation. Strength of muscles, e.g., quadriceps and gluteals, can be increased by isometric exercises. Therapy in a swimming pool can also attain similar results.
4. **Surgical** procedures are carried out to maintain the head of the femur within the acetabulum. Operation may be indicated in patients over age 6 years with severe involvement. Subtrochanteric or innominate **osteotomy** is usually performed.

AVASCULAR NECROSIS OF THE FEMORAL HEAD

Avascular necrosis, or **osteonecrosis,** of the femoral head is a pathologic process similar to Perthes' disease. However, avascular necrosis occurs in the adult after the epiphysis for the femoral head has joined the metaphysis.

Anatomy

The blood supply to the adult femoral head comes mainly from the capsular vessels. The capsule of the hip joint is attached (*see* Fig. 18–11B) anteriorly along the intertrochanteric line. It is attached to the posterior aspect of the femoral neck slightly proximal to the intertrochanteric crest. The blood vessels to the head of the femur penetrate the capsule and course along the neck of the femur (*see* Fig. 18–12). In dislocations of the hip or fracture of the femoral neck proximal to the attachment of the capsule, the blood supply to the head can be cut off.

Etiology

1. **Trauma.** Fracture of the neck of the femur or dislocation of the hip disrupts the blood supply along the capsule, especially along the posterior surface. Chances of avascular necrosis are greater if the fracture line is close to the articular surface.
2. **Idiopathic.** Many theories have been proposed to explain the interruption of blood supply:
   a. **Increased intraosseous pressure** results in decreased venous return, exudation of fluid, and further increase in pressure. This forms the basis for the operation of coring to decompress the bone marrow in treatment of this condition.
   b. **Fat embolism**—Avascular necrosis is associated with disorders of fat metabolism, and fat embolism may play some part in cutting off the blood supply.
   c. **Cytotoxicity**—e.g., in patients with history of **alcohol** abuse or treatment with **corticosteroid** preparations.
   d. Avascular necrosis may be associated with other conditions, e.g., sickle cell disease, caisson disease, gout, or Gaucher's disease.

Pathology

In avascular necrosis due to fracture, the portion of the head and neck proximal to the fracture becomes necrotic. In the idiopathic variety, a wedge-shaped area of the head loses its blood supply. The cellular elements in this region die. The **necrotic area** appears more dense on x-rays than the normal. It is usually located in the anterior and superior weight-bearing region of the head. The necrotic tissue is gradually replaced by a process called **creeping substitution.** A subchondral fracture followed by articular cartilage collapse ultimately leads to deformity of the head. The result of all these processes may be early degenerative arthritis of the hip joint. Pathologic stages and x-ray appearances are similar to those in Perthes' disease.

History

This condition usually affects males aged 30–60 years. Pain in the groin aggravated by weight-bearing is a common complaint. The onset of pain may be sudden and severe. History of injury, treatment with corticosteroid preparations, renal transplantation, or sickle cell disease may suggest the diagnosis.

Physical Examination

1. **Inspection.** The patient presents with **antalgic gait** with minimum time spent weight-bearing on the affected side.
2. **Range of motion. Active** and **passive** movements may be limited because of pain and muscle spasm.

Complication
Early degenerative arthritis is a common complication.

Differential Diagnosis
1. **Degenerative arthritis.** Plain x-rays help to distinguish between these two conditions.
2. **Stress fracture** of the femoral neck. The clinical presentation may be similar, and x-rays are negative in both conditions during the early stages (6–8 weeks). Technetium bone scan and **MRI** are helpful in early stages.

Investigations
1. **Plain x-rays** do not show changes for a few weeks. Pathologic and x-ray changes are similar to those in Perthes' disease.
2. Technetium **bone scan** shows decreased uptake in the affected area.
3. **MRI** may replace bone scanning as an investigation of choice during early stages.
4. **Pressure** within the marrow of the neck of femur is increased.
5. Intraosseous **venography** may show abnormal patterns.

Management
Medications and ancillary treatments, including NSAIDs, physical therapy, and non-weight-bearing walking, have *not* been successful in preventing deformity of head of the femur. **Surgical** modalities include:
1. **Decompression.** A core of bone, from the cortex of the femur to the necrotic region in the head, is removed. This operation is done before the collapse of the articular cartilage or subchondral fracture occurs and is supposed to prevent further progression of the disease.
2. Intertrochanteric or subtrochanteric **osteotomy** to change the weight-bearing area of the femoral head is done.
3. **Hemiarthroplasty** replaces the deformed head of the femur.
4. **Total hip replacement arthroplasty** is carried out when degenerative arthritis affects both the femoral head and acetabulum.

Bibliography

1. Busch MT: Slipped capital femoral epiphysis. Orthop Clin 18:637–647, 1987.
2. Ege Rasmussen K-J, Fanø N: Trochanteric bursitis: Treatment by corticosteroid injection. Scand J Rheumatol 14:417–420, 1985.
3. Hensinger RN: Congenital dislocation of the hip. Clin Symp 31(1):3–31, 1979.
4. Hensinger RN: Congenital dislocation of the hip. Orthop Clin North Am 18:597–616, 1987.
5. Herring JA: The treatment of Legg-Calvé-Perthes disease: A critical review of the literature. J Bone Joint Surg 76-A:448–458, 1994.
6. Landin LA, Danielsson LG, Wattsgard C: Transient synovitis of the hip. J Bone Joint Surg 69-B:238–242, 1987.
7. Larsen E, Johansen J: Snapping hip. Acta Orthop Scand 57:168–170, 1986.
8. Schapira D, Nahir M, Scharf Y: Trochanteric bursitis: A common clinical problem. Arch Phys Med Rehabil 67: 815–817, 1986.
9. Staheli LT, Coleman SS, Hensinger RN, et al: Congenital hip dysplasia. Instr Course Lect 33:350–363, 1984.
10. Thompson GH, Salter RB: Legg-Calve-Perthes disease. Ciba Clin Symp 38(1):2–31, 1986.

19

Knee

Arun J. Mehta, M.B., F.R.C.P.C.

The knee is the largest and most complicated synovial joint in the body. The joint surface, ligaments, and muscles are placed under tremendous stress during walking, squatting, running, and other activities. Problems such as injury, internal derangement, or degenerative arthritis commonly bring patients to a physician's office.

Differential Diagnosis

Pain
Pain in the knee may be diffuse or localized.
1. Pain in **front** of the knee may be due to:
   a. **Chondromalacia patellae.** Retropatellar pain that is aggravated by walking, running, or climbing stairs suggests chondromalacia patellae. The undersurface of the patella is tender, and the patient complains of pain on compression of the patella on femur.
   b. **Meniscus** (anterior horn) **tear.** Tenderness over the anterior joint line and a positive McMurray's test suggest tear of the anterior horn of a meniscus.
   c. **Prepatellar bursitis.** There is tender swelling over the patella.
   d. **Infrapatellar bursitis.** Tender swelling is located over the patellar tendon.
2. Pain over **medial side** of the knee may be due to:
   a. **Medial meniscus tear.** Symptoms may start after an episode of twisting injury. The patient complains of pain over the medial side of knee, effusion, and locking of the knee joint. Later, it becomes chronic and recurrent.
   b. **Degenerative arthritis.** The patient complains of pain over the joint line with some tenderness and small effusion. The pain is aggravated by weight-bearing activities. There may be some crepitus on movement. Plain x-rays show narrowing of the affected joint compartment with osteophytes.
   c. **Tibial collateral ligament injury** occurs when the tibia suffers a valgus and/or rotatory strain. There is pain and tenderness over the ligament. In complete tears, there is excessive lateral angulation of the tibia on femur.
3. Pain over **lateral side** of the knee may be due to:
   a. **Lateral meniscus tear** is not as common as the medial tear, and the symptoms are not as well-defined.
   b. **Degenerative arthritis** of the lateral compartment. The patient has pain over the lateral joint line, especially on weight-bearing. There may be a small effusion in the

joint and some crepitus on movement. Plain x-rays show narrowing of the affected joint compartment with osteophytes.

4. **Diffuse pain** in the knee may be due to:
   a. **Effusion** in the joint. Any acute, large swelling gives rise to diffuse pain. This may be due to inflammatory arthritis, hemarthrosis, or infection of the joint.
   b. **Degenerative arthritis.** When it affects both compartments of the knee joint, diffuse pain will result.

Swelling

1. **Localized** swelling is usually due to bursitis or a cyst in relation to a meniscus.
   a. Swelling in **anterior region** may be in relation to:
      i. **Suprapatellar bursa** is situated proximal to the patella and communicates with the main joint cavity.
      ii. **Prepatellar bursa** lies between the skin and patella.
      iii. **Infrapatellar bursa.** There are two infrapatellar bursae, a superficial one between the skin and patellar tendon and the deep bursa under the patellar tendon (*see* Fig. 19–2).
   b. **Lateral** or **medial** swelling
      i. **Cyst** in connection with a meniscus occurs more often with the lateral meniscus. A visible and/or palpable swelling is present, but this may be asymptomatic.
   c. **Posterior** swelling
      i. **Baker's cyst** is associated with degenerative arthritis of the knee.
2. **Diffuse** swelling is usually due to effusion in the joint. The swelling is noticeable at the sides of the patellar tendon, at the sides of the patella, or in the suprapatellar region.

Buckling

The knee **gives out,** or buckles, when the patient is walking, causing the patient to fall. This symptom may be due to weakness of the quadriceps, sudden pain, meniscus tear, subluxation of patella, or loose body.

Locking

The patient may complain of **locking** of the knee when suddenly he or she is not able to move the joint. It is usually accompanied by pain. This complaint may be a symptom of torn meniscus or due to a loose body in the joint.

Table 19–1 lists common knee problems according to the stage in life at which they occur.

Anatomy

The femoral condyles articulate with the tibial condyles and patella to form the knee joint. The fibula does not participate. The knee joint is a **modified hinge joint**. The large,

Table 19–1 Common Knee Problems According to Age

Children and adolescents	Apophysitis of the tibial tubercle
	Osteochondritis dissecans
	Chondromalacia patellae
Adolescents and young adults	Meniscus tear
	Sports-related injuries
	Ligamentous injuries
	Patellar problems
Adults >45 years old	Degenerative arthritis
	Degenerative meniscal tears

rounded femoral condyles glide and rotate on flat tibial plateaus. The patella glides in the groove between the femoral condyles. The long axis of the tibia is verticle to the ground, and both knees almost touch each other when we are standing. However, the femora are inclined about 10° away from the verticle to accommodate the pelvis. Because the female pelvis is wider, the femora are inclined more in females than in males. This angle between the axis of femur and tibia is called the physiologic valgus.

The fibrous **capsule** of the knee joint is attached at the articular margins of the femur and tibia. It is loose enough to allow flexion and extension movements. Anteriorly, the capsule is strengthened by the quadriceps tendon, patella, and patellar tendon (ligamentum patellae). On either side of the knee joint are tibial and fibular **collateral ligaments** to provide extra support. On the medial side, the thickened portion of the capsule is called the **tibial collateral ligament**. It is attached to the medial meniscus and restricts its mobility. The **fibular collateral ligament** is separate from the capsule.

Stability of the knee joint depends on the ligaments, capsule, and muscles and not on the shape of the bones. There are two important intra-articular ligaments within the fibrous capsule, i.e., anterior and posterior cruciate ligaments. These ligaments, when damaged, may lead to instability of the joint. The **anterior cruciate** is attached to the anterior portion of the intercondylar region of the tibia (*see* Fig. 19–6) and to the medial aspect of the lateral femoral condyle. It prevents the tibia from sliding anteriorly on the femur. The **posterior cruciate** is attached to the posterior part of the intercondylar region of tibia and goes anteriorly to the lateral aspect of the medial femoral condyle. It is the strongest ligament in the knee. It prevents the tibia from sliding backward on the femur and the knee from hyperextending. The posterior cruciate remains tight throughout the range of knee movements.

The **synovial membrane** lines the fibrous capsule and defines the cavity of the knee joint. Under normal conditions, there is very small amount of joint fluid, but large quantities of fluid can accumulate after injury, inflammation, or infection of the joint. There are two intra-articular semilunar cartilages, called the medial and lateral **menisci.** They are made up of fibrocartilage and fill some space between the femoral and tibial condyles. The menisci make the articular surfaces more congruous and are important in transferring weight from the femur to tibia. They are attached at their periphery to the margins of tibial condyles. Only the peripheral part of the menisci is supplied by blood vessels. Nutrition to the inner part of the meniscus is obtained from the synovial fluid.

There are many **bursae** around the knee joint. Some communicate with the main joint cavity, while others are isolated. These bursae facilitate movements of muscles and tendons. The **suprapatellar bursa** is an extension of the main joint cavity under the quadriceps tendon (*see* Fig. 19–2). It extends for 5–7 cm proximal to the upper border of the patella. When there is a moderate to large effusion in the joint, a swelling may be visible above the patella. This bursa then becomes palpable and fluid can be aspirated from it.

The **quadriceps muscle** is the main **extensor** of the knee joint and the most important muscle required in stabilization of the joint. Patients with quadriceps weakness walk with the knee in hyperextension, and getting up from a sitting position and going up and down stairs are very difficult. The quadriceps tendon has a large sesamoid bone called the patella. The patellar tendon is the continuation of the quadriceps tendon from the lower border of the patella to its insertion in the tibial tubercle. It is a broad and strong structure, and the central part of it can be used for reconstruction of other ligaments, such as the cruciate. The **hamstring muscles** in the back of the thigh are the main **flexors** of the knee.

The main movements taking place in the knee joint are **flexion** and **extension.** However, some **rotation** of the tibia on the femur is possible. The rotation cannot take place when the knee joint is fully extended because the ligaments are tight. The tibia rotates laterally during the last few degrees of extension and gets locked in full extension. Slight rotation of the tibia on the femur is possible after 20° of flexion. The flexion-extention movement is a complex movement involving gliding and rotation of the femoral condyles on the tibia.

History

The onset, duration, and progression of each symptom are queried. If it was related to any sports or other **injury,** details of the mechanism of injury, type of sport, and other are obtained. It is important to remember that **pain** in the knee may be **referred** from the hip joint. The hip joint should be examined in all cases of knee pain. Pain in the knee joint may be felt only during certain movements or activities, such as climbing stairs. Does the knee get **locked** in some position and prevent the patient from extending or flexing the joint? Does the knee feel **unstable?** It may give out at times because of sudden pain or weakness of the quadriceps muscle.

Physical Examination

1. **Inspection.** The inspection begins when the patient walks into the office. Observe the gait and how the patient sits down in a chair. Both lower extremities and lower back should be exposed for inspection of the knee. The knee is inspected in standing, sitting, and lying positions (**static**) and while walking (**dynamic**). Examination is carried out from the front, sides, and back. The two sides are compared for any differences. The tibiae are nearly parallel to each other and verticle when a person is standing (**alignment**). The knee joints touch each other. The femurs, however, are at an angle to accommodate the pelvis. Since the female pelvis is wider, the femurs are more inclined away from the verticle. **Deformities** like genu varum and genu valgum can be noticed from the front, whereas genu recurvatum is better observed from the side.

   The skin around the knee joint is inspected for any **bruise, abrasions, laceration,** or swelling. External signs of injury give a clue as to the mechanism of injury and internal structures damaged. A bruise over the lateral aspect of the knee after a car-pedestrian accident may suggest a tibial collateral ligament injury. Generalized **swelling** may be due to effusion in the joint. When there is a large effusion, the swelling is very obvious. A small amount of fluid in the joint obliterates the hollows on the sides of the patellar tendon. A localized swelling may be due to a bursa or a cyst in relation to a meniscus. The quadriceps **muscle atrophies** quickly when there is knee joint pathology, and it is more apparent in the lower thigh.

   Dynamic observation is done while the patient is walking. At heel strike, the knee is fully extended. It is slightly flexed during the stance phase. More flexion occurs in the late stance phase and early swing phase. The knee begins to extend in the late swing phase and terminates in full extension at the heel strike. The weight-bearing (stance phase) time on a painful extremity is cut down to reduce pain (**antalgic** gait). A stiff knee forces the patient to circumduct the leg and plantar flex the opposite foot more so that the affected extremity can clear the ground.

2. **Palpation.** An increase in **temperature** of the skin overlying the joint should be looked for before other tests are performed. Localized **tenderness** is helpful in pinpointing the pathology. **Anteriorly,** the suprapatellar pouch, superficial and deep surfaces of the patella, patellar tendon, tibial tubercle, and sites of prepatellar and infrapatellar bursae

should be palpated. This can be done with the knee fully extended and relaxed. The edge of the suprapatellar pouch can be rolled between the examining finger and the femur when it is thickened because of chronic inflammation. In a small effusion, the fluid can be squeezed from the suprapatellar pouch into the main joint cavity, and the hollows on the side of the patella are seen to fill up.

The subcutaneous surface of the **patella** is readily accessible for palpation. A prepatellar bursa may form between the skin and the bone. The undersurface of the patella can be palpated by displacing the patella medially and laterally when the quadriceps is relaxed. This may be tender in chondromalacia patellae. In recurrent dislocation of the patella, the patient may feel very apprehensive when the examiner tries to displace the patella laterally. The **patellar tendon** is the continuation of the quadriceps tendon from the lower pole of the patella to the tibial tubercle. This structure is easily palpable. The superficial bursa lies between the skin and tendon and the deep bursa is deep to the tendon (*see* Fig. 19–2).

The femoral condyles, collateral ligaments, joint line, and tibial condyles are palpated on the **sides.** The **femoral condyles** are easily palpable on both sides. The fibular and tibial **collateral ligaments** should be palpated for tenderness. The **joint line** is palpated with the knee flexed to 90°. The gap between the tibial and femoral condyles is easily felt anteriorly on either side of the patellar tendon. Tenderness along the joint line may indicate a problem with the meniscus, degenerative arthritis, or inflammation of the knee joint. The medial **tibial condyle** and anterior part of the lateral are accessible to palpation.

The **anserine bursa** is deep to the tendons inserting over the medial tibial condyle. The knee joint is covered by muscles and tendons over the **posterior** side and is not easily accessible. A synovial cyst (Baker's cyst) arising from the posterior aspect is sometimes palpable. The posterior structures can be palpated more easily after the knee is flexed.

3. **Range of motion.** Neutral position (0°) for the knee joint occurs when the femur and tibia are in the same coronal plane (Fig. 19–1). Normal range of flexion is about 135°. In full flexion of the knee, the heel touches the buttock.

  a. **Active.** A quick test for active ROM of the knee can be performed by asking the patient to squat from the standing position and get up. This may be difficult for elderly patients. This maneuver measures the ROM and strength of important muscle groups. The **quadriceps** is the most important muscle, and its strength is essential for walking, getting up from a sitting position, and going up and down the stairs. The patient, sitting on the examination couch with legs dangling over the edge, is asked to extend the knee against gravity. If there is significant weakness of the quadriceps, the patient may have trouble completing the last 10–20° of extension. This is called **quadriceps lag** or extension lag. It is important to correct this defect by quadriceps-strengthening exercises before the patient is allowed to walk without any walking aids.

  b. **Passive** movements are carried out when the patient is not able to perform full range of active movements. Flexion is tested with the patient lying prone. The leg is held just proximal to the ankle, and the knee is bent. There is about 10° of lateral and medial rotation of the tibia on femur when the knee is flexed >20°.

4. **Special Tests**

  a. **Effusion** in the joint. For small effusion, slide one hand over the suprapatellar bursa and squeeze fluid into the main joint cavity. The hollows on the sides of the patella and patellar tendons may fill up with fluid. Keep pressure on the suprapatellar bursa, and perform patellar tap and fluctuation tests.

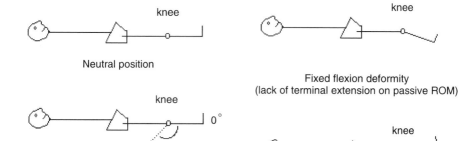

Neutral position

Fixed flexion deformity
(lack of terminal extension on passive ROM)

0°

135°

Normal range of flexion - extension 0° to 135°   Hyperextension (extension beyond neutral position)

Fig. 19–1   Examination of range of movements of the knee.

  i. **Patellar tap.** With two fingers, try to push the patella toward the femoral condyles. If there is fluid between the patella and the condyles, you will feel the patella hitting the femoral condyles.
  ii. **Fluctuation.** With one hand on the suprapatellar bursa, place the thumb of the other hand on one side and the index and middle fingers on the other side of the patella. Pressure by two fingers will push joint fluid and raise the thumb on the other side of the joint if there is fluid in the joint.
b. Measurement of **girth.**
  i. For effusion in the joint, the girth is measured about 2 cm proximal to the superior border of the patella, at the level of the suprapatellar bursa.
  ii. For quadriceps wasting, it is measured 10 cm proximal to the superior border of the patella and compared to the opposite side. It should be measured at the same level on both sides so that the girth can be compared for followup visits.
c. **Leg lengths** are measured to see if there is any discrepancy between the two sides.
d. Tests for **meniscus tear.**
  i. **McMurray's test** is performed with the patient lying on his back and the hips and knees flexed. The palm of one hand is on the front of the knee, and the other hand holds the heel. The leg is internally and externally rotated and then slowly extended with the leg in valgus and external rotation. Some examiners rotate the leg at various points during extension of the knee. A click may be heard or palpated over the medial or lateral joint line if the meniscus is torn.
  ii. **Steinmann test** is carried out with the patient sitting in front of the examiner with knees flexed to 90°. The examiner holds the leg as in McMurray's test. The leg is rotated while it is slowly extended. Pain or palpable click suggests meniscus tear or collateral ligament injury.
  iii. **Grind test** or **Apley test.** While the patient lies on his stomach, the knee is flexed to 90° and the heel is pressed down and rotated. This compresses the articular surfaces of the femoral and tibial condyles together and grinds the menisci. This maneuver is painful if the meniscus is torn or if there is degenerative arthritis of the knee joint.
e. **Pivot shift test** is positive in anterior cruciate ligament tear or tear of the posterior horn of the lateral meniscus. The patient is supine with the hip flexed 30° and knee 70°. The tibia is rotated internally and slowly extended with valgus stress. The lateral

condyle of the tibia subluxates anteriorly with a clunk when the knee comes up to 20–30° of flexion.

f. **Drawer sign.** The patient lies on the back with the hips and knees flexed and feet flat on the couch. The examiner holds the upper part of the leg with both hands and fixes the ankle with his or her elbow. The examiner pulls the patient's upper leg forward to test the anterior cruciate ligament and pushes it away to test for the posterior cruciate. The amount of movement of the tibia is compared with that in the normal leg.

g. **Lachman's test.** The drawer test is carried out with the knee flexed up to 20°.

h. Stress test for **collateral ligaments** is performed with the patient sitting at the edge of the examining table with legs dangling. The examiner sits facing the patient. One hand stabilizes the patient's thigh and knee, and the other holds the distal part of the leg. Varus or valgus stress is applied to the leg with the knee in full extension and 20° of flexion. The patient will complain of pain if there is partial tear of a collateral ligament, or there will be excessive movement in the direction of the stress if there is complete tear.

i. **Neurologic** examination

   i. **Sensation.** A branch of the femoral nerve supplies the front of the thigh. The lateral aspect of the thigh is supplied by the lateral cutaneous nerve of the thigh. The saphenous nerve innervates the medial aspect of the knee and leg and may be damaged in operations on the medial meniscus or tibial collateral ligament.

   ii. **Muscle strength** of the quadriceps (L3,4) and hamstrings (L5, S1) is tested.

   iii. **Knee reflex** is affected in femoral nerve or lumbar 3 or 4 nerve root involvement.

j. General **anesthesia** may be necessary for proper examination of the knee joint if the patient has a lot of pain and muscle spasm.

Investigations

1. **Plain x-rays.** Usually anteroposterior (AP) and lateral views are done. They are useful in diagnosis of degenerative arthritis, bony injuries, loose body, and chondrocalcinosis. In inflammatory arthritis, they are helpful in determining the extent of involvement of the bone, i.e., osteoporosis, bone cysts, joint space. In patients with patellar subluxation or dislocation, special views are ordered for evaluation of the patellofemoral joint (**sunrise** or **skyline** view). It helps in examination of the patellofemoral joint, its alignment, and shape of the femoral condyles. The **tunnel view** is useful when the history suggests a loose body in the knee joint. It shows the intercondylar area of the femur. **Weight-bearing** AP view helps in determining the joint space and hence the thickness of the articular cartilage. It is also helpful in assessment of deformity and instability of the knee. **Stress x-rays** are done if rupture of the collateral ligament is suspected.

2. **Aspiration** of joint fluid is done to rule out hemarthrosis, infection, or crystal-induced or inflammatory arthritis. It is especially useful in diagnosis and treatment of crystal-induced arthritis and infections.

3. **MRI** is useful in meniscus tears, ligament injuries, and osteochondritis dissecans. The need for invasive procedures such as arthrography is reduced considerably because MRI can provide much useful information.

4. **CT scan** is performed in complicated fractures around the knee.

5. **Arthrography.** The technique and interpretation of arthrography are very important in getting reliable results. In the hands of an expert, arthrography is useful for diagnosis of meniscus tears, anterior cruciate ligament tears, loose bodies, and osteochondral defects.

6. **Arthroscopy** is becoming increasingly popular and sophisticated. Meniscal and cruciate ligament tears can be diagnosed and repaired through an arthroscope. It also helps in diagnosis of difficult problems and for removing loose bodies.

Management

The following principles of conservative management are common to many knee conditions:

1. **Rest** in bed with the leg elevated on a pillow is provided initially for many traumatic and inflammatory disorders. Depending on the condition, an **elastic bandage** or **cast** helps in controlling swelling and allowing injured tissues to heal. The patient is gradually allowed to start walking non-weight-bearing, progressing to partial weight and then full weight-bearing with appropriate walking aids.

2. During the first 24–48 hours, **cold packs** are applied to the injured part to minimize swelling. Later, **hot packs** may be used before exercise to reduce pain.

3. Quadriceps muscle is very important for protecting the knee from further injury during walking, stair climbing, and other activities. **Isometric quadriceps exercises** should be started as soon as possible. These exercises should be taught before all elective knee operations and are resumed postoperatively as soon as the patient comes out of anesthetic. Later **ROM exercises** and exercises to strengthen quadriceps with weights or resistance are added.

4. A **brace** may be required to protect the knee if the knee joint is unstable or muscles are weak.

BURSITIS

Numerous bursae are found around the knee joint (Fig. 19–2). Inflammation in the anterior bursae is more common than in the posterior bursae. The patient may present with painful swelling and some limitation of function.

Anatomy

The **prepatellar** bursa is between the skin and the patella. There are two kinds of **infrapatellar** bursae. One is superficial to the patellar tendon, and the other is deep to it. The **suprapatellar** bursa is actually a synovial pouch that extends proximal to the patella and

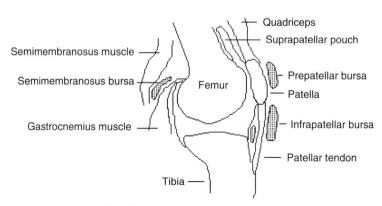

Fig. 19–2   Bursae around the knee joint.

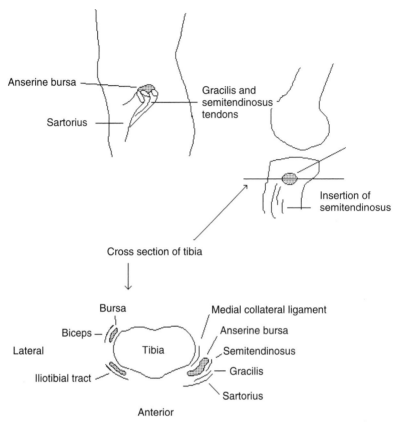

Fig. 19–3   Anatomy of anserine bursa.

under the quadriceps tendon. It is an extension of the cavity of the knee joint. The tendons of sartorius, gracilis, and semitendinosus insert in the medial condyle of the proximal tibia. The **anserine bursa** is between the bone and these tendons (Fig. 19–3).

Etiology
Chronic irritation by pressure or overactivity is the common cause for inflammation of a bursa around the knee. The prepatellar bursa is compressed between the hard floor and patella in activities involving kneeling, e.g., scrubbing floors. Bursitis of the prepatellar bursa was common in maids and was called **housemaid's knee.** The inflammation of the superficial infrapatellar bursa is called **clergyman's** or **carpet-layer's knee.**
   Infection of a bursa is the other cause of pain and swelling related to a bursa.

History
The patient presents with a **painful swelling.** He or she may have trouble bending the knee and kneeling. Walking and running may be difficult depending on the bursa involved.

Physical Examination
1. **Inspection.** A swelling is obvious in the prepatellar and superficial infrapatellar bursae. When other bursae are involved, the swelling may not be visible.
2. **Palpation.** Localized tenderness over the swelling is common when it is inflamed.
3. **Range of motion.** Active and passive ROM of the knee may be painful.

Differential Diagnosis
1. **Cellulitis** is not confined to the anatomic boundary of any bursa.
2. Infection or inflammation of the joint cavity (**septic arthritis**) results in effusion in the joint which gives rise to a much larger swelling.

Investigations
The fluid in the bursal sac can be aspirated to rule out infection.

Management
The activity that initiated the inflammation or aggravates the pain should be avoided. The fluid is aspirated, and a pressure bandage is applied. If there is no evidence of infection, a steroid preparation may be injected to reduce inflammation. Incision and drainage may be necessary for infection. A chronic bursa that has failed to resolve may need to be excised.

MENISCUS TEAR

Injuries to the medial and lateral menisci (also called **semilunar cartilages**) are a common problem in active young people involved in sports. These intra-articular semilunar fibrocartilaginous disks were at one time thought to be without any definite function. The whole meniscus was removed for a tear. However, it was found later that this approach may lead to early degenerative arthritis. Now, most surgeons prefer a more conservative approach and either repair the tear or try to remove only the torn part of cartilage.

Anatomy
The knee joint has two intra-articular fibrocartilaginous disks, called the medial and lateral menisci. These disks are shaped like a partial moon, and hence their name, semilunar. They cover the periphery of the tibial condyles and deepen the articular surface. Both are attached along their periphery to the tibial condyles. The medial meniscus is also attached to the capsule of the joint and the tibial collateral ligament. Because of this, it is less mobile and more vulnerable to injuries. The medial meniscus is torn twice as often as the lateral. The lateral meniscus, on the other hand, is not attached to the capsule or the fibular collateral ligament. The undersurface of the menisci is flat and conforms to the articular surface of the condyles of tibia. The femoral side of the menisci is curved to form a wedge between the tibial and femoral condyles (Fig. 19–4). A part of the body weight is transmitted through the menisci, and they act as shock absorbers. The thicker peripheral part is supplied by blood vessels, but the thinner central part is avascular and derives its nutrition from the synovial fluid. Tears in the vascular part have a better chance of healing.

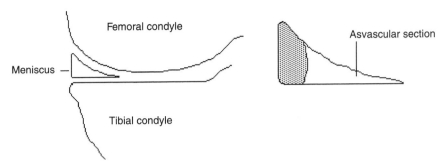

Fig. 19–4 The meniscus is situated between the femoral and tibial condyles. It is triangular in cross-section, with blood supply only to the lateral one-third. The medial two-thirds is avascular.

Medial Meniscus

Mechanism of Injury

The medial meniscus may get caught between the femoral and tibial condyles when the knee is flexed and the femur rotates forcefully on the tibia. This occurs when the foot is firmly planted on the ground and the person twists the body (Fig. 19–5). The peripheral attachment of the medial meniscus to the joint capsule and tibia is severed. This allows it to migrate within the joint and between the femoral and tibial condyles. The result is a torn meniscus. The tibial collateral ligament may also be torn at the same time. The anterior part of the meniscus is injured when the knee is flexed slightly and the posterior part injured when the knee is in full flexion.

Pathology

Most tears secondary to **trauma** are longitudinal. When the tear is extensive, the central part may be displaced toward the intercondylar region. These extensive longitudinal tears are also described as "bucket handle" tears. When a part of the cartilage gets caught be-

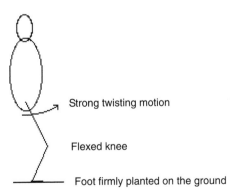

Fig. 19–5 A strong twisting motion of the body with the knee flexed and feet firmly planted on the ground is the common mechanism of injury to the meniscus.

tween the femoral and tibial condyles, the patient is not able to flex or extend the knee, and the knee is said to be "locked."

Degenerative changes in the menisci are very common in people over 40 years of age. Fissures, fibrillation, and transverse tears may occur without any history of injury. After the cartilage is removed by the surgeon, a new one is formed. The reformed cartilage is not as elastic as the original. The swelling that occurs after an injury is due to **effusion** in the joint. Effusion is a reaction of the synovial membrane to injury. Hemarthrosis occurs if there is associated injury to a ligament or synovial membrane. Injury to ligaments like the tibial collateral and posterior cruciate may occur with the tear of the medial meniscus.

History
The details of how the initial injury occurred should be obtained. Information on the type of sport, position of the lower extremity, and movement of the body helps in determining the structures that may be injured. Some patients hear or feel a **snap** or tearing sensation in the knee and develop severe **pain.** He or she is not able to walk on the affected leg. The pain is felt over the medial aspect of the knee joint. **Swelling** develops in few hours. The pain and swelling may subside within a week or two without treatment.

Later, the patient may give a history of recurrent episodes of **locking** of the knee in flexion, pain, and swelling of the joint. These episodes are brought on by activity similar to that precipitating the first episode or something much less strenuous, e.g., walking. The patient is not able to flex or extend the knee from a "locked" position. The patient may complain of the knee giving-way or buckling (**instability**) while walking. This may be due to sudden pain, quadriceps weakness, or a torn cruciate ligament.

Physical Examination
1. **Inspection.** Observation of the knee may show obliteration of the hollows on the sides of the patellar tendon or swelling in the suprapatellar area because of **effusion. Wasting** of the quadriceps muscle may be visible in the thigh.
2. **Palpation** along the joint line elicits **tenderness.** The tenderness is more anterior if the anterior horn of the meniscus is affected. The posterior joint line is not easily accessible to palpation. If the tibial collateral ligament is sprained, tenderness may be anywhere from the medial femoral condyle to the medial tibial condyle.
3. **Range of motion.** All active and passive movements are restricted when the patient visits during an episode of locking. The patient may complain of pain during the terminal few degrees of extension if the anterior horn of the meniscus is involved or during last few degrees of flexion if the posterior horn is torn.
4. **Special tests** are performed as described at the beginning of this chapter.
   a. **Patellar tap** and **fluctuation** are positive when there is effusion in the knee joint.
   b. During **McMurray's test,** movement of the cartilage may be felt by the fingers over the joint line. The patient experiences some pain, too.
   c. **Compression** and **distraction tests** of Apley's may be positive.

Differential Diagnoses
1. **Rupture of the tibial collateral ligament** can occur with a torn medial meniscus or as an isolated injury. In partial rupture, tenderness extends vertically along the ligament beyond the joint line. In complete rupture, there is excessive valgus of the leg when the thigh is fixed and valgus strain is applied to the leg. Rupture of the posterior cruciate, tibial collateral ligament, and medial meniscus may occur in the same patient after a severe injury.

2. **Loose body** in the joint can present with locking of the knee, effusion, and pain. Usually, physical examination is negative in patients with a loose body. Plain x-rays are useful in diagnosis.
3. **Degenerative joint disease** may present with pain, tenderness over joint line, and crepitus on movement. There is no history of locking. The pain is worse on getting up in the morning and at the end of the day. Plain x-rays are useful in confirming degenerative joint disease.
4. **Pes anserine bursitis** presents with pain and tenderness over the medial aspect of the proximal tibia at the level of tibial tubercle.

Investigations
1. **MRI** is a very useful, reliable, noninvasive test for lesions of the meniscus. Its sensitivity and specificity are >90%. The information provided is helpful in selecting the operative procedure.
2. **Arthroscopy** is useful in cases where diagnosis is difficult. Operations for meniscus repair can be carried out through the arthroscope.
3. **Arthrography.** Injection of radio-opaque dye in the joint was performed more often before MRI and arthroscopy became available.

Course
Chronic meniscus tear with recurrent attacks of pain, locking, and swelling can lead to early onset of degenerative arthritis.

Management
If the knee joint is locked, it should be reduced within 24 hours. Sometimes, the joint unlocks itself with bedrest. If it does not, the joint should be manipulated. Conservative measures, as mentioned at the beginning of this chapter, are followed. The decision to operate depends on the patient's age, type of tear (bucket handle or horizontal), mechanism of injury, associated ligament injuries, duration and severity of symptoms, and functional impairment.
Goals of treatment are:
  1. Reduce knee joint if it is locked.
  2. Control swelling and pain.
  3. Maintain ROM.
  4. Increase muscle strength, especially of quadriceps.
  5. Return to normal activities.
1. **Medications** are prescribed mainly to control pain.
2. **Ancillary**. Ice packs, skin traction, aspiration (if there is a large effusion), and compression bandage are prescribed as an iniital treatment. Isometric quadriceps exercises are started as soon as possible. Gentle passive ROM exercises and walking with appropriate aids, non-weight-bearing on the affected side, are added later. The program of exercises is increased from active ROM, to gradually increasing weight-bearing, and finally to exercises against resistance. Special exercises to achieve specific skills required in the individual patient's sports or occupation are then prescribed. If at any time pain and swelling recur, the new activity or exercise is curtailed.
3. **Surgical.** Operation is recommended when there is a history of locking, recurrent episodes of pain, effusion, and instability or after conservative measures have failed. Significant numbers of patients develop degenerative arthritis after removal of the whole meniscus (**total meniscectomy**). Patients with problems secondary to a degen-

erated meniscus should be treated conservatively, because long-term follow-up results after operation are not as good as those for traumatic tears.

Surgical options include:
a. Repair of meniscus
b. Partial meniscectomy
c. Total meniscectomy

Lateral Meniscus
The lateral meniscus is smaller than the medial and is not attached to the fibular collateral ligament. It is more mobile and is not torn as often as the medial meniscus. The symptoms of lateral meniscus tear are vague, and pain is not well-localized, making this injury more difficult to diagnose. Chronic recurrent episodes of medial meniscus tear may ultimately affect the lateral meniscus, too.

Cyst of the Meniscus
Cystic degeneration of the meniscus can present with dull aching pain that is aggravated by activity. It is more common in lateral meniscus. A swelling may be palpable along the joint line. The cyst should be removed by operation if it is symptomatic.

Calcification of the Meniscus
Deposition of calcium in the meniscus is sometimes visible on plain x-rays as a fine line within the joint space. This may be seen in calcium pyrophosphate dihydrate crystal deposition disease.

LIGAMENT INJURIES

Ligaments of the knee joint prevent abnormal or excessive movement. They stabilize the joint in a passive way, whereas muscles do it by active contraction. Injury and laxity of the ligaments make it difficult to perform some activities and lead to early degenerative arthritis.

Anatomy
Two important ligaments on either side of the knee are the **tibial collateral** and **fibular collateral** ligaments (Fig. 19–6). They prevent excessive valgus and varus movements of the knee. The anterior and posterior cruciates are two intra-articular ligaments that also contribute to stabilizing the knee joint. Both of these ligaments are within the fibrous capsule (intra-articular) but are extrasynovial (not bathed by synovial fluid).

Pathology
Injuries to the ligaments are classified into three grades. Grades I and II are partial ruptures, and Grade III is complete rupture. The partial ruptures are treated conservatively, whereas Grade III may require surgical intervention. The ruptured fibers of the ligament heal by scar tissue. After complete rupture, the ligament is not as strong as the original tissue and is usually longer than before the injury. It may not be able to prevent abnormal movements during routine activities, such as walking, or more strenuous activities, such as running or playing football.

History
Swelling immediately after injury suggests hemarthrosis. Injury to the fibrous capsule, synovial membrane, or intra-articular structure (bone or ligament) is the usual cause of blood in the joint cavity.

Investigations
1. **Plain x-rays** help to rule out associated fractures and assess the extent of degenerative changes.
2. **Stress x-rays** are done to diagnose complete rupture of ligaments.
3. **MRI** is a good noninvasive test for diagnosis of ligament injuries.
4. **Arthroscopy** is useful in evaluating intra-articular ligament ruptures and repair of certain varieties of ruptures.

Complications
Chronic instability and **degenerative arthritis** are the common complications following a ligament injury.

Management
The treatment of a ligament injury should be decided after considering the following four points:
1. **Patient's goals.** What would the patient like to achieve after the treatment program is finished? Does he want to go back to playing football? Will he be satisfied with walking around, if necessary with a brace?
2. **Duration of injury.** Acute injuries in young athletes are treated in a very different manner than long-standing injuries. The severity and extent of degenerative changes will dictate the type of management and operation that is best for a patient.
3. **Severity of injury.** If one ligament is ruptured, other structures may be able to compensate, and the patient can be treated conservatively. As more structures are damaged, it becomes difficult for the remaining structures to compensate and provide stability to the joint. **Partial rupture** of one ligament is usually treated conservatively.
4. **Motivation** of the patient is very important in following a rigorous rehabilitation program. The outcome depends very much on the patient's compliance and motivation. Conservative management of an acute injury is similar to that outlined at the beginning of this chapter.

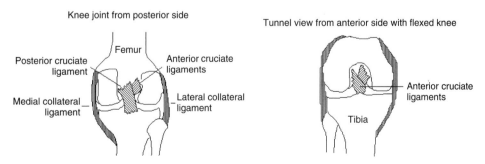

Fig. 19–6 Ligaments of the knee joint.

Tibial Collateral Ligament

The tibial collateral ligament is the most frequently injured ligament of the knee. It may be associated with injuries to the medial meniscus, joint capsule, and anterior cruciate ligament.

Anatomy

The tibial collateral ligament is attached proximally to the medial epicondyle of the femur. Distally, it is inserted into the medial aspect of the tibial condyle at the level of the tibial tubercle about 4–5 cm distal to the joint line. The fibers of the ligament are almost vertical. It prevents the tibia from excessive valgus movement.

Mechanism of Injury

Valgus strain on a flexed and externally rotated tibia is the usual mechanism of injury. This can occur in sports and activities when the body rotates to the opposite side of the leg, which is fixed on the ground. The tibial collateral ligament may also rupture when a car bumper hits against a pedestrian's leg from the lateral side.

Pathology

The ligament may rupture at its femoral or tibial attachment or in the middle. The medial capsule of the joint, medial meniscus, and anterior cruciate ligament may be damaged at the same time. If the medial capsule is torn, blood and synovial fluid accumulate inside the joint cavity.

History

The patient complains of pain over the medial aspect of the knee.

Physical Examination

1. **Inspection.** Abrasions over the lateral aspect and a bruise over the medial aspect of the knee may be present.
2. **Palpation. Tenderness** over the medial femoral condyle is the most common finding.
3. **Range of motion.** All movements are painful during the acute stage. Later, pain is aggravated by valgus stress.
4. **Special tests.** It is important to distinguish between partial and complete rupture of the ligament by **stress tests** and **stress x-rays.** The knee joint does not open up on valgus stress in partial ruptures. The examination may have to be carried out under anesthesia because of pain and muscle spasm. If only the tibial collateral ligament is ruptured, the medial joint space opens up on valgus stress with the knee flexed to 20°. If it opens up with the knee fully extended, then one of the cruciate ligaments is injured, too.

Differential Diagnoses

It may be very difficult to diagnose which structure is damaged and to what extent. All attempts should be made to distinguish between a partial and complete tear and all other associated injuries by investigations mentioned above. The injury may affect the tibial collateral ligament, medial meniscus, medial joint capsule, and anterior or posterior cruciate ligaments.

Management

Partial tears are usually managed conservatively (see the beginning of this chapter). Complete tears are treated according to the patient's expectation of functional outcome, motivation, and severity and duration of injury.

Surgical. Compete tears of the middle of the ligament usually require reconstruction of the ligament.

Fibular Collateral Ligament

Injuries to this ligament are not as common as those to the tibial collateral ligament.

Anatomy

The fibular collateral ligament extends from the lateral femoral condyle to the head of the fibula. It is separate from the fibrous capsule of the joint and is not attached to the lateral meniscus. In addition to the fibular collateral ligament, the knee joint is supported on the lateral side by the fibrous capsule, iliotibial tract, and expansion from the popliteus muscle.

Mechanism of Injury

Since the medial side of the knee joint is protected by the opposite leg, the knee is not forced into varus deformity very often, and the fibular collateral ligament is not damaged as frequently as the tibial collateral.

Pathology and clinical features are similar to those of the tibial collateral ligament, but on the lateral side. On varus stress, the joint opens up on the lateral side.

Management

The principles of management are similar to those for the tibial collateral ligament.

Anterior Cruciate Ligament

Anatomy

The anterior cruciate ligament (ACL) is attached to the anterior part of the intercondylar area of the tibia. Its proximal end is inserted in the medial side of the lateral condyle of the femur. It is directed upward, backward, and laterally. The ACL prevents the tibia from gliding forward on the femur and limits hyperextension and rotation. It is not as strong as the posterior cruciate ligament.

Mechanism of Injury

Isolated injury of the ACL occurs when the proximal end of the tibia is hit from the front and pushed backward. This ligament can also be damaged together with the tibial collateral by a strong rotatory force pushing the tibia into valgus and external rotation.

Pathology

Hemarthrosis is common after cruciate ligament tears because they are intra-articular structures. Usually, the midportion of the ligament is ruptured.

History

The patient complains of pain in the knee joint immediately after injury. He or she has difficulty in walking and develops a swelling soon after. In chronic tears, the patient may complain of the knee "giving way."

Physical Examination

Special tests. The tibial collateral ligament is taut in full extension and prevents anterior slide of the tibia on the femur. It is relaxed in slight flexion of the knee, and that is why the **Lachman's test** is more sensitive than the **anterior drawer test** for rupture of ACL. Abnormal movement on the anterior drawer test with the tibia in external rotation suggests rupture of the ACL, whereas the same finding with the tibia in internal rotation indicates anterior and posterior cruciate ligament tears.

The **pivot shift test** is also positive in ACL tears. The examiner may get a false-negative result if there is a large effusion in the joint or a lot of muscle spasm.

Differential Diagnoses

Injury to the ACL may be accompanied by damage to the tibial collateral ligament, medial meniscus, and medial joint capsule. MRI and arthroscopy may help in determining the extent of the injury.

Management

Isolated ACL tear can be treated conservatively by intensive rehabilitation. If a brace and strong quadriceps do not stabilize the joint, a reconstructive procedure is considered. Surgical repair can be done if the rupture has taken place near its bony attachment. A reconstructive procedure may be required if the ligament is torn in the middle.

Posterior Cruciate Ligament

Anatomy

The posterior cruciate ligament (PCL) is very strong. It arises from posterior part of the intercondylar area of the tibia and inserts in the lateral side of the medial femoral condyle of the femur. It is taut during full range of flexion of the knee and prevents posterior slide of the tibia on the femur. The PCL prevents hyperextension, adduction, and abduction and also limits rotation of the tibia.

Mechanism of Injury

It takes a severe injury to rupture this ligament. The combination of external rotation and valgus or internal rotation and varus stress on a flexed knee is needed to rupture the PCL. This ligament also can be ruptured when a dashboard hits the front of the tibia in car accidents (dashboard injury). Its rupture is usually accompanied by injury to one of the collateral ligaments or anterior cruciate.

Physical Examination

Special tests. The **posterior drawer** test is positive.

Management

Associated injuries, such as meniscus or collateral ligament tears, may require surgical repair. Hemarthrosis should be aspirated. Ice packs, compression bandage, and rest are part of the initial line of treatment. Isometric quadriceps exercises are started as soon as possible. Later, gentle ROM exercises are added. Other measures as mentioned at the beginning of this chapter are carried out. Each patient should be assessed for any instability. A brace, which prevents the type of instability that the patient has, is prescribed.

Surgical. If conservative measures fail and the patient is interested in following vigorous sports activities, surgical reconstruction should be considered.

FRACTURES

Fractures of the Patella

Anatomy
The patella is the largest sesamoid bone in the body and is attached to the quadriceps tendon. It glides in the intercondylar groove of the femur during flexion and extension of the knee. It is subcutaneous and prone to injury.

Mechanism of Injury
1. **Direct trauma**—e.g., the knee hits the dashboard in a car collision, or a blunt object hits the front of the knee.
2. **Indirect trauma**—Very forceful contraction of the quadriceps muscle can fracture a patella.

Classification of Fractures
1. **Comminuted** fracture of the patella usually occurs after direct trauma.
2. **Transverse** fracture occurs after an indirect trauma.

History
The type of injury gives a clue to the type of fracture. There is severe pain and swelling around the front of the knee joint. The patient usually is unable to walk or extend the knee.

Physical Examination
1. **Inspection. Abrasions** over the patella are seen in direct injury to the knee. **Swelling** is secondary to hemarthrosis or hematoma.
2. **Palpation.** There is marked tenderness over the patella. A gap may be palpable in transverse fractures of the patella.
3. **Range of motion.** All movements are very painful, and active extension of the knee may be impossible.

Investigations
Anteroposterior and lateral x-rays of the knee and tangential views of the patella usually give enough information.

Complications
Degenerative arthritis of the patellofemoral joint is common after fractures of the patella. **Stiffness** of the knee can occur after immobilization in a cast.

Management
Undisplaced fracture can be treated conservatively. If there is a large, painful effusion in the joint, it is aspirated. A plaster **cast** is applied and the joint immobilized. A displaced

transverse fracture is treated by open reduction and **internal fixation** by wires or screw. A badly comminuted fracture in an elderly patient may require **excision of the patella.** Exercises to improve ROM and quadriceps strength help the patient regain function.

Other Fractures

Fractures of the shaft of femur, supracondyle, and condyle are beyond the scope of this book. Fractures involving the articular surface require very accurate reduction. Adherence of quadriceps to femur, knee stiffness, and later, degenerative arthritis of the knee are common complications of these fractures. Fracture of the lateral condyle of the tibia occurs more frequently than the medial fracture. Ligaments of the knee may be damaged at the same time.

DISLOCATIONS

Dislocation of the Patella

Subluxation and dislocation of the patella are more common than dislocation of the knee joint. It requires much more violent force to dislocate a knee joint.

Anatomy

The patella is maintained in the intercondylar groove of the femur by the large lateral condyle of the femur, active contraction of the vastus medialis muscle, and the fibrous capsule of the knee joint on the medial side of the patella. The quadriceps muscle tries to pull the patella laterally. The magnitude of this force depends on the Q-angle (Fig. 19–7).

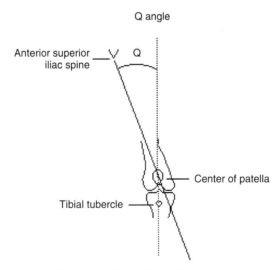

Fig. 19–7   Measurement of Q-angle. A line is drawn from the anterior superior iliac spine to the center of the patella. A second line is drawn from the center of patella to the tibial tubercle. The angle between these two lines is called the Q-angle.

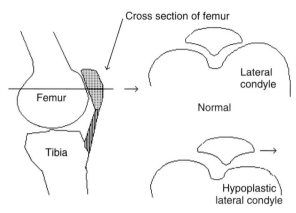

Fig. 19–8 The lateral condyle of the femur is larger than the medial condyle and prevents lateral displacement of the patella. The patella is more likely to dislocate when the lateral condyle is hypoplastic.

Mechanism of Injury
Factors predisposing to subluxation or dislocation of the patella include:
1. **Increased Q-angle.** This is more common in females because of their wider pelvis. Subluxation of the patella is more common in females, too.
2. Poorly developed lateral condyle of the femur (Fig. 19–8).
3. **Weakness of vastus medialis**
4. **Laxity of ligaments**
5. **Patella alta.** When the patella is too high (above the level of lateral condyle), there is no bony structure to prevent it from being pulled laterally. The patellar tendon is much longer than normal (Fig. 19–9).

Pathology
The patella is usually displaced laterally.

History
A dislocated patella occurs commonly in adolescent girls. The patient complains of sudden severe pain and locking of the knee. It happens when the knee is flexed and the tibia is externally rotated. The first episode requires much more force, but subsequent dislocations can occur more easily. The knee joint may swell after each episode.

Physical Examination
1. **Inspection.** Subluxation of the patella usually reduces by itself. Except for some **tenderness,** there are no physical signs that can be elicited. In dislocation, the patella can be observed in an abnormal, **lateral position.** There may be **atrophy** of the vastus medialis muscle as compared to the normal side. This muscle is seen as a bulge on the medial side of the upper pole of the patella when the knee is fully extended against resistance.
2. **Palpation.** Abnormal position of the patella is confirmed by palpation before the dislocation is reduced. There is tenderness over the patella and surrounding soft tissues.
3. **Range of motion.** As long as the patella is dislocated from its normal position, the knee joint cannot be flexed or extended.

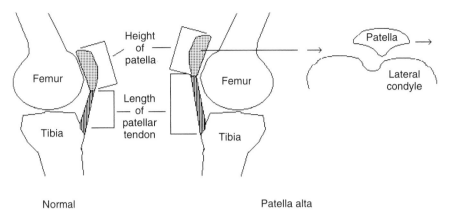

Normal   Patella alta

Fig. 19–9 The height of the patella and length of the patellar tendon are nearly equal. If the patellar tendon is longer than the vertical height of the patella, then the patella rides high on the femur (patella alta). In patella alta, the patella rides high on the femur and is proximal to the condyles of femur. There is no lateral condyle to prevent lateral dislocation of patella. Patella alta is one of the predisposing causes of dislocation of patella.

4. **Special tests.** Any attempt by the examiner to dislocate the patella is resisted by the patient and produces a facial expression known as an **apprehension sign.** With one hand, the examiner pushes the patella laterally, while with the other hand, he or she flexes the knee. At a certain point during this maneuver, the patient's facial expression becomes anxious, and the patient resists any further flexion.

Differential Diagnoses
Torn anterior horn of the meniscus or a loose body can present with a history of the knee giving-way or locking.

Investigations
1. **X-rays.** Tangential views of the patella help in determining any abnormality of the patellofemoral joint and the lateral condyle of the femur.
2. **MRI.** Movement of the patella in the intercondylar groove of the femur can be observed by dynamic MRI. The patellar and femoral surfaces should be congruent in a normal person.

Course
The initial episode of dislocation requires a great amount of force. Each subsequent recurrence occurs with less force. **Degenerative arthritis** of the patellofemoral joint may result after years of recurrent dislocations.

Management
The dislocation of the patella is reduced as soon as possible, and a pressure bandage is applied. Ice packs help to reduce swelling and pain. Isometric quadriceps exercises are started. Movements of the knee joint and weight-bearing are discouraged initially.

Further episodes are prevented by avoiding activities that precipitate subluxation or dislocation. Quadriceps strength should be maintained by regular exercises. If recurrent dislocation or subluxation still occur, surgical correction by lateral soft tissue release with tightening of the medial side may be considered.

Dislocation of the Knee Joint

Knee dislocation is not common. It takes a great force to dislocate the knee joint, and when dislocation occurs, it is usually accompanied by injury to blood vessels and nerves.

INFECTIOUS ARTHRITIS

Infectious arthritis is also known as **septic arthritis,** pyogenic arthritis, bacterial arthritis, or septic joint. The knee is the most commonly affected joint. Nearly half of all infections in the joints occur in the knee.

Etiology

1. In **children,** the lower femoral epiphysis is intra-articular, and osteomyelitis can spread to infect the joint. *Staphylococcus aureus* is the most common organism in infants and young children, as well as the elderly.
2. The knee is the most commonly affected joint due to **gonococci** in sexually active individuals, and infectious arthritis should be at the top of the list of differential diagnoses for a **young adult** presenting with a hot, tender, and swollen knee joint.
3. Bacteria may originate from some other source (e.g., tooth abscess) and infect a joint by the **hematogenous** route. **Intravenous drug abuse** is another cause of infectious arthritis.
4. In **older patients,** the etiology may be a complication of previous arthroplasty or rheumatoid arthritis. **Immunosuppressed** patients and those with other chronic illnesses, such as diabetes mellitus, alcoholism, or malignancy, are also prone to develop infectious arthritis of the knee.
5. The knee joint is very superficial and can be infected by a **puncture wound** or a laceration.

Pathology

Proteolytic enzymes are released by leukocytes in the synovial fluid. These enzymes destroy the articular cartilage, collagen fibers, and chondrocytes. Increased vascularity leads to marked osteoporosis in the juxta-articular bone. If infection is not controlled, the joint is completely destroyed very quickly.

History

The patient presents with a **painful, swollen joint.** History of **fever** with **chills** may or may not be present. These symptoms may be minimal in the elderly and immunosuppressed patients. A child will refuse to walk or stand (**loss of function**) on the affected extremity because of pain.

Physical Examination

1. **Inspection.** The knee joint is **swollen** and skin over it is **erythematous.**

2. **Palpation.** The skin is **warm** and **tender** to touch.
3. **Range of motion.** All movements are painful and markedly **restricted.**

Differential Diagnoses
1. **Gout** or other crystal-induced arthritis can be distinguished by examination of the joint fluid for crystals.
2. Presence of organisms in the joint fluid helps in diagnosing infection in a patient with flareup of **rheumatoid arthritis.**
3. **Traumatic** conditions are distinguished by joint fluid examination and plain x-rays.

Investigations
1. Fluid should be **aspirated** (as an emergency procedure) from any joint suspected of infection. The joint fluid in infections is very thick and opaque. **Gram stain** shows the presence of polymorphonuclear leukocytes and bacteria to confirm the diagnosis. The WBC is usually >50,000/mm^3 with 90% polymorphonuclear cells. Gram stain of the joint fluid may be negative in gonococcal infection. Urethral, cervical, pharyngeal, or rectal culture is more likely to be positive in gonococcal infections. For proper treatment, **culture** and **sensitivity tests** are carried out. Appropriate culture medium should be used for anaerobic, gonococcal, mycobacterial and other unusual infections.
2. **X-rays** initially may show only some **soft tissue swelling.** Bony changes may take up to 2 or 3 weeks to appear. Juxta-articular **osteoporosis** occurs after a week or two, and destruction of bone occurs later. It is very important *not* to wait for x-ray changes for diagnosis of infectious arthritis.

Course
Morbidity and mortality are related to the delay in diagnosis and initiation of appropriate treatment. The infection may spread locally and systemically to form sinuses and septicemia.

Complications
1. **Joint stiffness** can occur because of fibrosis.
2. Pus may track and burst through skin, forming a **draining sinus.**
3. **Toxemia** and **death** can result, especially in the elderly, frail, and immunosuppressed.

Management
Infection of a joint should be treated as an emergency. Joint fluid is aspirated as soon as it accumulates. Appropriate antibiotics are given intra-articularly and/or intravenously.

   Surgical. Incision and drainage may be necessary if all pus cannot be aspirated or infection cannot be controlled by needle aspiration.

RHEUMATOID ARTHRITIS

The knee joint may be involved early in rheumatoid arthritis. Sometimes, the patient may present with knee pain and swelling before other joints are affected. Pain and effusion may lead to wasting of the quadriceps and flexion contracture of the knee. The patient may complain of painful swelling in the popliteal region. The thickened synovial membrane in chronic rheumatoid arthritis is palpable 2–3 inches above the upper border of the patella. It can be rolled between the examiner's fingers and the femur. Long-standing effusion and inflammation produce ligamentous laxity, which may lead to joint instability and valgus or varus deformity.

The knee joint is superficial and easily accessible for aspiration of joint fluid and intra-articular injections. Infection of the knee joint occurs more frequently than infection of other joints in patients with rheumatoid arthritis and should be ruled out in acute exacerbation of a single joint in a patient with rheumatoid arthritis.

DEGENERATIVE JOINT DISEASE

Degenerative joint disease (DJD) of the knee is a very common problem. Pain in the knee on weight-bearing and at night is a common complaint.

Etiology
The cause of most degenerative arthritis of the knee is unknown (idiopathic). Obesity, torn meniscus, injury to the knee joint, deformity, and recurrent subluxation or dislocation of the patella are common predisposing factors for secondary DJD of the knee.

Pathology
The degenerative process may affect the patellofemoral, medial, or lateral tibiofemoral compartments of the knee joint. In recurrent dislocation of the patella, the patellofemoral arthritis is more prominent. The medial tibiofemoral compartment is more often involved than the lateral. This leads to narrowing of the medial joint space and varus deformity of the knee.

History
Degenerative arthritis of the knee is very common in people over age 45 years and is especially common among obese women. The onset is insidious. **Pain** in the knee on weight-bearing is the usual presenting symptom for DJD of the tibiofemoral joint. Pain is aggravated by overuse, such as long walks, running, or going up and down stairs. Patients with patellofemoral arthritis complain of pain on activities involving active contraction of the quadriceps, e.g., going up or down stairs. The patient also complains of **morning stiffness** which may last for 15–30 minutes.

Physical Examination
1. **Inspection.** There may be genu varum or valgum **deformity** due to unequal involvement of the medial or lateral compartment of the knee joint. A mild to moderate amount of **effusion** in the joint may also be present. In some patients, a swelling may be seen in the popliteal fossa which is due to a synovial cyst (Baker's cyst) that communicates with the main cavity of the knee joint.
2. **Palpation.** There may be **tenderness** over the joint line in arthritis of the medial or lateral compartment of the tibiofemoral joint. In patellofemoral joint disease, the tenderness is on pressure over the patella.

3. **Range of motion.** A mild flexion **contracture** with limitation of flexion is seen in long-standing cases. **Crepitus** is palpable on movement of the joint.

Differential Diagnoses

Chondromalacia patellae and DJD of the patellofemoral joint have very similar signs and symptoms but occur in very different age groups. Slowly progressive **monarticular inflammatory arthritis** may be difficult to differentiate during early stages of the disease.

Investigations

Plain x-rays show irregular **narrowing of the joint space** because of thinning of the articular cartilage. This may involve the patellofemoral joint or the medial or lateral compartment of the knee joint. The tibiofemoral joint space (thickness of articular cartilage) is assessed by x-rays taken in the weight-bearing position. A tangential view is ordered for patellofemoral arthritis. **Subchondral sclerosis** and **osteophyte** formation are other radiologic signs of DJD. Sharp joint margin described as **spiking** is an early sign. This may be seen at the upper and/or lower end of the patella on lateral x-rays or on the tibial spine in anteroposterior view.

The **joint fluid** is viscous and may contain up to 5,000 WBCs/mm^3.

Course

The disease may be slowly progressive, or after reaching a certain stage, it may become stationary.

Management

The x-ray changes do not necessarily correlate with the symptoms. Management depends on the severity of symptoms and their effect on the patient. Conservative measures should be tried first. **NSAID**s are started together with instructions in a home program of local **heat, quadriceps exercises,** and use of a **cane** in the opposite hand. If the patient is overweight, instruction in proper **diet** is useful. **Elastic support** or a knee brace may help relieve some pain. If this does not work, an intra-articular **injection of steroid** preparation usually gives temporary relief.

Operation may be considered if night pain interferes with sleep or walking distance is significantly limited despite a trial of conservative measures. Surgical options include:
1. **Arthroscopic** debridement or removal of loose bodies
2. **Arthroplasty** of one or both compartments or of the patellofemoral joint
3. **Excision of patella** if only the patellofemoral joint is affected
4. **Arthrodesis** of the joint in young adults with severe arthritis

CHONDROMALACIA PATELLAE

Chondromalacia is a pathology term that means softening of the cartilage. It has become a clinical diagnosis and is mainly used for patients presenting with anterior knee pain and tenderness over the undersurface of the patella.

Anatomy

The articular surface of the patella has a ridge that fits in the intercondylar groove of the femur. The patella glides up and down during flexion and extension of the joint.

Etiology

1. **Primary** or idiopathic when there are no predisposing causes
2. **Secondary** to direct trauma, recurrent subluxation of patella, or abnormal tracking of patella in the intercondylar groove of femur

Pathology

The changes of chondromalacia start around the central ridge over the articular surface of the patella. They are more marked over the medial facet of the patella. The cartilage becomes yellow and soft. Fine **fissures** appear which become large, and the cartilage begins to break-down. Pieces of cartilage become loose and float around in the joint cavity. Changes of **degenerative arthritis** (erosion of the cartilage and osteophytes) may appear later.

History

Pain in front of the knee is the main complaint. It may be diffuse and vague. The pain is aggravated while climbing stairs or sitting for long periods (e.g., while watching a movie). The articular surfaces of patella and femur are pressed together during these activities. Pain brought on by sitting is relieved by extending the knees. The patient may complain of **locking** if there is a loose body in the joint.

Physical Examination

1. **Palpation.** The knee joint should be fully extended and well-supported so as to relax the quadriceps muscle. The patella is pushed toward the medial and lateral side with one hand, and the undersurface of the patella is palpated by the other hand. (Since the lateral condyle is larger and projects farther than the medial, it is easier to push the patella toward the medial side). **Tenderness** on this exam suggests abnormal cartilage.
2. **Range of motion.** One hand is placed on the patella, and the knee joint is flexed and extended. If the articular surface of the patella is abnormal, **crepitus** may be palpated during this maneuver.
   a. **Active**—The patient complains of pain under the kneecap when asked to extend the knee against resistance.
3. **Special tests.** The Q-angle (*see* Fig. 19–7) may be >20° in patients with tendency to subluxate the patella.

Differential Diagnoses

Tear of the anterior horn of the meniscus, prepatellar or infrapatellar bursitis, or jumper's knee should be ruled out.

Investigations

1. **Plain x-rays** are normal in early stages. Changes of degenerative arthritis may be seen later.
2. **Arthroscopy** is diagnostic. Therapeutic procedures such as shaving the cartilage can be carried out through an arthroscope.

Course

Spontaneous remission may occur in some patients, after many years. In a few patients, symptoms of chondromalacia progresses to degenerative arthritis of the patellofemoral joint.

Management

For idiopathic chondromalacia, conservative measures are followed. Painful activities are avoided. Isometric quadriceps **exercises** and, later, short arc quadriceps exercises help in strengthening the muscle. Specific surgical procedures, e.g., **lateral soft tissue release,** may be required for recurrent subluxation of the patella. The degenerated cartilage may be shaved off through an **arthroscope** if conservative measures fail. Excision of the patella or replacement arthroplasty is considered for severe patellofemoral degenerative arthritis.

COMMON PERONEAL NERVE PALSY

The common peroneal nerve is frequently injured or involved in peripheral neuropathy. There is weakness of the dorsiflexors of the foot, and the patient presents with a foot drop.

Anatomy

The sciatic nerve divides into common peroneal and tibial nerves. The separation of nerve fibers of these two divisions occurs in the hip region, but they are enclosed in a common fibrous sheath. The nerves separate from each other near the proximal part of the popliteal fossa. Because of this anatomic arrangement, injury of the sciatic nerve in the hip region may present with predominant involvement of only common peroneal nerve fibers. The tibial component may be injured minimally or not at all.

The common peroneal nerve passes deep to the medial side of the biceps femoris to the posterior aspect of the head of the fibula. It then winds around the neck of the fibula and divides into superficial and deep branches. The **superficial branch** supplies the peroneus longus and brevis muscles, whereas the **deep branch** innervates the anterior tibial, extensor hallucis longus, and extensor digitorum longus muscles.

Etiology

External pressure on the common peroneal nerve as it winds around the neck of the fibula is the usual cause of peroneal nerve palsy. The nerve is more susceptible in **diabetics** and alcoholics. The nerve may be damaged by a **tight cast,** while sitting with the legs crossed, while the patient is in a coma, or during prolonged bedrest. The common peroneal component may be damaged in **operations on the hip joint** or injuries in that region. The cause of peroneal nerve palsy may not be apparent in many cases (**idiopathic**).

History

The patient presents with a **foot drop** because of weakness of the dorsiflexors of the foot. He or she walks with a high stepping gait in order to clear the ground. There may be history of tripping and falling because of difficulty in clearing objects (such as rugs) on the floor.

Physical Examination
1. **Inspection.** The **shoe** on the affected side may show scuff marks over the front end.
2. **Special tests.** Neurologic examination reveals **weakness** of the dorsiflexors and evertors of the foot. One group of muscles (dorsiflexors or evertors) may be weaker than the other. **Sensation** of the skin over the lateral aspect of the distal leg and dorsum of the foot may be diminished.

Differential Diagnoses
The possible causes of foot drop are covered in Chapter 20. Sometimes, sciatic nerve injury may predominantly affect the common peroneal division. **Electromyography** of the hamstring, gastrocnemius, and other lower extremity muscles may help in localizing the lesion. Injury to the sciatic nerve occurs after fractures around the hip joint or in operations such as arthroplasty of the hip.

Investigations
Electromyography and nerve conduction studies help in confirming the clinical diagnosis and in determining the extent, severity, and site of lesion.

Course
The course depends on the severity, duration, and etiology of the lesion. A total involvement of the nerve with wallerian degeneration of most of the fibers may take from 18 months to 2 years to recover, if it recovers at all. A **neurapraxia** (physiologic block to nerve conduction) which develops on a operating room table may recover in a few weeks.

Complications
1. A patient with a foot drop may **fall** because the foot gets caught on a rug or step.
2. **Equinus deformity** of the foot may develop if the foot drop is of long duration.

Management
Every attempt should be made to **prevent** peroneal nerve palsy by padding the vulnerable site over the head of the fibula during casting, anesthesia, and prolonged bedrest. If it occurs, the cast should be changed. A plastic or metal **brace** (ankle-foot orthosis) will help the patient walk better. Spontaneous improvement occurs in most cases. **Physical therapy** helps maintain ROM of the foot and ankle joints. Exercises to strengthen muscles are prescribed as nerve recovery takes place.

LOOSE BODIES

The knee is the most common site for free-floating intra-articular loose bodies. They present with a history of sudden severe pain and locking of the joint.

Etiology
1. **Degenerative joint disease.** An osteophyte may break loose and float around in the joint.

2. **Chip fracture.** A small fragment of bone and articular cartilage, e.g., fracture of tibial spine, can form a loose body.
3. A piece of **meniscus** can separate and form a loose body.
4. **Osteochondritis dissecans** is avascular necrosis of the subchondral bone. The necrosed bone with attached articular cartilage may separate from the femur and form a loose body. The etiology of this condition is unknown, but it may be due to injury. The medial femoral condyle is traumatized by the tibial spine and starts the process of avascular necrosis. It occurs in adolescents and young adults. The pathology is very similar to that of avascular necrosis of the head of the femur.
5. **Inflammatory** or **infectious arthritis.** Fibrinous loose bodies may form in rheumatoid arthritis or tuberculosis of the knee joint.

Pathology
The articular cartilage covering a loose body can survive and even grow in synovial fluid. The loose body can get trapped between the femoral and tibial condyles, damage the articular cartilage, and lead to degenerative arthritis.

History
Osteochondritis dissecans may be asymptomatic in the beginning. The initial symptoms vary with the etiology of the loose body. Patients complain of **locking** of the joint while walking or running. There is sudden, severe **pain,** and the patient is not able to flex or extend the knee. This is different from the locking due to torn meniscus in which only extension is limited. The joint **swells** later on. There may be deep, dull pain in the joint between episodes of locking.

Physical Examination
1. **Palpation.** Sometimes, the patient is able to palpate the loose body along the joint line or in the suprapatellar pouch. It moves around and can disappear within the joint space (sometimes called joint mouse).
2. **Range of motion** is limited only during the episode of locking.

Differential Diagnoses
The list of differential diagnoses is the same as that mentioned under Etiology.

Investigations
1. **Plain x-rays.** Routine anteroposterior and lateral views may not show the loose body. Intercondylar or **tunnel view** is ordered if a loose body is suspected. This view is also helpful in showing the defect due to osteochondritis dissecans in the femoral condyle. The sesamoid bone fabella, in one of the tendons of origin of the gastrocnemius muscle, is frequently mistaken for a loose body.
2. **MRI** is useful in the early diagnosis of osteochondritis dissecans.
3. **Arthroscopy** is done to find out if the articular cartilage and avascular bone are attached or loose. A loose body can also be removed through an arthroscope.

Complications
Degenerative arthritis may result from continuous trauma to the articular cartilage.

Management

The patient is advised to avoid running and other sports that might precipitate an attack of locking. If there is a moderate amount of fluid in the joint, it is aspirated. Quadriceps exercises are helpful in maintaining stability of the joint. An operation is considered when there is history of recurrent locking and effusion. The loose body is removed if it is small, or it is fixed with pins if it is a large piece from osteochondritis dissecans.

THE QUADRICEPS MUSCLE

The extensor mechanism of the knee joint is very important for proper function of the lower extremity. It is essential for rising from the sitting position, normal walking, jumping, running, and going up and down stairs. Weakness or injury of the quadriceps muscle and its tendon will affect all these functions.

Anatomy

The quadriceps muscle is made up of four muscles that arise from the femur and pelvis: rectus femoris, vastus medialis, vastus intermedius, and vastus lateralis. They make up the main muscle mass in the front of the thigh. All the muscles come together and form the quadriceps tendon. It seems to insert into the upper pole of the patella, but actually the patella is a sesamoid bone within this tendon. It continues at the lower border of the patella as the patellar tendon and inserts into the tibial tubercle. The femoral nerve (made up of lumbar 2, 3, and 4 roots) supplies the quadriceps muscle. This muscle is a powerful extensor of the knee joint.

Etiology

Quadriceps weakness may be due to:
1. **Femoral nerve palsy** as seen in diabetics
2. **Knee pathology** and/or effusion in the knee joint
3. **Disuse atrophy** after immobilization in a cast or prolonged bedrest
4. **Muscular dystrophy** in children

Mechanism of Injury

1. **Powerful contraction** of the quadriceps muscle can rupture the muscle. In an elderly person, the tendon may rupture when he or she tries to regain balance after stumbling.
2. **Direct injury,** e.g., fall on the knee, can fracture the patella and disrupt the extensor mechanism. The quadriceps muscle may rupture from a direct trauma against the thigh.

Pathology

The extensor mechanism may be damaged at the level of:
1. Quadriceps muscle
2. Quadriceps tendon proximal to the patella
3. Fracture of the patella
4. Patellar tendon at its origin at the lower pole of the patella, at its insertion into tibial tubercle, or between these two sites

History

The patient complains of sudden **severe pain** in the thigh or knee depending on the site of rupture. He or she is unable to walk or get up from the sitting position.

Physical Examination

1. **Inspection.** A **swelling** and **bruise** appears soon after injury.
2. **Palpation.** There is **tenderness** at the site of injury. A gap in the quadriceps muscle, between fragments of patellar fracture, or patellar tendon may be palpable.
3. **Range of motion.** All movements of the knee are painful at the time of injury.
   a. **Active** extension of the knee is very weak or impossible.
   b. **Passive**—After the initial pain subsides, passive movements of the knee should be full.

Differential Diagnoses

Appropriate x-rays are taken to rule out fractures.

Investigations

Plain x-rays usually give all the information necessary for management.

Complications

Rupture of the quadriceps muscle can lead to myositis ossificans. Permanent weakness of the extensor mechanism may cause difficulty in athletic activities, rising from the sitting position, or going up and down stairs.

Management

Rupture of the muscle is treated conservatively with ice packs, rest, and a cast. Complete rupture of the patellar tendon or fracture of the patella may need surgical repair. Rehabilitation therapy is prescribed to increase ROM of the knee, quadriceps strength, and walking with appropriate aid.

Jumper's Knee

Repeated contraction of the quadriceps sometimes leads to partial tear or tendinitis of the patellar tendon near the lower pole of the patella. This condition occurs in basketball and volleyball players. They present with **pain** over the patellar tendon or the lower pole of patella which is aggravated by activity. There is well-localized **tenderness.** The pain is reproduced by active contraction of the quadriceps muscle against resistance. Treatment consists of avoiding the activity which brought on the symptoms, local ice packs, rest, and NSAIDs.

APOPHYSITIS OF THE TIBIAL TUBERCLE

This condition is also known as **Osgood-Schlatter's disease**.

Anatomy

The patellar tendon is inserted into the tibial tubercle. The tubercle is formed by a part of the upper tibial epiphysis or a separate apophysis which unites with the main shaft of tibia at around 20 years of age.

Etiology
The exact etiology is unknown, but it may be the result of chronic repetitive strain on the immature apophysis or partial avulsion and avascular necrosis.

Pathology
The pathologic findings are very similar to those of avascular necrosis of the epiphysis of the femoral head. There is fragmentation of the apophysis, followed by spontaneous healing.

History
The condition is more common in males between 10–15 years of age. They complain of pain over the tibial tubercle which is aggravated by running, jumping, or kneeling. This condition is self-limiting.

Physical Examination
1. **Inspection.** Slight **swelling** may be noticed in the painful area.
2. **Palpation.** There is **tenderness** over the tibial tubercle.

Investigations
Lateral x-ray may show fragmentation of the apophysis.

Management
The patient is advised to avoid activities that aggravate pain. It may remain painful for a year or two.

Bibliography

1. Cooper DE, Arnoczky SP, Warren RF: Meniscal repair. Clin Sports Med 10:529–548, 1991.
2. Dunn JF: Osgood-Schlatter disease. Am Fam Physician 41:173–176, 1990.
3. Feagin JA Jr: The office diagnosis and documentation of common knee problems. Clin Sports Med 8:453–459, 1989.
4. Jackson AM: Recurrent dislocation of patella [editorial]. J Bone Joint Surg 74-B:2–4, 1992.
5. Kanuus P: Nonoperative treatment of acute knee ligament injuries: A review with special reference to indications and methods. Sports Med 9:244–260, 1990.
6. Mink JH, Deutsch AL: Magnetic resonance imaging of the knee. Clin Orthop 244:29–47, 1989.
7. Schenck RC Jr, Heckman JD: Injuries of the knee. Clin Symp 45(1):2–32, 1993.
8. Simmons E Jr, Cameron JC: Patella alta and recurrent dislocation of patella. Clin Orthop 274:265–269, 1992.
9. Terry GC: Office evaluation and management of the symptomatic knee. Orthop Clin North Am 19:699–713, 1988.

20

Foot

Arun J. Mehta, M.B., F.R.C.P.C.

The foot is constructed to bear the weight of the body during standing and walking. In rare instances, it can perform some of the functions of the hand—e.g., children born without the use of their hands may be able use their feet to pick things up, write, or even play a musical instrument. However, for most of us, the foot provides stable support by its strong ligaments and the shape of its bones. During walking and running, the foot takes the initial impact, adapts to uneven surfaces, and provides push-off to propel the body. The stress endured by the foot is much more than the body weight, especially in activities like running and jumping.

Differential Diagnosis

Pain
A. **Pain in the forefoot.** The forefoot consists of metatarsals and phalanges. Much of the body weight is borne by the heads of the first and fifth metatarsals.
   1. **Callus.** Pain occurs over a thickened area of the skin. It is worse after the patient walks a long distance.
   2. **Degenerative joint disease** of the first metatarsophalangeal (MTP) joint. The patient complains of pain and tenderness over the joint with limitation of movements. This condition is secondary to trauma, rheumatoid arthritis, or hallux valgus deformity. Limitation of dorsiflexion of the first MTP joint with pain on walking may be due to **hallux rigidus.**
   3. **Hallux valgus** with bunion. There is valgus deformity of the big toe with swelling over the medial aspect of the first MTP joint.
   4. **Stress fracture** of the metatarsal. Pain in the forefoot develops after an unusual activity, e.g., basic training in the army. On examination, localized tenderness is seen over the metatarsal just proximal to the metatarsal head. X-rays may be negative initially.
   5. **Gout** presents with very painful inflammatory arthritis of the first MTP joint. Other joints may also be involved.
   6. **Morton's neuroma.** The patient complains of pain in the forefoot radiating down to one or two toes with tenderness between two metatarsals. The pain is aggravated by squeezing the metatarsals together.
B. **Pain in midfoot**
   1. **Avascular necrosis** of the navicular bone
   2. **Tendinitis** affecting the peroneus longus, tibialis anterior, or tibialis posterior tendons

C. **Pain in bottom of the heel**
  1. **Plantar fasciitis** presents with chronic recurrent pain and tenderness near the anterior end of calcaneum.
  2. **Fracture of the calcaneum.** History of a fall from a height and local tenderness over the calcaneum are present. It may be accompanied by a compression fracture of a vertebra.
D. **Pain in the back of the heel**
  1. **Retrocalcaneal bursitis.** There is tenderness and pain behind the heel after an unaccustomed activity, such as running or jumping.
  2. **Rupture of tendo Achillis.** The patient complains of sudden, severe pain behind the lower third of the leg. He or she is unable to stand on the toes or walk. There may be a palpable gap in the Achilles tendon.
E. **Diffuse pain in the foot**
  1. **Peripheral neuropathy.**—The patient may complain of burning pain in the feet with no relation to activity. The pain is usually bilateral and worse at night. A history of diabetes or alcohol abuse are common causes.
  2. **Peripheral vascular disease.** Pain due to vascular insufficiency is brought on by walking a definite distance and relieved by rest. The pain is usually felt in the calf and leg. However, patients with impending gangrene of the foot complain of very severe, diffuse pain in the foot. It is usually preceded by a long history of intermittent claudication. The toes or whole foot may be cold to touch and of dusky color, with very poor capillary return.
  3. **Reflex sympathetic dystrophy** presents with severe burning pain after an injury. Hyperesthesia and hyperemia are common findings on examination.

Foot Drop
A. **Unilateral foot drop.** The patient is not able to pull the foot up against gravity. It may be due to:
  1. **Stroke.** There may be a history of involvement of the upper extremity, face, or speech to suggest the diagnosis of a cerebrovascular accident.
  2. **Fifth lumbar radiculopathy.** Pain radiating down from the gluteal region to the foot, with weakness of the foot dorsiflexors and diminished sensation near the webspace between the big and second toe, is commonly seen in L 4–5 disc prolapse and radiculopathy.
  3. **Common peroneal nerve palsy** may be due to direct pressure on the common peroneal nerve at the neck of the fibula. It is usually not painful.
  4. **Peripheral neuropathy** sometimes affects one side more than the other initially, and the patient may present with unilateral foot drop.
B. **Bilateral foot drop**
  1. **Peripheral neuropathy.** Weakness of the dorsiflexors of both feet occurs, with tingling, numbness, weakness, and atrophy of muscles of both feet and hands. Diabetes and alcohol abuse are common causes.

Foot Deformity
Several neurologic conditions may present with deformities of foot:
1. Cerebral palsy
2. Cerebrovascular accident
3. Peripheral neuropathy
4. Charcot-Marie-Tooth disease

Anatomy

The foot is divided into three parts:

1. **Hindfoot** consists of the talus and calcaneum. The talus articulates with the tibia and fibula to form the **ankle** joint. It is a hinge joint with movements in one plane. The talus also articulates with the calcaneum at the subtalar joint. This joint takes part in the composite movements of inversion and eversion. Body weight passes through the tibia, talus, and calcaneum to the ground.
2. **Midfoot** is made up of the navicular, cuboid, and three cuneiform bones. The midfoot forms the dome of the longitudinal **arch.**
3. **Forefoot** consists of the metatarsals and toes.

History

Pain in the foot is a very common symptom. Its **onset, duration,** and **progression** are noted. The **location** of pain may give an important clue as to the diagnosis. It is necessary to know the relation of pain to the time of day and **activity.** Pain due to trauma, infection, and inflammatory arthritis is present at rest and made worse by weight-bearing. Neuropathic pain is worse at night. Fifth lumbar or first sacral **nerve root pain** is felt in the gluteal region, back of the thigh, leg, and foot. Pain due to overuse is worse after any activity such as running. Standing and walking aggravate pain in most of the conditions. Has the **gait** changed because of problems with the foot? How has it changed? Rheumatoid arthritis usually affects the feet, hands, elbows, shoulders, neck, and knees. Inquire about involvement of other joints. The soft tissues of the feet are involved in Reiter's disease.

Physical Examination

Inspection

Inspection of the foot starts when the patient enters the examination room. The **gait** is observed for any evidence of pain. Later, the walking pattern is examined without shoes. The patient is asked to remove shoes and socks, undress from the waist down, and wear a short gown. The patient sits on the examination couch, and the examiner sits across at a lower level. The foot is inspected in **non-weight-bearing** and **weight-bearing** positions from following viewpoints:

1. **Top.** The **color** and appearance of the **skin** and **nails** are noted and compared with the opposite side. Diffuse swelling (**edema**) of the foot is best seen over the dorsum. The toes normally point $10°$–$15°$ externally. Count the number of toes and see if they are all present—sometimes a missing toe is not obvious. Look for any **deformity** of the foot.
2. **Plantar surface. Callosity** or abnormal thickening of the skin is usually found over the heads of the metatarsal bones. Look for any foreign body or an infected open wound, especially in diabetics with peripheral neuropathy.
3. **Medial side.** The longitudinal **arch** of the foot extends from the heel to the head of the first metatarsal. It is flattened in **pes planus** (flatfoot) and exaggerated in **pes cavus.**
4. **Back.** When the patient stands, the heel should be directly under the ankle joint and leg. The Achilles tendon lies in the center with medial and lateral malleoli on either side. The tip of the lateral malleolus is lower and more posterior than the medial malleolus.

Palpation

Palpation of the foot should proceed systematically to elicit **temperature,** tenderness, and characteristics of any swelling. In peripheral vascular disease, the skin is cold, whereas in infection and inflammatory arthritis, there is increased warmth around the affected area. **Localized tenderness** is very important in pinpointing the pathology. All anatomic structures are palpated, especially the first MTP joint, heel, insertion of tendo Achillis, and ankle joint. The thickness of the plantar skin and **fat pad** under the skin gives some indication as to the cause of pain.

Range of Motion

Movement is examined at the first MTP, ankle, and subtalar joints. The foot lies at a right angle to the leg, and ROM is measured from this as the neutral position (0°). **Dorsiflexion** is the movement when the foot or toes are pulled up toward the head, and **plantar flexion** occurs when the foot is pushed away. There is some confusion regarding the meaning of the terms *pronation* and *supination* and *eversion* and *inversion*. The foot is rotated toward the outer or inner side, and these movements take place at multiple joints.

1. **Active.** Movements **against gravity** and **against resistance** help in determining the strength of muscles and in localizing the lesion to a particular nerve root or peripheral nerve. Weakness of dorsiflexion of the foot and big toe suggests a peroneal nerve or fifth lumbar nerve root problem. The plantar flexors of the toes and foot are supplied by the posterior tibial nerve and mainly first sacral nerve root. **Functional range** is tested by asking the patient to stand on the toes and heels
2. **Passive.** Movements are tested if active ROM is abnormal. See Table 20–1.

Special Tests

1. **Circulation**
   a. **Skin color.** In patients with peripheral vascular disease, the skin blanches when the leg is elevated and becomes cyanotic when the leg is dependent.
   b. **Capillary return.** When pressure is applied to the nail, it blanches. The pink color returns very quickly after the pressure is removed. In peripheral vascular disease, it takes much longer for the pink color to return.
   c. **Skin temperature.** The tips of the toes are cold when there is insufficient blood flow.
   d. **Arterial pulsation. Dorsalis pedis artery** is palpated over the dorsal aspect of the proximal foot. It lies between the tendons of the extensor pollicis longus and extensor digitorum longus. The **posterior tibial artery** is palpated between the medial malleolus and the heel over the medial aspect of the proximal foot.
2. **Neurological examination** is done to localize the lesion at the level of cauda equina, nerve root, plexus, or peripheral nerve. This should include sensation, muscle strength, and reflexes.
3. **Gait.** A preliminary examination of gait is done when the patient walks into the examination room. More detailed observations are made when the patient is asked to walk with and without shoes to determine different conditions.
   a. **Antalgic gait.** Any abnormal gait pattern due to a painful condition, e.g., a callosity, or degenerative joint disease of the hip or knee is called antalgic gait. The patient tries to minimize pain by staying on the painful side for the shortest period of time. He or

Table 20–1   Passive ROM of Foot Joints

Joint	Dorsiflexion	Plantar flexion
First MTP	70°–90°	20°–30°
Ankle	20°	50°

she reduces the weight-bearing (stance) phase of the gait on painful side. If a painful corn is on the sole of the foot, he or she tries to keep that part off the ground.

b. **High stepping gait** is secondary to a foot drop. The dorsiflexors of the foot are weak and unable to lift the toes off the ground. To compensate for this, the patient lifts the thigh and leg more to clear the ground. This gait is seen in hemiplegics, common peroneal nerve palsy, or peripheral neuropathy.

4. **Shoes.** How long has the patient had this pair of shoes? Does he or she have many different varieties of shoes? Are they comfortable? Inquire about the **type** of shoes commonly worn—e.g., high heels, narrow pointed toes, dress shoes with a very stiff sole, tennis shoes.

a. General **shape** of the shoe. Is it deformed?

b. **Size.** A proper-fitting shoe is important for comfort and in preventing callosities. Most women's shoes are too narrow in front, leading to callus formation over the fifth and first metatarsal heads. Compare the size of the shoe with the foot by placing the shoe next to the sole. Callosities develop over the dorsal surface of toes if there is not enough space in the toebox. The counter of the shoe should fit well around the heel.

c. **Scuff marks.** Are there scuff marks near the toes (indicates foot drop) or near the counter?

d. **Wear.** Is there **uneven wear** over one side of the heel (very common) or sole? Spasticity after a stroke can result in the front and outer aspect of the sole wearing much faster.

Investigations

1. **Plain x-rays** are useful in diagnosis and in determining the severity of pathology. They are especially useful for diagnosing conditions of the bone and joint.
2. **Radionuclide bone scan** is necessary for early diagnosis of stress fracture, avascular necrosis, or reflex sympathetic dystrophy.
3. **CT scan** may be required in patients with complicated fractures.
4. **MRI** is useful in delineating tendon ruptures, early osteomyelitis, and other soft tissue problems.

CONGENITAL CLUBFOOT

Talipes equinovarus is the most common variety of clubfoot deformity. There is plantar flexion at the ankle and foot, inversion of the foot, and adduction deformity at the forefoot.

Anatomy

In the normal foot, the long axis of calcaneum lines up with the cuboid and fifth metatarsal bones, and the axis of the talus lines up with that of the medial cuneiform and first metatarsal (Fig. 20–1). In talipes equinovarus, there is subluxation of the talonavicular joint. The angle between the long axis of talus and calcaneum is reduced. Thus, the foot is plantar-flexed and turned inward.

Etiology

The exact cause of clubfoot is not known, but two factors, **genetic** and **intrauterine pressure,** are blamed for its occurrence. The genetic factor is presumed to be an autosomal dominant trait with reduced penetrance. Clubfoot may be associated with:

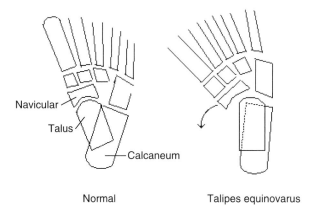

Normal   Talipes equinovarus

Fig. 20–1 In talipes equinovarus, there is subluxation of the talonavicular joint. The angle between the long axis of talus and calcaneum is reduced.

1. **Spina bifida.** X-rays of the spine should be done to rule out spina bifida, which may not be always obvious.
2. **Arthrogryposis.** Multiple joints are involved with stiffness, dislocations, and deformities.
3. Other neurologic conditions, e.g., cerebral palsy or Friedreich's ataxia

Pathology
There are **contractures** of ligaments of the joints, especially on the medial and plantar aspect of the foot. The muscles and tendons are small and short. The **navicular** bone is **subluxed** medially and toward the plantar surface. Initially, the bones are normal in shape but later become **deformed,** especially the navicular and talus. The deformity affects multiple joints. At the ankle, there is plantar flexion due to a tight Achilles tendon. There is inversion at the subtalar, talonavicular, and other midfoot joints. The metatarsals are plantar-flexed and adducted in relation to the midfoot.

History
The deformity should be diagnosed at birth or soon after. Boys are affected more often than girls (ratio of 2:1).

Physical Examination
1. **Inspection.** The plantar surface of the foot is rotated medially into **inversion,** and the forefoot is pulled into **varus** (Fig. 20–2). The foot is also in **plantar flexion** (equinus). The deformity is described as **talipes** (clubfoot) **equino** (plantar flexion) **varus** (of the forefoot and heel).
2. **Palpation.** Soft tissues, such as the plantar aponeurosis and Achilles tendon, are palpated to see how difficult it is to correct the deformity. The severity of clubfoot is determined by the stiffness of the soft tissues.
3. **Range of motion. Passive** movement is attempted to correct the varus deformity of the forefoot and equinus of the foot.

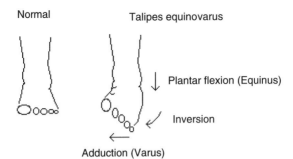

Normal   Talipes equinovarus

Plantar flexion (Equinus)

Inversion

Adduction (Varus)

Fig. 20–2   Talipes equinovarus deformity as seen from the front. There is plantar flexion, inversion, and adduction of the forefoot.

4. **Special tests.** Neurologic exam is done to rule out spinal cord, cauda equina, and peripheral nerve diseases.

Course
If not treated, and sometimes despite treatment, the patient may develop **fixed deformity.** Later, painful callosities and degenerative arthritis occur in the affected foot. Adults with talipes equinovarus deformity walk on the outer aspect of the foot with a stumbling gait.

Differential Diagnosis
Other congenital deformities of the foot include:
1. **Metatarsus adductus.** Only the metatarsals are turned medially.
2. **Metatarsus primus varus.** The first metatarsal is displaced medially.
3. **Talipes calcaneovalgus.** The foot is everted and dorsiflexed.

Investigations
On **plain x-rays** of a normal foot, the talus, navicular, medial cuneiform, and first metatarsal lie in a straight line (Fig. 20–1). In talipes equinovarus, the navicular is subluxed medially and inferiorly. The distal bones, medial cuneiform, and first metatarsal follow the navicular.

Management
Early diagnosis and treatment are absolutely essential for good outcome. Treatment should be started within a few days of birth. Despite good early treatment, half of the patients may require surgery. Any patient suspected of having a foot deformity should be referred to a specialist.
1. **Ancillary**
   a. **Manipulation** and **cast.** The deformities are corrected in following order:
      i. Forefoot adduction
      ii. Inversion of the hindfoot
      iii. Equinus at the ankle
         The corrected position is then maintained by cast.
   b. **Splinting** helps maintain the correction. There is a great tendency to relapse, and so regular followups are important.

2. **Surgical.** Many different kinds of operations are available. Tight soft tissue structures over the medial aspect of the foot are cut to allow correction of the deformity. Some tendons may require lengthening or their insertion transferred to achieve proper muscle balance. In very severe deformity with bony changes, operation of **triple arthrodesis** is done. A wedge of bony tissue is removed from the convex lateral side, and the foot is fused in the corrected position.

INJURIES TO LIGAMENTS

Lateral Ligament
Partial and complete tears of ligaments of the ankle joint are very common. It is very important to diagnose the severity of trauma and formulate a plan for management accordingly. The duration of disability varies considerably.

Anatomy
The ankle joint is a **hinge joint** with movements taking place only in one axis. The movements are **plantar flexion** and **dorsiflexion.** There are two strong ligaments, the lateral and medial (deltoid ligament) collateral, which stabilize the ankle joint (Fig. 20–3). These ligaments and the bony configuration of the ankle prevent excessive lateral and medial twisting movements (inversion and eversion) at the ankle joint. The medial collateral ligament is stronger than the lateral.

Mechanism of Injury
Ligament injuries are common in **sports** involving running and jumping. The foot is twisted while landing on the ground. This injury can also happen during walking on uneven ground. The lateral ligament is injured if the foot is turned in (**inverted**), and the medial ligament is injured if the foot is **everted.** Injury to the lateral ligament is much more common.

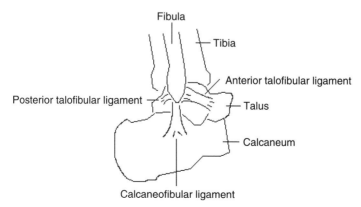

Fig. 20–3 The lateral collateral ligament of the ankle has three parts: anterior talofibular, calcaneofibular, and posterior talofibular.

Pathology
The fibers of the ligament involved are torn. The lateral ligament is injured in the vast majority of cases. The injury is classified according to severity into grade I (mild), II (moderate), or III (severe). In grade III, the ligament is completely torn, whereas in grades I and II, the ligament is only partially torn. There is bleeding in the surrounding tissues. Hemarthrosis occurs if the capsule of the joint is torn. The ligamentous tissue takes 6–8 weeks to heal.

History
The patient develops **pain** immediately after twisting the ankle. If the foot is twisted inward, (as is usually the case), pain and **swelling** are observed over the lateral aspect of ankle. The patient is not able to walk or run.

Physical Examination
1. **Inspection. Swelling** appears over the injured ligament. The size of this swelling depends on the severity of trauma and how it is treated. Deformity results only if there is fracture or dislocation. **Bruise** is seen several days after the injury.
2. **Palpation.** There is **localized tenderness** over the injured ligament. The extent of the tender area depends on the severity of the injury.
3. **Range of motion**
   a. **Active**—All active movements are painful.
   b. **Passive**—Inversion is especially painful.
4. **Special tests.** The **anterior drawer test** is similar to the drawer test for the knee. The leg is held with one hand and the heel with the other. The heel is pulled forward while the leg is kept fixed. If the anterior talofibular ligament is ruptured, the heel can be moved forward relative to the leg.

Course/Complications
Rupture of a ligament can take a long time to heal. Return to full function can take even longer. Complications include:
1. **Chronic instability** of the ankle can result after complete rupture of a ligament. The patient feels that the ankle is not stable while weight-bearing on the affected side.
2. **Recurrent strain** or injury to the same ligament may occur as a result of incomplete healing or inadequate treatment.

Differential Diagnosis
Fractures around the ankle joint should be ruled out by x-rays.

Investigations
1. **Plain x-rays** are ordered to rule out fractures. Anteroposterior, lateral, and oblique views are usually done.
2. **Stress x-rays** help to show complete rupture of the ligament. Under anesthesia, the heel is inverted to see if the superior surface of the talus remains congruent with the articular surface of the tibia (Fig. 20–4).

Management
Treatment is controversial, but the trend is toward a conservative approach. The duration of immobilization depends on the severity of the injury. It is determined by the initial swelling, tenderness, bruising, and instability. The torn ligament needs to be protected from

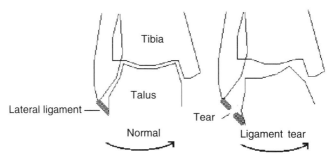

Fig. 20–4   Stress test for lateral ligament rupture.

further injury until it heals, which may take 2–8 weeks. Later, if the pain and tenderness persist, the period of immobilization or support may be extended. **Rehabilitation** to regain ROM in the ankle and other joints of the foot, strength of muscles, and agility requires specific and prolonged therapy. Conservative (nonsurgical) treatment with aggressive rehabilitation is recommended for most patients.
1. **Ancillary.** Some orthopedic surgions treat even complete tears conservatively.
    a. Initial treatment consists of **RICE** (rest, ice pack, elevation, and compression bandage). Weight-bearing on the affected leg is not permitted. The other alternatives are strapping or cast with the heel in slight eversion if the lateral ligament is injured.
    b. Rehabilitation procedures are started as soon as possible, with gentle ROM exercises, gradually increasing weight-bearing, and later, exercises to strengthen muscles, especially the evertors of the ankle.
2. **Surgical** repair is done for:
    a. Complete tears with instability
    b. Chronic instability

Medial Ligament Sprain
Sprains of the medial ligament are not very common. The mechanism of injury is similar but opposite to that of the lateral ligament. The foot is twisted laterally while walking, running, or jumping. Pain, swelling, and tenderness are over the medial aspect. The treatment principles are similar to those for the lateral ligament tears.

STRESS FRACTURE OF THE METATARSAL

Stress fracture is also known as **march fracture,** or **march foot,** as well as **fatigue fracture.** The patient presents with pain in the metatarsal region after an unusually long walk or run.

Etiology
During normal walking, a lot of body weight is transferred through the head of the first metatarsal to the ground during the push-off phase. If the first metatarsal is shorter than the second, then the head of the second metatarsal bears an extra amount of stress during walking or running. A stress fracture may develop after an unusually long march or run.

Pathology
The fracture fragments are not displaced. Healing occurs with callus formation.

History
Onset of **pain** in the middle of forefoot after an unusual activity is the usual presentation, although it may start insiduously after a moderately severe activity. There is constant pain which is aggravated by weight-bearing.

Physical Examination
1. **Inspection.** Some swelling may develop over the dorsum of the forefoot. No deformity is seen because there is no displacement of fracture fragments.
2. **Palpation.** Exquisite **tenderness** over the distal shaft of metatarsal is elicited. A **swelling** may be palpable at the fracture site a few weeks after the onset of pain.
3. **Range of Motion.** Active and passive movements of the metatarsophalangeal (MTP) joint are painful and may be restricted.

Investigations
1. **Plain x-rays** may not show the fracture during early stages because the fracture line is very fine (Fig. 20–5A). If the x-rays are negative and pain persists, x-rays should be repeated after 2–3 weeks. The fracture line or exuberant callus formation (Fig. 20–5B) becomes more apparent.
2. **Bone scan** shows increased uptake in the involved area at an early stage and may help in early diagnosis.
3. **MRI** can also help in early diagnosis of a stress fracture.

Management
1. **Medications.** Analgesics are prescribed to relieve pain.
2. **Ancillary**
   a. A **walking cast** is applied when there is severe pain. The cast can be removed when the pain subsides.
   b. **Exercises** to improve intrinsic muscle strength and increase ROM are prescribed after the cast is removed.
   c. Metatarsal bar just proximal to the metatarsal heads helps reduce weight-bearing stress over them.
   d. Proper **shoes** with arch support help distribute body weight properly.

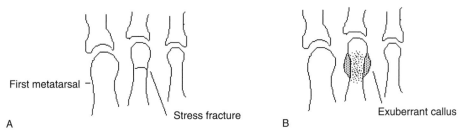

Fig. 20–5 Radiographic stages of stress fracture. *A,* Early, the stress fracture may not be visible on x-rays. After a few weeks, a very faint line across the shaft of the metatarsal is seen. *B,* A month or more after the onset of symptoms, exuberant callus forms at the fracture site.

RUPTURE OF ACHILLES TENDON

Diagnosis of rupture of the Achilles tendon can be missed in >50% of cases. Sudden, severe pain in the back of the heel during activity involving strong contraction of the gastrocnemius-soleus muscle is characteristic of rupture of this tendon.

Anatomy
The tendon of the gastrocnemius and soleus muscles (Achilles) inserts into the posterior aspect of the calcaneum. It is a very strong tendon that lifts the entire body weight when we push off on each step while walking or when we stand on our toes. The main action of the gastrocnemius and soleus muscles is to plantar-flex the ankle.

Mechanism of Injury
Sudden, strong contraction of the gastrocnemius-soleus muscle may rupture the Achilles tendon. This may happen while running or jumping.

Pathology
Rupture occurs 2–5 cm proximal to the insertion of the tendon into the calcaneum. It can happen more easily in a previously degenerated tendon. The tendon can heal if the two ends are kept in close proximity for 6–8 weeks.

History
The patient complains of sudden severe **pain** behind the ankle joint. It starts during any activity involving running or jumping, such as tennis or basketball. Sometimes, rupture happens when the patient misses a step and tries to stop himself or herself from falling. The patient starts to **limp** and has difficulty walking or is unable to walk at all immediately after this episode.

Physical Examination
1. **Inspection.** A **swelling** may appear behind the ankle joint. A bruise is noticed 12–24 hours later.
2. **Palpation.** There is localized **tenderness** over the tendon. A **defect** in the tendon may be palpated. This becomes more apparent when the foot is gently dorsiflexed while palpating the tendon.
3. **Range of motion**
   a. **Active** plantar flexion is painful and **weak.** The patient is not able to stand on the affected foot and lift the heel off the ground.
   b. **Passive** dorsiflexion is painful.
4. **Special tests. Thompson's test.** The patient lies prone and bends the knee on the affected side to 90°. The calf muscle is squeezed by the examiner. If the Achilles tendon is intact, the foot will plantar-flex. If the Achilles tendon is ruptured, the foot will not move.

Course
The tendon heals over a period of time, even if it is not treated. However, some weakness of plantar flexion remains, and the patient may have difficulty with running and jumping.

Differential Diagnosis

1. **Partial rupture** of Achilles tendon may be very difficult to differentiate from a complete rupture. A palpable gap in the tendon is good evidence of a complete rupture. Sometimes, this gap is not palpable because of hematoma.
2. **Tendinitis** of Achilles tendon is usually a chronic, painful condition with exacerbations related to activity. Pain is not as severe, and the Thompson's test is not positive.

Investigations

1. **Plain x-rays** are useful in excluding fractures.
2. **MRI** shows the actual defect in the tendon.

Management

Management is controversial. Some surgeons recommend surgical repair for most patients, while others restrict it to young athletic patients who are involved in vigorous physical activity.

Ancillary. Conservative treatment consists of immobilization in a cast with the foot in plantar flexion. The cast may extend above the knee, with the knee in flexion to relax the gastrocnemius muscle. A similar cast is also required after a surgical repair. The cast is kept on for 6–8 weeks. Physical therapy is started to regain mobility of the ankle and foot and later strength of the muscles.

Surgical repair of the tendon is followed by cast immobilization and physical therapy.

RHEUMATOID ARTHRITIS

Inflammation of the joints of the foot is very common in rheumatoid arthritis.

Pathology

Soft tissue inflammation affects synovial membranes of the joints, tendon sheaths, and bursae. The **metatarsophalangeal** (MTP) and **proximal interphalangeal** (PIP) **joints** of the foot are commonly affected, with deformities of these joints occurring later in the course of the disease. The **tendon sheaths** of posterior tibial, flexor hallucis longus, peronei, and anterior tibial tendons are commonly involved. Among the **bursae,** the retrocalcaneal bursa is the one that is commonly affected.

History

MTP joints of the toes are involved early and frequently. The ankle, midfoot, and hindfoot joints are not affected as frequently as those of the forefoot. **Pain** in the region of inflammation is the main complaint. It is aggravated by weight-bearing, especially during an exacerbation of the disease, making every step painful. Deformities of the toes and foot develop later.

Physical Examination

1. **Inspection. Swelling** around the inflamed joints may vary over time. It is observed easily around the first MTP and ankle joints. Painful **calluses** develop over the plantar aspect of the heads of the metatarsals and dorsal aspect of PIP joints. The following **deformities** are common:

   a. **Hallux valgus** with bunion. The big toe is pulled toward the second toe and develops a soft tissue swelling over the medial aspect of the metatarsal head.

   b. Dorsal and lateral **subluxation** of proximal phalanges of the second to fourth toes leads to clawing of the toes.

   c. Loss of plantar arches of the foot gives rise to **flatfoot** deformity.

2. **Palpation.** There is **tenderness** over inflamed synovium during acute exacerbations.

3. **Range of motion.** All movements are restricted and painful when joints are inflamed.

   a. **Active** movement against resistance is painful when the tendon sheath is affected. If the posterior tibial tendon sheath is inflamed, then inversion of the foot against resistance gives rise to pain over the medial aspect of the ankle.

   b. **Passive.** Gentle passive movements are not as painful.

4. **Special tests.** The **gait** is slow with small steps.

Investigations

Plain x-rays of the foot are useful in diagnosis and management. Early changes of **soft tissue swelling** and **periarticular osteoporosis** occur around MTP joints. **Erosions** are more common over the medial aspect of metatarsal heads. Later, lateral and dorsal **subluxation** of MTP joints is seen.

Management

1. **Medications** are the same as those used in the treatment of rheumatoid arthritis (see Chapter 4).

2. **Ancillary**

   a. **Shoes** should be wide enough to accommodate the foot and have a high toebox if there is clawing of the toes. They should be light with soft uppers and a soft sole. If there are painful calluses over metatarsal heads, a metatarsal bar just proximal to them may help alleviate some pain. For a markedly deformed foot, a custom shoe with molded insole may be indicated.

   b. Appropriate use of canes, crutches, or a walker can relieve some weight-bearing stress. However, it puts more strain on the upper extremity joints.

3. **Surgical** procedures are carried out when conservative measures fail to relieve pain due to deformities and calluses. Common operations are for severe hallux valgus and claw toes. Arthroplasty can relieve pain due to secondary degenerative arthritis in the MTP joints.

PLANTAR FASCIITIS

Pain in the heel over its medial aspect at the origin of the plantar fascia is a very common problem.

Etiology

With each step, the longitudinal arch of the foot flattens and stretches the plantar fascia. Repeated trauma of the plantar fascia being stretched at its origin results in chronic inflammation. Plantar flexion deformity due to tight Achilles tendon, cavus deformity of the foot, or short lower extremity puts more stress on the plantar fascia. Plantar fasciitis may be precipitated by any of these conditions.

Pathology
A bony spur seen on x-rays at the anterior end of the calcaneum is the body's reaction to the inflammation. The inflammation near the attachment of the plantar fascia is the cause of pain.

History
Pain is felt over the anterior and medial aspect of the plantar surface of the heel. It starts gradually and is usually of long duration. Pain is aggravated by walking or running.

Physical Examination
1. **Palpation. Tenderness** over the anterior end of the calcaneum is characteristic (Fig. 20–6).
2. **Range of Motion**
   a. **Passive.** Pushing the metatarsal heads upward or extension of the toes causes pain near the origin of the plantar fascia.
3. **Special tests.** Standing on heels and toes may be painful.

Differential Diagnosis
Similar symptoms can be due to a **foreign body** or an **abscess** in the heel.

Investigations
Lateral **x-ray** of the foot may show a bony spur growing from the anterior end of the calcaneum. The bony spur does not always correlate with severity of pain.

Management
Conservative measures, including stopping the activity that precipitated the pain, wearing a good pair of running shoes, exercises to stretch the plantar fascia, and NSAIDs, are tried

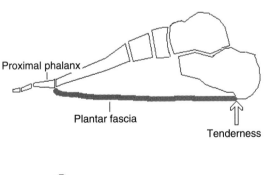

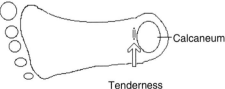

Fig. 20–6   Anatomy of plantar fascia and the site of palpable tenderness in plantar fasciitis.

first. Later, orthotics and local injection may be tried. If nothing has helped and the pain is still incapacitating, surgical treatment may be considered.
1. **Medications**
   a. **NSAIDs**
   b. Local injection of **steroid** preparation in the inflamed area
2. **Ancillary**
   a. Stop activities that might have precipitated the problem, e.g., running.
   b. **Exercises** to stretch the plantar fascia and gastrocnemius—soleus muscle
   c. **Ultrasound** therapy over painful area
   d. Good running **shoes** with soft heel and arch support
   e. **Heel cups** and special **orthotics** to relieve pressure over the heel
3. **Surgical** release of the plantar fascia is the last resort.

HALLUX VALGUS

In various conditions, the big toe is pushed laterally toward the second toe. The head of the first metatarsal becomes prominent and develops a bursa over the medial aspect. This bursa may get inflamed and painful.

Etiology
Hallux valgus deformity may be the result of:
1. Narrow pointed shoes
2. Rheumatoid arthritis
3. Metatarsus primus varus—a congenital deformity with a shortened, adducted first metatarsal

Pathology
In the normal foot, the axis of the big toe is nearly parallel to that of the first metatarsal. There is similar relationship between the first and second metatarsal. In hallux valgus, the big toe is deviated toward the second toe. The head of the first metatarsal becomes prominent and develops a bursa over its medial aspect (Fig. 20–7). This bursa may get inflamed or infected, and the skin over it becomes thickened. The articular cartilage over the exposed

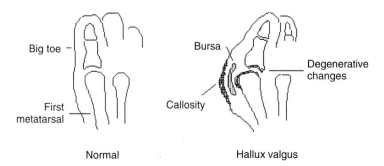

Fig. 20–7 Pathologic features of hallux valgus.

part of head of first metatarsal degenerates, and the metatarsophalangeal (MTP) joint develops degenerative arthritis.

History
Pain over the medial aspect of the first MTP joint is usually the first symptom. This pain may result from a callosity or inflamed bursa. Walking becomes difficult, and running is impossible. Later, the bursa may burst and discharge pus. If the second toe develops hammertoe deformity, the callus over the dorsum of this toe becomes painful.

Physical Examination
1. **Inspection.** The big toe is deviated toward the second at the MTP joint. There is a prominence over the medial aspect of the head of the first metatarsal due to bony overgrowth, bursa, and callus formation. Redness and tenderness are present if the bursa is inflamed.
2. **Palpation.** The head of the first metatarsal is felt under the callosity and bursa over the medial aspect.
3. **Range of motion.** Active and passive **abduction** of the big toe at the MTP joint are restricted in late cases because of contractures of soft tissues on the lateral side of the big toe. (The axis of the second toe is considered as neutral for movements of abduction and adduction of the toes.) Flexion and extension at this joint are restricted later when degenerative arthritis develops.

Course
Initially, the deformity is correctable. Later, soft tissue contractures over the lateral aspect of the MTP joint do not allow the big toe to be brought in line with the metatarsal. The bursa becomes inflamed, and infection may spread as cellulitis or burst to form a discharging sinus. The deformed big toe may push the second toe to produce hammertoe deformity.

Investigations
Plain **x-rays** help to determine the extent of degenerative arthritis and deviation of the first metatarsal. The joint space is narrowed with spur formation in degenerative arthritis.

Management
Ancillary. During the early stage, the deformity can be corrected by pushing the big toe medially:
1. The structures over the lateral aspect of the big toe are stretched manually to correct the deformity.
2. The patient performs exercises to strengthen the adductors of the big toe.
3. A dynamic splint is prescribed to correct the deformity.
4. Proper shoes which accommodate the distal foot are essential. The portion of the shoe over the bursa can be stretched to relieve pressure.

Surgical. Many operations are devised for this condition. Selection of the operation depends on the patient's problems and the surgeon's preferences. Two of the procedures are:
1. **Excision arthroplasty** of the first MTP joint. The proximal part of the proximal phalanx is removed, the bursa excised, and the bony prominence of the head is trimmed (Fig. 20–8).
2. **Osteotomy** of the first metatarsal is performed to correct its varus deformity.

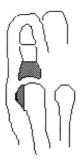

Fig. 20–8 Excision arthroplasty. The operation consists of removal of the proximal half of the proximal phalanx, medial part of the head of the first metatarsal, and the bunion. A false joint forms between the metatarsal head and the remaining proximal phalanx.

HALLUX RIGIDUS

Pain in the metatarsophalangeal (MTP) joint of the big toe develops with severe limitation of dorsiflexion and degenerative changes on x-rays.

Anatomy
The MTP joint of the big toe is dorsiflexed (extended) to about 50°–75° during the push-off stage of normal walking (Fig. 20–9).

Etiology
The exact etiology is not known. Hallux rigidus is believed to be a form of primary degenerative arthritis affecting the MTP joint, or it may be secondary to trauma.

Pathology
The articular cartilage is destroyed. **Osteophytes** form near the joint margins and especially over the dorsal aspect of the joint. A callosity or bunion may form over the exostosis on the dorsal aspect of the MTP joint.

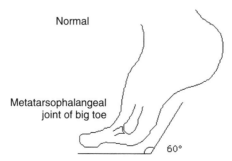

Normal

Metatarsophalangeal
joint of big toe

60°

Fig. 20–9 Normal range of extension (dorsiflexion) at the MTP joint of the big toe is 0°–90°. During the push-off stage of walking, considerable extension is necessary for smooth, painless gait.

History

A minor injury may precede the onset and subsequent exacerbations. The MTP joint becomes **painful** and **swollen.** The pain is aggravated at each step during the pushoff phase because dorsiflexion of the MTP joint is restricted.

Physical Examination

1. **Inspection.** During the early stages, there may be swelling due to inflammation and effusion in the joint. Later, a callus or bursa develops on the dorsal aspect. During normal gait, the body weight is borne by the calcaneum, head of the fifth metatarsal, and then the head of the first metatarsal. Patients with hallux rigidus avoid weight-bearing on the head of first metatarsal because of pain. After the weight is transferred from the calcaneum to the head of the fifth metatarsal, push-off occurs, and the medial aspect of the forefoot does not touch the ground. The push-off phase is short and jerky.
2. **Palpation.** There is tenderness in the region of the first MTP joint.
3. **Range of motion**
   a. **Active.** Movements at the MTP joint are restricted because of pain and muscle spasm.
   b. **Passive.** Dorsiflexion is markedly restricted. Gentle passive plantar flexion is usually full.

Course

Exacerbations and remissions may occur depending on the severity of inflammation. As the disease progresses, limitation of dorsiflexion of the MTP joint gets worse.

Differential Diagnoses

Other common problems of MTP joint, including **gout,** should be excluded.

Investigations

Plain x-rays show irregular narrowing of the joint space, subchondral sclerosis, and osteophyte formation. Lateral view may show a large osteophyte over the dorsal aspect of the MTP joint (Fig. 20–10).

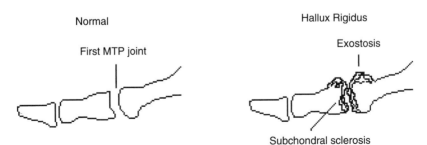

Fig. 20–10 Lateral x-rays of the foot show narrowing of the joint space of the first MTP joint, subchondral sclerosis, and osteophyte formation over the dorsal aspect (exostosis).

Management
1. **Medications.** NSAIDs help some to reduce inflammation.
2. **Ancillary.** A rocker-bottom **shoe** with metatarsal pad helps avoid dorsiflexion at the first MTP joint.
3. **Surgical.** Depending on the patient's problems and goals, different surgical procedures such as excision, arthroplasty, replacement arthoplasty, or arthrodesis can be recommended.

DEFORMITIES OF THE TOES

Deformities of toes have been described by different nomenclature in various textbooks. Flexion deformity of a distal interphalangeal (DIP) joint is called the **mallet toe,** whereas flexion deformity of the proximal interphalangeal (PIP) joint is called a **hammertoe. Clawing of toes** occurs in neurologic conditions when hyperextension deformity is seen in the metatarsophalangeal (MTP) joint with flexion at the interphalangeal joints of the toes. (Fig. 20–11).

Etiology
The toes may be deformed because of **tight shoes** or secondary to another deformity such as a **cavus foot.** Deformities are also seen in **neurologic conditions** in which there is weakness of the intrinsic (small) muscles of the foot. Peripheral neuropathy (e.g., diabetic neuropathy) is an example.

Pathology
In the early stages of disease, the deformities are correctable. **Contractures** develop in the ligaments of the involved joints and tendons later. **Callosities** are formed because of abnormal pressure on the skin.

History
Most of the deformities of the toes develop slowly over years. The patient usually goes to see a physician because of pain due to callosities.

Physical Examination
1. **Inspection.** Clawing, hammertoe, and mallet toe can be distinguished on inspection. Other associated deformities, such as cavus of the foot, should be sought. There is

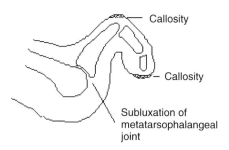

Fig. 20–11 Claw toe deformity and sites of callus formation due to abnormal pressures.

wasting of small muscles of the foot in neurologic conditions like peripheral neuropathy.
2. **Palpation** of the skin is carried out to confirm callosities and elicit any **tenderness.**
3. **Range of motion**
   a. **Passive.** An attempt is made to correct the deformity and check for contractures of ligaments and tendons.
4. **Special tests.** Neurologic exam is done, especially if there is clawing of the toes, to rule out peripheral neuropathy, cauda equina lesion, or spinal cord lesions.

Investigations
1. **Plain x-rays** are done before surgery to determine the condition of the joints and bones.
2. **Urine** and **blood** tests are done to rule out diabetes.

Management
Ancillary
1. **Taping** of toes is done when the deformity can be corrected by the examiner.
2. **Shoes** with high toebox to accommodate the deformity and relieve pressure on the callosity are prescribed.
   Surgical correction is recommended when conservative measures fail, and the patient has to limit his or her activities because of pain.

INGROWN TOENAIL

Infection near the corner of a toenail is a common condition. It usually affects the big toe, giving rise to pain and discharge.

Anatomy
The nail is formed by nail matrix at the base and grows distally. It protects deeper tissues and is covered on three sides by skinfolds. The distal edge is free to grow.

Etiology
Tight shoes and poor hygiene are usually blamed for the onset of infection. The anterior corner of the nail grows and digs into the soft tissue surrounding the nail. (Fig. 20–12). Irritation from this leads to infection.

Pathology
The infection may lead to swelling of the skinfold and pus formation. In diabetic patients or those with poor blood supply, the infection is more likely to spread and become cellulitis of the foot.

History
Pain over the distal corner of a toenail is the initial symptom. Every step on the affected side aggravates the pain. Pain may be minimal in diabetics with peripheral neuropathy. Throbbing pain which is worse at night is a sign of abscess formation.

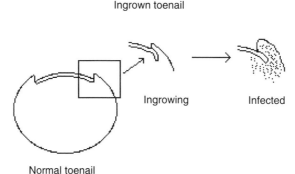

Fig. 20–12   Pathology of ingrown toenail.

Physical Examination

1. **Inspection.** The skin near the corner of the nail is swollen and red. There may be purulent discharge. If untreated, the abscess may spread under the nail.
2. **Palpation.** The inflamed area is markedly tender.

Complications

Infection may spread, especially in diabetics, and cause cellulitis of the foot.

Differential Diagnosis

Trauma to a toe is painful and tender and may lead to infection later.

Investigations

Tests to rule out diabetes, especially in persons with chronic, recurrent infections, should be carried out.

Management

1. **Prevention.** Diabetic patients are advised not to wear tight, ill-fitting shoes. The toenails should be trimmed so that the corners are right angles and the front edge is straight (Fig. 20–13). Prompt treatment of early stages of infection in a diabetic patient is very important.
2. **Medications.** Antibiotics are required when infection spreads to more proximal areas or when infection occurs in a diabetic patient.
3. **Ancillary**
   a. **Rest** is the most difficult part of treatment to carry out. Walking should be avoided and especially walking with shoes. Slippers or thongs are preferable for use at home.
   b. **Hydrotherapy.** The affected foot is immersed in warm water with Epsom salt or iodine preparation added to it. Soaking the foot for 15–20 minutes, two or three times a day, helps to relieve vascular congestion and pain.
4. **Surgical** treatment is necessary when there is pus under the nail. The extent of surgery depends on the spread of infection. The following procedures may be done:

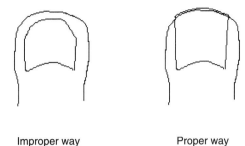

Improper way   Proper way

Fig. 20–13   The corner of the nail should be allowed to grow beyond the fold of skin near the lateral side. This will prevent the nail from digging into the nailfold and getting infected.

    a. Removal of nail spicule that is digging into soft tissue
    b. Partial excision of the nail. A quarter or third of the nail is removed.
    c. Excision of whole nail, if abscess has spread and lifted the nail off its bed.

PLANTAR DIGITAL NEUROMA

Plantar digital neuroma is also known as **interdigital neuroma,** Morton's metatarsalgia, or **Morton's neuroma.** Severe burning pain in the region of the metatarsal radiating to the toes is the usual complaint.

Anatomy
The plantar digital nerves are branches of the lateral and medial plantar nerves, which run between the metatarsals and supply the toes. The nerves between the third and fourth and between the second and third metatarsals are most commonly involved. The digital nerves divide into two branches to supply the adjacent sides of two toes.

Etiology/Pathology
Pressure of tight shoes is believed to cause inflammation (**neuritis**) which later leads to fibrosis in and around the nerve. A **fusiform swelling** may form proximal to the division of the nerve into its two terminal branches (Fig. 20–14).

History
The patient complains of **pain** in the distal part of the foot (**metatarsalgia**). It is severe and burning in character and felt over the plantar aspect. The pain may radiate distally into the contiguous sides of the toes supplied by the digital nerve. It is usually brought on by walking with tight shoes and is relieved by removing the shoe and rest. Sometimes, the pain continues even at night.

Physical Examination
1. **Inspection.** The foot looks normal on inspection.
2. **Palpation.** Firm pressure by a finger on the dorsum of the foot and a thumb over the

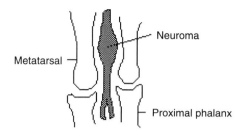

Fig. 20–14   Interdigital neuroma between two metatarsals.

plantar aspect, between the distal shafts of third and fourth metatarsals, reproduces pain (**tenderness**). The neuroma is located just proximal to the metatarsal heads between the shafts. Side-to-side compression of metatarsals also reproduces the pain (Fig. 20–15). The neuroma is usually not palpable as a swelling. Sensory exam may reveal diminished sensation (**hypesthesia**) in the distribution of the affected nerve.

Investigations
1. **X-rays** help to rule out stress fracture.
2. **MRI** may show the neuroma as a swelling in connection with the digital nerve.

Management
1. **Ancillary**
   a. Most **shoes** do not accommodate the forefoot adequately, especially women's shoes. Shoes wide enough for the forefoot should be tried before any other treatment.
   b. **Rest** to involved structures is provided by avoiding walking.
   c. If these two measures do not work or the condition is chronic, local **injection of steroids** is given to relieve inflammation. The steroids are infiltrated around the tender area in the intermetatarsal region and not into the nerve itself.
2. **Surgical. Excision** of the neuroma is undertaken if all conservative measures fail to relieve symptoms. The sensation in the toes supplied by that nerve is lost.

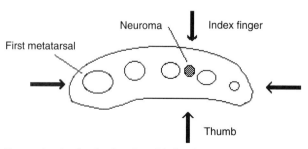

Fig. 20–15   Deep palpation by the thumb and index finger over the neuroma is tender. The pain is also reproduced by squeezing the first and fifth metatarsals together.

THE FOOT IN DIABETES

A large number of diabetics develop foot problems. Some end up with amputation of the foot or leg. Proper management of diabetes and its complications can avoid or delay amputation.

Pathology
Diabetics are more prone to develop **atherosclerosis** of large blood vessels and microangiopathy of smaller ones. **Peripheral neuropathy** is another common complication of diabetes. Patients with diminished pain sensation are more likely to neglect minor injuries which then develop into spreading **infection** or large **ulcers**. Peripheral neuropathy can lead to **neuropathic** (Charcot) **joints** and **deformities** of the foot. This, in turn, gives rise to abnormal pressure on the skin, callus formation, and skin breakdown. Inadequate blood supply and abnormal metabolism interfere with healing.

History
The patient may present with symptoms of peripheral neuropathy, vascular insufficiency, or one of their complications. **Tingling** and **numbness** of stocking and glove distribution are very common. Some complain of a painful or unpleasant sensation or that their feet are cold. An **ulcer** with foul-smelling discharge is another way that a diabetic may present. **Pain** and swelling of the foot with **fever** usually indicate spreading infection.

Physical Examination
1. **Inspection.** The weight-bearing areas of the foot should be carefully observed for **ulcers.** Skin breakdown is common over the heads of the metatarsals on the sole, heel, or dorsal aspect of the proximal interphalangeal (PIP) joint of a toe with clawing. The base is usually necrotic tissue. Surrounding skin may be thickened. Redness of the surrounding skin, diffuse swelling of the foot, and purulent discharge indicate infection. Involvement of the motor nerves in peripheral neuropathy causes weakness of the intrinsic muscles of the foot. Unopposed action of the extrinsic muscles leads to **clawing of the toes** and cavus deformity of the foot. The neuropathic process destroys the joints of the midfoot and ankle. The transverse and longitudinal arches of the foot are flattened.
2. **Palpation.** Tenderness may be present when there is infection.
3. **Range of motion** may be restricted because of muscle weakness, soft tissue contractures, or neuropathic joints.
   a. **Active.** A foot drop indicates weakness of the dorsiflexors of the foot. The patient is not able to actively dorsiflex the foot against gravity.
4. **Special tests.** Dorsalis pedis and posterior tibial pulses should be palpated to determine the status of peripheral vessels.

Differential Diagnoses
Conditions that give rise to neuropathic joints, peripheral vascular disease, and peripheral neuropathy should be considered in the differential diagnoses. Diabetes is the most common cause of neuropathic joints in the United States.

Investigations

1. Plain **x-rays** help in diagnosing complications, such as osteomyelitis and neuropathic joints, and in determining severity of deformities.
2. **Doppler** studies are done to evaluate the circulatory status.
3. **Culture** and **sensitivity** testing of discharge from the ulcer are important for treating infections.

Course

Once the skin breaks down, the infection is very likely to spread. This outcome can be avoided to some extent by vigorous treatment of the ulcer. The course of neuropathic joints is also progressive, with increasing deformity which may lead to ulceration, infection, and amputation.

Complications

1. **Peripheral neuropathy** may involve sensory, motor, and sympathetic nerves. Patients may develop paresthesias, diminished sensation, muscle weakness, and foot deformity.
2. **Peripheral vascular disease**
3. **Ulceration** of the skin
4. **Infection** may spread from subcutaneous to deeper tissue planes and bone.
5. **Neuropathic joints** with gross destruction and deformities

Management

Good control of diabetes is an essential part of the management. Treatment of each complication is considered below:

A. **Peripheral neuropathy** presents with unpleasant sensations, e.g., pain and paresthesias in the foot.
1. **Medications. Carbamazepine** (Tegretol) has been used for pain secondary to peripheral neuropathy.
2. **Ancillary.** Transcutaneous electrical nerve stimulation (TENS) helps in relieving pain in some patients.

B. **Skin ulcer** is very common in diabetics.
1. **Prevention** of skin breakdown by educating the patient is one of the most important services that can be provided. Following points should be stressed:
   a. Inspect the soles and heel every day for redness or ulcer.
   b. Wash feet daily, dry them thoroughly, and apply skin lotion to keep them soft.
   c. Wear thick socks. Wash socks every day and dry them before putting them on. There should be no wrinkles in the socks. If they get wet because of perspiration, change them.
   d. Shoes should be long and wide enough to fit the feet. New shoes should be worn for short periods. Before putting on shoes in the morning, feel for any nails projecting inside.
   e. Corn and callus should be treated. Any blister or skin breakdown should be reported to a physician immediately.
2. **Ancillary.** Once an ulcer has developed, it needs to be kept clean and protected from further injury and pressure.
3. **Surgical** debridement is carried out whenever there is necrotic tissue.

C. **Infection** in a diabetic foot should be treated vigorously.
1. **Medications.** Appropriate antibiotics are started. Intravenous antibiotics are necessary for osteomyelitis or severe spreading infections.

2. **Ancillary.** The foot is protected from further injury.
3. **Surgical.** Incision and drainage is performed when there is pus.
D. **Neuropathic joints** present with progressive deformities of the foot.
  1. **Ancillary.** Custom-molded **shoes** are prescribed. A weight-relieving **brace** helps the foot by passing the weight-bearing stress to more proximal areas.
  2. **Surgical** procedures such as arthrodesis are not recommended because bones do not fuse very easily in patients with neuropathic joints.

AVASCULAR NECROSIS

Avascular Necrosis of the Navicular
This condition is also known as **Köhler's disease.**

Anatomy
The navicular bone is at the dome of the longitudinal arch of the foot (Fig. 20–16). It articulates with talus on the proximal side and distally with the three cuneiform bones. It is located over the medial aspect of the midfoot. Among the tarsal bones, the navicular is the last bone in the foot to ossify.

Etiology
The exact etiology is not known. The navicular bone is subjected to a lot of mechanical stress during weight-bearing activities, and this may be related to interference with its blood supply.

Pathology
Areas of bone necrosis develop when blood supply to the bone is cut off. Later, the necrotic tissue is removed and new blood vessels form. The navicular is reformed usually to its normal shape and size in about 3 years.

History
Avascular necrosis of the navicular is more common in boys. The common age group is between **3–8 years. Pain** in the foot is the usual presenting symptom. It is aggravated by weight-bearing.

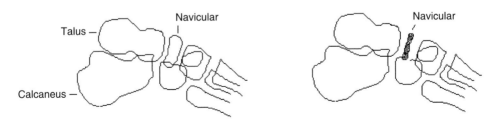

Fig. 20–16 Lateral x-rays of the foot show increased density of the navicular bone with fragmentation. The bone is smaller in anteroposterior dimension, and there is increased space between adjacent bones.

Physical Examination
1. **Inspection.** The child walks on the lateral aspect of the foot and **limps** because of pain. There may be some swelling over the medial aspect of the dorsum of the midfoot.
2. **Palpation.** Tenderness is localized over the navicular bone.
3. **Range of motion.** Movements of the foot are painful during the acute stage.

Differential Diagnoses
Infection and **fractures** should be ruled out.

Investigations
Plain **x-rays** show increased density and reduced anteroposterior dimension of the navicular (Fig. 20–16).

Management
Ancillary. During the acute stage, when the child has a painful limp, a below-knee walking **cast** is applied. It is removed after 3–6 weeks when pain subsides. The foot is protected by **arch supports,** steel shank in the sole, and medial heel wedge.

Aseptic Necrosis of the Head of the Metatarsal
This condition, also known as **osteochondrosis,** Freiberg's disease, or **Freiberg's infraction,** produces pain, swelling, and tenderness over the head of the metatarsal. On x-rays, the affected head of the metatarsal looks fragmented, and the metatarsophalangeal (MTP) joint later develops degenerative arthritis.

Etiology
Inadequate blood supply, trauma, infection, and endocrine imbalance are some of the hypotheses put forward to explain this condition.

Pathology
The head of the second metatarsal is affected more often than any other. Part of the epiphysis becomes necrotic and collapses. The head of the metatarsal becomes deformed. Fragments of articular cartilage may form loose bodies in the joint. Degenerative arthritis develops as a result of irregular joint surface and loose bodies.

History
The onset is usually between the ages **13–18 years.** The patient complains of **pain** in the forefoot with swelling over the dorsum. Pain is aggravated by walking. There is no history of trauma in most cases.

Physical Examination
1. **Inspection.** There may be some **swelling** near the base of the second toe.
2. **Palpation. Localized tenderness** is elicited over the head of the affected metatarsal during the acute phase.
3. **Range of motion.** Active and passive movements of the MTP joint are restricted because of pain.

Course
After the initial symptomatic phase, pain and swelling subside. There may be a period of many years before pain due to degenerative arthritis develops.

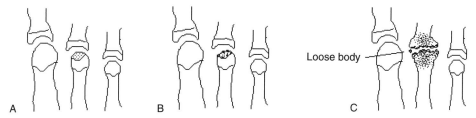

Fig. 20–17 Progression of aseptic necrosis of the metatarsal head. *A,* There is increased density of the affected part of the metatarsal head on x-rays. *B,* Fragmentation and flattening of the head occur later. *C,* The head of the metatarsal and base of the proximal phalanx are flattened. Subchondral sclerosis and irregular joint space narrowing develop later. There may be loose bodies in the joint.

Investigations

Plain x-rays of the foot may be difficult to interpret during the early stages of disease. The necrotic part of the bone looks more **dense** because of relative radiolucency of the surrounding bone (Fig. 20–17A and B). The necrotic area collapses, and joint space between the metatarsal head and proximal phalanx is increased. Later, the head becomes flattened and enlarged. Small fragments of the bone are seen as **loose bodies** in the joint cavity. Still later, the articular surface of the proximal phalanx become irregular, and changes of **degenerative arthritis** are observed (Fig. 20–17C).

Management

1. **Medications. Analgesics** are prescribed for pain relief.
2. **Ancillary**
   a. A short leg **cast** is applied, and the patient is asked to walk non-weight-bearing on the affected side until pain subsides. A walking cast may be enough if the symptoms are not very severe.
   b. After the cast is removed, a **metatarsal bar** helps relieve some strain on the metatarsal head.
   c. Later, when degenerative changes develop in the joint, the patient may benefit by using a **rocker-bottom shoe.**
3. **Surgical.** Some surgeons recommend excision arthroplasty of the MTP joint if there is no relief of symptoms. This approach is controversial.

Bibliography

1. Alexander IJ, Johnson KA, Parr JW: Morton's neuroma: A review of recent concepts. Orthopedics 10:103–106, 1987.
2. Birrer RB, DellaCorte MP, Grisati PJ: Common Foot Problems in Primary Care. Philadelphia, Hanley & Belfus, 1992.
3. Boulton AJ: The diabetic foot. Med Clin North Am 72:1513–1530, 1988.
4. Crawford AH, Gabriel KR: Foot and ankle problems. Orthop Clin North Am 18:649–666, 1987.
5. Harrelson JM: Management of diabetic foot. Orthop Clin North Am 20:605–619, 1989.
6. Kwong PK, Kay D, Voner RT, White MW: Plantar fasciitis: Mechanics and pathomechanics of treatment. Clin Sports Med 7:119–126, 1988.
7. Lassiter TE, Malone TR, Garrett WE: Injury to lateral ligaments of the ankle. Orthop Clin North Am 20: 629–640, 1989.
8. McGuire T, Kumar VN: Rehabilitation management of the rheumatoid foot. Orthop Rev 16:671–676, 1987.
9. WU KK: Morton's interdigital neuroma: A clinical review of its etiology, treatment, and results. J. Foot Ankle Surg 35:112–119, 1996.

Index

Page numbers in *italics* indicate figures; numbers folowed by "t" indicate tables.